W9-AHA-315

Handbook of Physical Medicine and Rehabilitation
The Basics

Handbook of Physical Medicine and Rehabilitation
The Basics
Second Edition

Edited by
SUSAN J. GARRISON, M.D.
Associate Professor
Department of Physical Medicine and Rehabilitation
Medical Director, Rehabilitation Center
The Methodist Hospital
Houston, Texas

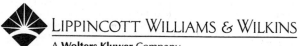
LIPPINCOTT WILLIAMS & WILKINS
A **Wolters Kluwer** Company

Philadelphia · Baltimore · New York · London
Buenos Aires · Hong Kong · Sydney · Tokyo

Acquisitions Editor: Robert Hurley
Developmental Editor: Joanne Bersin
Production Editor: Melanie Bennitt
Manufacturing Manager: Benjamin Rivera
Cover Illustrator: Marjory Dressler
Compositor: Circle Graphics
Printer: R. R. Donnelley–Crawfordsville

© 2003 by LIPPINCOTT WILLIAMS & WILKINS
530 Walnut Street
Philadelphia, PA 19106 USA
LWW.com

Printed in the USA

Library of Congress Cataloging-in-Publication Data

Handbook of physical medicine and rehabilitation, the basics / edited by
  Susan J. Garrison.—2nd ed.
      p. ; cm.
   Includes bibliographical references and index.
   ISBN 0-7817-4434-2
   1. Medicine, Physical—Handbooks, manuals, etc. 2. Medical
rehabilitation—Handbooks, manuals, etc. I. Garrison, Susan J.
   [DNLM: 1. Physical Medicine—Handbooks. 2. Rehabilitation—
Handbooks. WB 39 H23654 2003]
   RM700.H15 2003
616′.03—dc21
                                                        2002043397

---

10 9 8 7 6 5 4 3 2 1

Contents

Contributing Authors

Theresa Frasca Berner, M.O.T., O.T.R./L. *Rehabilitation Team Leader, The Ohio State University Medical Center, Columbus, Ohio*

Donna M. Bloodworth, M.D. *Associate Professor, Department of Physical Medicine and Rehabilitation, Baylor College of Medicine, Houston, Texas*

Michael L. Boninger, M.D. *Associate Professor, Department of Physical Medicine and Rehabilitation, University of Pittsburgh, Pittsburgh, Pennsylvania*

Diana D. Cardenas, M.D. *Professor, Department of Rehabilitation Medicine, University of Washington, Seattle, Washington*

Andy S. Chan, M.D. *Assistant Professor, Department of Physical Medicine and Rehabilitation, Baylor College of Medicine, Houston, Texas*

John Cianca, M.D. *Assistant Professor, Baylor College of Medicine; Director of Sports and Human Performance Medicine, Human Performance and Rehabilitation, Houston, Texas*

David X. Cifu, M.D. *The Herman J. Flax, M.D. Professor and Chairman, Department of Physical Medicine and Rehabilitation, Virginia Commonwealth University, Richmond, Virginia*

Gary S. Clark, M.D. *Assistant Clinical Professor, Department of Rehabilitation Medicine, Kaleida Health/Buffalo General Hospital, Buffalo, New York*

Gerald Felsenthal, M.D. *Clinical Professor, Department of Epidemiology and Prevention Medicine, University of Maryland School of Medicine, Baltimore, Maryland*

Gerard E. Francisco, M.D. *Clinical Associate Professor, Department of Physical Medicine and Rehabilitation, University of Texas, Houston, Texas*

Ramakrishna K. Gadi, M.D. *Chief Resident, Department of Physical Medicine and Rehabilitation, Virginia Commonwealth University Hospitals, Richmond, Virginia*

Susan L. Garber, M.D., O.T.R., F.A.O.T.A., F.A.C.R.M. *Associate Professor, Department of Physical Medicine and Rehabilitation, Baylor College of Medicine, Houston, Texas*

Fae H. Garden, M.D. *Associate Professor, Department of Physical Medicine and Rehabilitation, Baylor College of Medicine, Houston, Texas*

Susan J. Garrison, M.D. *Associate Professor, Department of Physical Medicine and Rehabilitation; Medical Director, Rehabilitation Center, The Methodist Hospital, Houston, Texas*

Theresa Gillis, M.D. *Department of Physical Medicine and Rehabilitation, Virginia Commonwealth University, Richmond, Virginia*

Steve M. Gnatz, M.D. *Marianjoy Rehabilitation Hospital, Wheaton, Illinois*

Martin Grabois, M.D. *Professor and Chairman, Department of Physical Medicine and Rehabilitation, Baylor College of Medicine, Houston, Texas*

Phala A. Helm, M.D. *Professor, Department of Physical Medicine and Rehabilitation, University of Texas Southwestern Medical Center of Dallas, Dallas, Texas*

Sally Ann Holmes, M.D. *Assistant Professor, Department of Physical Medicine and Rehabilitation, Baylor College of Medicine, Houston, Texas*

Cindy B. Ivanhoe, M.D. *Department of Physical Medicine and Rehabilitation, Baylor College of Medicine, Houston, Texas*

Jennifer J. James, M.D. *Clinical Assistant Professor, Department of Physical Medicine and Rehabilitation, University of Washington, Seattle, Washington*

Kenneth Kemp, M.D. *Department of Physical Medicine and Rehabilitation, Baylor College of Medicine, Houston, Texas*

C. George Kevorkian, M.D. *Associate Professor, Department of Physical Medicine and Rehabilitation, Baylor College of Medicine, Houston, Texas*

Karen J. Kowalske, M.D. *Associate Professor and Chair, Department of Physical Medicine and Rehabilitation, University of Texas Southwestern Medical Center, Dallas, Texas*

Thomas A. Krouskop, M.D. *Department of Physical Medicine and Rehabilitation, TIRR-Baylor College of Medicine, Houston, Texas*

Charles E. Levy, M.D. *Associate Professor, Department of Orthopedics and Rehabilitation, University of Florida, Gainesville, Florida*

John J. Nicholas, M.D.   *Professor, Department of Physical Medicine and Rehabilitation, Temple University School of Medicine, Philadelphia, Pennsylvania*

Maureen R. Nelson, M.D.   *Clinical Associate Professor, Department of Physical Medicine and Rehabilitation, Baylor College of Medicine, Houston, Texas*

Gulapar Phongsamart, M.D.   *Department of Physical Medicine and Rehabilitation, Medical College of Wisconsin, Milwaukee, Wisconsin*

Elliot J. Roth, M.D.   *The Paul B. Magnuson Professor and Chairman, Department of Physical Medicine and Rehabilitation, Northwestern University Feinberg School of Medicine, Chicago, Illinois*

Jay V. Subbarao, M.D.   *Clinical Professor, Department of Orthopedic Surgery and Rehabilitation, Loyola University Medical Center, Maywood, Illinois*

Margaret A. Turk, M.D.   *Professor, Department of Physical Medicine and Rehabilitation, SUNY Upstate Medical University, Syracuse, New York*

Carlos Vallbona, M.D.   *Professor, Department of Family and Community Medicine, Baylor College of Medicine, Houston, Texas*

Michael J. Vennix, M.D.   *Assistant Professor, Department of Physical Medicine and Rehabilitation, Baylor College of Medicine, Houston, Texas*

Jacqueline J. Wertsch, M.D.   *Professor, Department of Physical Medicine and Rehabilitation, Medical College of Wisconsin, Milwaukee, Wisconsin*

Foreword

In my welcoming Foreword to the birth of the First Edition of this new generation of books in 1995, I wrote that its "conception and birth were inevitable." My glowing praise of its editor, authors, purpose, and format could be attributed by skeptics to my pride as its "godfather," but I now gloat that I was right, absolutely right! That newborn lived up to all my expectations including one that I didn't mention—even books grow older.

Although the first edition was lively and graceful in youth, and even in middle age, like all creatures, this lovely creation grew older and was ready for its regeneration. Here it is.

This second edition makes LIP for the passage of time. True to its heritage, it will insure that all students of physical medicine and rehabilitation (the clan with which I'm proud to be a member) will have a constant companion that they can love and trust. Once more, I'm proud to be its "godfather," certain that the family is back to glowing health.

John Basmajian, O.C., O. Ont.,
MD, DScC, LLD, FRCPC,
FRCP(Glasgow), FRCP(Edinb),
FAFRM / FRCP(Austral), HonDip, St.L.Col.
McMaster University
Hamilton, Ontario

Preface

It is always gratifying to have a pet project that is successful. The *Handbook of Physical Medicine and Rehabilitation Basics,* First Edition, has been such a project. Originally conceived as simply handouts for the medical students and residents at our Physical Medicine & Rehabilitation program at Baylor College of Medicine, the book became a national and international best-seller. It has now been translated into at least five different languages.

However, no matter how basic an approach one takes about medical topics, the very nature of scientific process dictates that, over time, some elements will change. The analogy can be made with boiling water. One can heat water in the sun, over an open fire, using electrical energy, a gas-stove top, or even in a microwave oven. The water still becomes warmer using energy transfer, although the methods by which the heating is accomplished may differ, due to advances in technology or simply by the application of energy in a different form. The basics of the practice of PM&R have not changed greatly in the past few years, but we have learned to apply some basic knowledge in new ways. It is therefore appropriate to revise and update.

In creating this second edition of the handbook, I simply tried to take something that was already good and improve it. In doing so, I attempted to broaden the expertise of the chapter authors by using physiatrists from across the United States, in combination with those here at Baylor, whenever possible. We have kept the same format, that is, alphabetized by diagnosis. In this edition, we have added chapters regarding the use of wheelchairs and geriatric rehabilitation. The chapters have been updated in content and suggested readings. The index has been purposely expanded to enhance quick retrieval of information at the bedside or during rounding.

It has been a rewarding experience to revise this popular book. As you read this, we are already working on the third edition. This second edition would not have been possible without the input and patience of all of the authors. Thank you so much for participating in this project.

This edition has also benefited from the input of many secretaries during a time of frequent change in my administrative office staff. Thank you to Chris Robinson, who was key in the first edition and planning for the second. I also thank Omega Miller, who was with us through the completion of this project. I sincerely appreciate the feedback from the numerous PM&R residents and medical students over the years; we frequently used the handbook at bedside during rounds to clarify teaching points. Of course, there would be no book if it had not been for the dogged determination of the editors at Lippincott Williams & Wilkins. Thank you to Joanne Bersin for your determination.

Make this handbook your starting point to trigger further questions, discussion, and reading in the field of PM&R. The more we know, the better we can serve our patient population.

Susan J. Garrison, M.D.

Handbook of
Physical Medicine
and Rehabilitation
The Basics

Physical Medicine and Rehabilitation: Philosophy, Patient Care Issues, and Physiatric Evaluation

Ramakrishna K. Gadi and David X. Cifu

PHILOSOPHY

Physical Medicine and Rehabilitation (PM&R) involves the diagnosis and treatment of physical and functional disorders. The rehabilitation model differs from the traditional medical model in several ways. Management of disability rather than treatment of disease is emphasized. The physician is considered a teacher or facilitator rather than merely a "knower" or a "doer"; the patient is an active, rather than passive, participant. PM&R employs an interdisciplinary team approach, in which specialists exchange information and ideas about various problems. The traditional model uses a more fragmented multidisciplinary approach of multiple specialists working independently on specific problems. The goals of the rehabilitation model are improvement of function and adjustment to disability rather than disease cure.

Commonly used terms in PM&R include impairment, disability, and handicap. Impairment signifies the residual limitation resulting from disease, injury, or a congenital defect, such as loss of motor strength of the legs after spinal cord injury. Disability signifies the inability to perform a functional skill, such as walking. Handicap signifies the interaction of a disability with the environment, such as being unable to enter a restaurant because it is not wheelchair accessible.

HISTORY

The origins of physical medicine can be traced through the centuries-old tradition of employing physical agents such as heat, cold, and water for medical benefit and specifically to the 1890 introduction of therapeutic diathermy, a type of deep heating using shortwaves. The principles of medical rehabilitation were initially formulated during treatment of soldiers in 1919 following World War I. The merging of PM&R into a single field began in the 1920s, gained momentum in the 1930s, and was spurred on by World War II. By 1947, PM&R was officially sanctioned as a specialty by the American Board of Medical Specialties. Physiatry, from the Greek *physio* meaning "nature," is the shortened name of the specialty; the physiatrist (pronounced fiz"e-at' rist) is a PM&R physician.

Board qualification in PM&R requires a 1-year medical, surgical, or pediatric internship followed by 3 years of PM&R residency. Fellowships in PM&R are generally 1 year and include pediatrics, head injury, spinal cord injury, sports medicine, electrodiagnosis, pain, and research. Board certification requires successful completion of both a written and oral examination. Currently, there are approximately 1,200 PM&R residents in over 80 accredited residency programs nationwide. Since 1947, over 6,500 physicians have been certified as Diplomates of the American Board of Physical Medicine and Rehabilitation; over half of these have been certified in the last 10 years.

Physiatry has evolved over the years to provide its practitioners the opportunities to treat a variety of patients. Not only do physiatrists provide rehabilitative services in the acute setting but also in the subacute and long-term arenas as directors of skilled nursing facilities and nursing homes. Furthermore, outpatient practice has diversified vastly to include specialization in musculoskeletal, electrodiagnostic, chronic pain, interventional, holistic and alternative medical approaches, and others. The PM&R physician has many tools in his or her armamentarium.

PATIENT CARE ISSUES

Interdisciplinary Team

Use of the interdisciplinary team in patient management distinguishes PM&R practice from other medical specialties. The team works together to evaluate and identify problems, set therapeutic goals, and provide intervention. The patient's diagnosis and the therapeutic setting, such as inpatient or outpatient, determines the degree of interdisciplinary involvement as well as the specific team members who comprise the team.

These may include the following:

Dietician. The dietician evaluates nutritional status, recommends appropriate diet based on personal and team assessments, and councils the patient and family on dietary modifications.

Occupational therapist (OT). The OT emphasizes fine motor skills; evaluates and trains patient in activities of daily living (ADLs) skills (dressing, hygiene, bathing, eating); provides range of motion (ROM), strengthening, endurance, and coordination exercises for the upper extremities and cervical area; assesses driving skills; and recommends orthoses (braces) for the upper extremities, adaptive equipment (modified utensils, reachers), and home modifications as needed.

Physiatrist. The physiatrist evaluates medical and functional status, manages medical care, orders therapies, and usually coordinates total rehabilitation and physical medicine efforts.

Physical therapist (PT). The PT emphasizes the gross motor skills; evaluates and trains the patient in mobility, such as wheelchair and gait; teaches balance and transfer skills involving moving from one fixed position to another, such as from bed to chair; provides ROM, strengthening, endurance and coordination exercises for limbs and trunk; provides physical modalities including superficial and deep heat, cold, hydrotherapy, electrical stimulation, and traction; and recommends specific orthoses and adaptive equipment such as wheelchairs and gait aids.

Prosthetist/orthotist. The prosthetist/orthotist designs, fabricates, and fits prostheses (artificial limbs) and orthoses (braces and splints).

Psychologist. The psychologist assesses emotional, intellectual, and perceptual functioning; councils and provides psychotherapy to patient and family; and provides the team with recommendations for care.

Recreational therapist (RT). The RT assesses the patient's interests and skills, incorporates leisure time activities into the rehabilitation program, and assists in the patient's community reintegration.

Rehabilitation nurse. The rehabilitation nurse manages the nursing care team, serves as an educational resource to other (nonrehabilitation) nursing personnel, instructs patient and family in functional skills, and reinforces skills learned in therapy.

Social worker. The social worker evaluates a patient's living situations; discusses financial and living arrangement options; provides emotional support to patient, family, and team; and serves as a liaison between patient and family and the team.

Speech pathologist. The speech pathologist evaluates and treats problems with communication and swallowing and assists with cognitive retraining.

Vocational counselor. The vocational counselor evaluates the vocational interests, training, and skills; provides counseling concerning returning to work; and serves as a liaison between the patient and prospective employers.

Others. Professionals who may be a part of the team (depending on the clinical milieu) include respiratory therapist, child life specialist, horticultural therapist, music therapist, dance therapist, animal-assisted therapy specialist, chaplain, rehabilitation dentist, audiologist, and pharmacist.

Rehabilitative Care Settings

PM&R is involved in the care of patients with a variety of diagnoses. These include amputation, arthritis, traumatic brain injury (TBI), burns, cancer, cardiopulmonary disease, chronic pain, fractures, pressure ulcers, sports injury, stroke, musculoskeletal (acute) pain, neuromuscular disease, congenital deformities, childhood onset disabilities, peripheral and central nervous system dysfunction, osteoporosis, disabilities related to aging, polytrauma, spinal cord injury, and generalized deconditioning resulting from any factors. The settings in which each of these is typically managed and the interdisciplinary team members usually involved are summarized in Table 1.1.

Future Trends

The future of physiatry, although difficult to predict, will certainly include a greater emphasis on the rehabilitation concerns of the geriatric population and the severely disabled. This is due to a number of factors:

- Overall increased life expectancy—the proportion of individuals 65 years and older in U.S. society is projected to increase from 12% in the 1990s to 20% in 2030.
- The percentage of so-called old-old individuals, 85 years and older, in the geriatric population will increase from 39% at present to 50% in the year 2030.

Table 1.1.   Rehabilitative Care Settings

Setting	Rehabilitation Category	Team Members
Inpatient rehabilitation • Free-standing facility, general or specialized • Unit within an acute care hospital, usually general rehabilitation	Amputation, arthritis, brain injury, cancer, cardiopulmonary, musculoskeletal, CNS dysfunction, fractures, geriatrics, neuromuscular, pediatrics, peripheral neuropathy, polytrauma, SCI, stroke. Patient demonstrates lack of independence in mobility, ADLs, and/or communication.	Physiatrist, OT, PT, social worker, psychologist, dietician, RT, speech pathologist, pharmacist, prosthetist/orthotist, nurse, vocational counselor, and other specialty therapists
Inpatient consultation • Acute care facility including psychiatry • Skilled nursing facility • Nursing home	Same as above, as well as chronic pain, and generalized deconditioning. Patient may not yet be a candidate for inpatient rehabilitation due to medical/surgical instability.	Physiatrist, consulting physician, appropriate therapists, social worker, prosthetist/orthotist, pharmacist, and dietician
Outpatient rehabilitation • Free-standing comprehensive outpatient rehab facility • Affiliated with acute care facility (PT/OT/speech departments)	Same as above, and chronic pain, industrial injuries, and sports medicine. Patient has progressed through inpatient rehab or does not require inpatient hospitalization for treatment.	Physiatrist, social worker, therapists, prosthetist/orthotist, vocational counselor

ADLs, activities of daily living; CNS, central nervous system; OT, occupation therapy; PT, physical therapy; RT, recreational therapist; SCI, spinal cord injury.

- The population of "oldest-old," 85 years and older, by the year 2050 will have increased nearly seven times compared with the population in 1920. Individuals of these advanced age groups are more prone to have multiple diseases and require more functional support. To allow an enhanced quality of life, more extensive and comprehensive interventions are required.
- Survivability of the severely disabled has vastly increased in recent years, because of technologic advances in care. This has resulted in an increasing proportion of dependent individuals, capable of living near-normal lifespans, who will require extensive intervention.

Other Practice Settings

PM&R physicians focus on prevention, diagnosis, and treatment of disability and maximization of function. A variety of practice settings are used to achieve these ends. Today, many physiatrists are focusing on musculoskeletal rehabilitation and its benefits to their patients. This focus includes treatment of common disorders such as back and shoulder pain. Many center on interventional physiatry with the use of peripheral joint, epidural, and facet injections. Some use acupuncture to treat disorders such as chronic pain, myofascial pain, and fibromyalgia, as well as many other disorders.

PHYSIATRIC EVALUATION

Chief Complaint

Record the chief complaint in the patient's own words. This gives important clues in assessing the patient's perceptual status, intellectual level, and concerns regarding existing illnesses and dysfunction.

Medical History and the Review of Systems

Regardless of medical specialty, the basic elements of medical history taking are the same. In PM&R, the history should also reflect on the extent to which the chief complaint affects the patient's physical and functional independence. In certain situations, this information may require the corroboration of the patient's primary caregiver.

In reviewing organ systems, remember that any illness or disability affects multiple areas. Carefully address each of these. Create a comprehensive problem list, listing active and inactive problems. (See example, Table 1.2.)

Use patience in taking a history from a patient with a communication disorder, such as a stroke, cerebral palsy, or head injury. Speech difficulties are far more frustrating to the patient than to the physician. Assistance from a speech therapist or a family member may be helpful.

Vocational and Social History

Document the patient's social and vocational history in detail. The social history gives insight into social dynamics and available support systems, which will affect the patient's reintegration into society. The vocational history provides a guideline for possible retraining to return the patient to the workforce or to assist in vocational or recreational activities. See Table 1.3.

Table 1.2.   Medical Rehabilitation Patient Problem List

1. Left hemiplegia secondary to right CVA, thrombotic, on (*date*)
2. Functional dependence secondary to #1
3. Urinary incontinence secondary to #2
4. History of hypertension, medication controlled
5. History of coronary artery disease with angina pectoris
6. History of glaucoma with decreased visual acuity
7. History of urinary tract infection (resolved)
8. Status post cholecystectomy (inactive)

CVA, cerebrovascular accident.

Functional History and Evaluation

Loss of function results from an illness or an injury; the disability must be assessed in terms of the patient's independent functioning at home, at work, or at school and compared with premorbid functioning. The key functions include the following:

- Self-care (feeding, grooming, bathing, dressing, and toileting)
- Sphincter control (bladder and bowel)
- Mobility/transfers (bed, chair, toilet and shower)
- Locomotion (wheelchair, ambulation and stair-climbing)
- Social cognition (social interaction, problem solving, and memory)
- Communication

Degrees of dependence and independence can be briefly described as follows:

- Fully independent
- Independent within assistive device or modification of the environment
- Stand-by assistance required (supervision by another person) in some, or most, of daily functioning
- Physical assistance required in some, or all, of daily functioning
- Fully dependent

Various scales have been developed for a more uniform evaluation of function. The Functional Independence Measure (FIM) as-

Table 1.3.   Social/Vocational History

Support system
Premorbid personality
Premorbid life style
Educational level
Substance abuse
Work history (type, place, abilities)
History of avocational (recreational) interests

sesses activities of self-care, mobility, locomotion, communication, and social cognition on a 7-point scale from fully independent to fully dependent. It is the most widely used global (general) scale of function. There are more task specific scales that can be used, including the Barthel Index, the Katz Index, the Kenny Index, and the Klein-Bell ADL Scale.

Physical Examination

The physical examination in its key elements (inspection, palpation, and auscultation) does not differ from that of any other specialty. It is, however, more problem-focused in its attempt to determine how the existing disability affects the functioning of other organ systems and to what extent the body compensates for impaired or lost function of any organ systems.

The physical examination should include the following:

I.   Vital signs
II. Mental status examination
    A. Alertness
    B. Logical thinking
    C. Understanding and following instructions
    D. Recent and immediate recall
    E. Hostile or threatening behavior
    F. Confabulations
III. Neuromuscular examination: DOCUMENT PATIENT POSITION! (lying, sitting, or standing)
    A. Inspection
        1. Joint alignment (contractures, hypomobility, or deformity)
        2. Muscle bulk (atrophy or hypertrophy)
        3. Muscle activity (clonus or increased tone at rest)
        4. Body posture (leaning, imbalance)
        5. Cranial and peripheral nerve assessment (muscle asymmetry, posturing)
    B. Palpation
        1. ROM (active and passive)
        2. Joint stability
        3. Muscle tone (both active movement and passive stretch)
        4. Muscle strength (Table 1.4)
        5. Altered perception of touch, pain, temperature, and proprioception
        6. Deep tendon reflexes (scale of 0 to 4+)
        7. Presence of abnormal reflex (Babinski, Kernig, bulbocavernosus)
        8. Cerebellar examination (synchronous action of muscle groups with volitional movement, nystagmus, imbalance)
IV. Functional examination
    A. Bed mobility (turning from side to side)
    B. Sitting
        1. Coming from supine to sit
        2. Static (supported) versus dynamic (unsupported)

Table 1.4.   Muscle Strength[a]

Grade	Assessment
0/5 (absent)	No evidence of muscle contraction
1/5 (trace)	Visible contraction but no joint movement
2/5 (poor)	Full range of motion with gravity eliminated
3/5 (fair)	Full range of motion against gravity
4/5 (good)	Full movement against moderate resistance
5/5 (normal)	Full movement against strong resistance

[a]This does not apply to the strong antigravity muscles, which are too powerful to be assessed by manual examination. Tiptoe or heel walking is a better way of assessing the gastrocnemius and tibialis anterior muscles, respectively.

C. Transfers
  1. From sit to stand
  2. From bed to other surface
  3. Type, that is, standing pivot
  4. Document equipment, such as sliding board
D. Gait
  1. Document assistive device, if any:
    a. Hand used
    b. Appropriate sequencing
    c. Condition of device
  2. Observe ambulation from front, side, and rear
  3. Note abnormalities such as wide or narrow base of support, prolonged or shortened stance phase, hip hiking, circumduction, Trendelenburg gait (indicating pelvic stabilizer weakness)

Electrodiagnosis

Electrodiagnosis is a diagnostic tool that augments the clinical examination, specifically with regard to the neuromuscular system. It consists of needle examination of a muscle (electromyography), which determines the presence of any involuntary muscle activity at rest (fibrillations, sharp ways, fasciculations), reflecting a muscle membrane's instability; the presence or absence of motor units, action potentials, and their recruitment patterns; and quantification and configuration of motor unit action potentials.

Nerve conduction studies (NCS) are performed to evaluate the conductibility of a peripheral nerve, including proximal and distal nerve segments, functional integrity of the neuromuscular junction, a quantitative reflex evaluation, and sensory/visual/auditory parameters (evaluating peripheral and central nerve pathways).

The most important points to remember are that the electrodiagnostic study is only an adjunct to the clinical examination not a substitute; it is much easier for the electromyographer to assist in making a diagnosis if the referral includes a tentative diagnosis and the reason for requesting the study. Refer to Chapter 9, EMG.

SUGGESTED READINGS

Delisa JA, ed. *Rehabilitation medicine: principles and practice.* Philadelphia: JB Lippincott, 1988:3–24.

Delisa JA, Martin GM, Currie DM. *Rehabilitation medicine: past, present and future.*

Erickson RP, McPhee MC. Clinical evaluation. In: Delisa JA, ed. *Rehabilitation medicine: principles and practice.* Philadelphia: JB Lippincott, 1988:25–65.

Grabois M. Evaluation of disability. In: Halstead LS, Grabois M, eds. *Medical rehabilitation.* New York: Raven Press, 1985:13–32.

Halstead LS. Philosophy of rehabilitation medicine. In: Halstead LS, Grabois M, eds. *Medical rehabilitation.* New York: Raven Press, 1985:1–6.

Halstead LS, Grabois M. Rehabilitation specialists. In: Halstead LS, Grabois M, eds. *Medical rehabilitation.* New York: Raven Press, 1985:7–12.

Itoh M, Lee MHM. The epidemiology of disability as related to rehabilitation medicine. In: Kottke FJ, Stillwell GK, Lehmann JF, eds. *Krusen's handbook of physical medicine and rehabilitation.* Philadelphia: WB Saunders, 1982:199–217.

Acute Pain

Steve M. Gnatz

DEFINITION

Pain is the most common reason for which patients seek treatment by physicians. Biologically, the pain signal represents potentially dangerous tissue damage. Pain is a warning to the organism to stop or escape from damaging activity and allows regenerative processes to work. However, pain is a complex interplay of peripheral nerve, spinal cord, and brain processes that are incompletely understood. If, for unknown reasons, the pain signal continues despite the removal of the painful stimulus, pain loses its adaptive value and may result in significant physical and psychosocial disability.

Most acute pain can be eliminated by discontinuing the source of tissue damage, resting the damaged part, and using simple analgesia. Physical medicine techniques enhance physical recovery from many painful conditions, particularly if simple measures have not eliminated the pain or if significant loss of function has occurred.

NEUROANATOMY AND NEUROPHYSIOLOGY OF PAIN PATHWAYS

Most nociceptor afferent input is transmitted from the peripheral pain sensors through the small (0.1 to 1.0 μm diameter) unmyelinated C fibers to the central nervous system (CNS). Some pain impulses, particularly thermal and mechanical pressure stimuli, reach the CNS through myelinated A-delta fibers (1 to 4 μm diameter). Peripheral stimuli enter the dorsal horn of the spinal cord where most of the C fibers synapse in the substantia gelatinosa (lamina II). Pain impulses ascend the spinothalamic and spinoreticular tracts to project on the lateral and medial thalamic nuclei and the brainstem, respectively (Fig. 2-1). Projection of these impulses to the sensory cortical areas brings the pain to consciousness and makes locating it in the body possible. Substance P, an 11-amino acid peptide, has been identified as a peripheral neurotransmitter in the dorsal horn of the spinal cord. Endogenous opioids, such as beta-endorphin and enkephalins in the CNS and periphery, inhibit pain.

EPIDEMIOLOGY

Pain is a universal phenomenon. Everyone experiences pain during his or her lifetime. At least 80% of the population at some time will have low back pain, the most common cause of worker absence and loss of productivity in industrialized countries. Neck pain may be present in up to 50% of the population at some time in life, and up to 20% of the female population experiences fibromyalgia. About 1.6% of the population has an ongoing problem with temporomandibular joint pain. See Table 2.1 for common symptoms of craniomandibular dysfunction.

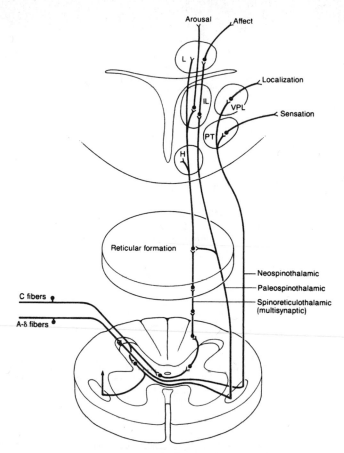

Fig. 2-1. Pathways of pain sensation, from the periphery to the central nervous system. H, hypothalamus; IL, intralaminar thalamic nuclei; L, limbic system; PT, posterior thalamic nuclei; VPL, ventral posterolateral thalamic nuclei. (From Walsh N et al. Treatment of the patient with chronic pain. In: DeLisa JA. *Rehabilitation medicine*, 2nd ed. JB Lippincott, 1993:975, with permission.)

ETIOLOGY AND PATHOPHYSIOLOGY

Acute pain can usually be linked to a precipitating event, usually traumatic. Possible causes are in Table 2.2.

One should assume that all pain is real. However, remember that pain is subjective; there can be no objective measurement of it. Pain that is incapacitating to one may be inconsequential to another person or to the same person under different circumstances. All pain perception is individual.

In general, the longer pain persists, the less likely complete resolution becomes. This assumes that adequate workup for etiologic

Table 2.1.   Common Symptoms of Craniomandibular Dysfunction

- Jaw symptoms
  Painful movement and limited opening
  Clicking, popping, or other joint noise
  Locking open or closed
- Headaches
  Usually muscle-contraction type
  Areas involved: temporal, occipital, or generalized
  May present with vascular or migraine-like symptoms
- Ear symptoms
  Tinnitus, fullness in the ears, hearing loss
  Vestibular dysfunction, vertigo, dizziness, nausea
- Eye symptoms
  Pain behind the eyes, blurring of vision, photophobia
- Facial, neck, and upper back pain
  Generally described as tightness, soreness, stiffness
  May be sharp, hyperesthetic (can mimic neuralgia,
  radiculopathy)
- Other
  Sinus pressure, stuffiness
  Tooth and gum complaints
  Autonomic phenomena, sweating, lacrimation
  Swallowing difficulty

and contributing factors has been performed and that perpetuating factors have been controlled as much as possible. Patients who are adaptable, educable, and willing to take responsibility for aspects of treatment within their control generally have better outcomes than those with significant psychosocial issues, lack of insight, or secondary gain motives.

GENERAL GUIDELINES FOR ASSESSMENT OF THE PATIENT WITH PAIN

- Obtain a complete medication and treatment history. Do not repeat a previously unsuccessful treatment, unless it was implemented incorrectly.
- Review previous diagnostic tests, operative reports, therapists' notes, consultants' notes, and recorded psychosocial information.
- Have the patient complete a pain diagram.
- Use a pain rating scale.
- Identify an acute traumatic event, if possible.
- Characterize pain using the mnemonic PQRST: Provocative and palliative factors, Quality, Region-radiation, Severity, and Temporal characteristics. Pain can be diffuse and difficult for the patient to describe.
- Obtain pain descriptors that help identify a specific pain syndrome.
- Observe the patient walking, sitting, and moving both when unaware of being observed and when being directed.
- Assess what, if any, psychosomatic overlay is present. Identify depression if suspected.

Table 2.2.   Etiologies of Acute Pain

Trauma
Overuse syndrome
Improper body mechanics
"Microtrauma"
Systemic or localized disease process
    Degenerative
    Inflammatory
    Infectious
    Malignant

- Organize the proper workup for diagnosis.
- Develop a rational treatment plan based on the established diagnosis. It is better to leave a patient undiagnosed than to make an erroneous diagnosis.
- Differential diagnoses of commonly seen musculoskeletal pain problems are listed in Table 2.3.

FUNCTIONAL EVALUATION

Obtain a history of the patient's current and past social situation, including vocational, family, and interpersonal stresses. Characterize the extent of disability by noting current functional limitations in activities of daily living, exercise endurance, and dependence on adaptive equipment. Record litigation status and other aspects of potential secondary gain, which may impede recovery.

PHYSICAL EXAMINATION

The physical examination is a directed neuromuscular and joint examination. Identify the painful structures and document variations from the normal that may interfere with function. Although details of the examination are specified by the history, certain elements are constant. Seek alterations in muscle strength, sensation, and deep tendon reflexes. Patients often cannot participate in manual muscle testing because of the resulting pain. "Giveway" weakness is not always associated with poor cooperation on the patient's part.

Search carefully for dermatomal or root level dysfunction of sensory and reflex systems. These hard neurologic signs are difficult to produce voluntarily. However, muscle atrophy resulting from immobility may contribute to decreased deep tendon reflexes.

Examine joint structures for effusion, decreased range of motion (ROM), and deformity; palpate tendons and ligamentous structures.

Palpate muscle to evaluate for trigger points or tight bands of muscle that, when deeply palpated, cause referred pain in a specific pattern. Figure 2-2 demonstrates common tender muscle areas related to fibromyalgia. Instruct the patient to perform specific maneuvers such as a straight leg raising test (patient supine, leg raised from horizontal), Tinel's sign (tap over median nerves of wrist), or the Finkelstein test (thumb wrapped up in fist, wrist

Table 2.3.   Differential Diagnosis of Commonly Seen Musculoskeletal Pain Problems

- Bone
  Fracture (acute traumatic, stress, compression)
  Dislocation
  Metastatic lesion
  Other intrinsic bone lesion (bone cyst, osteoma, hemangioma, etc.)
  Infection
- Joint
  Cartilaginous dysfunction (tear, degeneration, inflammation, dislocation)
  Synovial fluid (gout, pseudogout, infection, etc.)
  Ligaments (tear, stretch, contracture)
  Capsule, bursae (inflammation, contracture)
  Osteophytic spurring, osteoarthritis
- Muscle, tendon
  Overstretch, tear, rupture
  Contracture
  Weakness, fatigue
  Inflammation, intrinsic muscle disease
  Trigger points, tender points (myofascial pain/fibromyalgia)
  Inflammation of tendon sheath (tenosynovitis)
- Nerve
  Compression (nerve roots, peripheral entrapments)
  Stretch (brachial plexus, etc.)
  Direct trauma
  Inflammation
  Neuropathy (diabetic, EtOH, etc.)
- Biomechanical, kinesiologic
  Postural abnormality
  Overuse, unequal or imbalanced strength
  Gait abnormality
  Anatomic variation (unequal leg lengths, etc.)

EtOH, ethanol.

ulnar deviated) to aid in the clinical confirmation of the suspected diagnosis. Other tests are listed in Table 2.4.

TREATMENT

Treatment of acutely painful conditions differs from the treatment of chronic pain. In acute pain management, resting the damaged structure is essential for recovery. This contrasts with the management of chronic pain, in which the patient usually needs mobilization because of underuse of affected areas. Contracture of collagenous structures, including tendon, ligament, and joint capsules, occurs rapidly in patients with painful ROM. These may require gentle passive range of motion (PROM) to avoid the vicious cycle of pain, immobility, contracture, and increased pain. Similarly, atrophy of immobilized muscle should be avoided, if possible, through the use of isometric exercise.

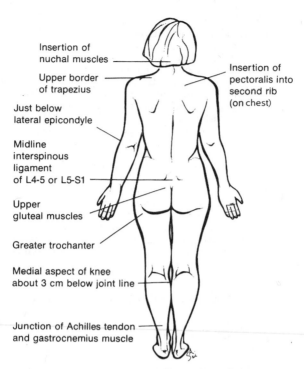

Insertion of nuchal muscles

Upper border of trapezius

Just below lateral epicondyle

Midline interspinous ligament of L4-5 or L5-S1

Upper gluteal muscles

Greater trochanter

Medial aspect of knee about 3 cm below joint line

Junction of Achilles tendon and gastrocnemius muscle

Insertion of pectoralis into second rib (on chest)

Fig. 2-2.   Typical locations of tender points in fibromyalgia.

Table 2.4. Other Tests	
Category	Uses/Examples
Physical quantitative testing	Cybex/Stress test
Diagnosis-specific laboratory data	Rheumatoid factor, ANA, CPK, sedimentation rate
Radiographic evaluation Routine	Identify fractures, bone and joint pathology
MRI	Identify muscle, tendon, ligament abnormalities
Electrodiagnostic testing (EMG/NCV)	Evaluation of the neuromuscular system, nerve entrapments, radiculopathy, myopathy, or myositis

ANA, antinuclear antibody; CPK, creatinine phosphokinase; EMG, electromyography; MRI, magnetic resonance imaging; NCV, nerve conductor velocity.

Physical Modalities

The physical modalities of heat, cold, electricity, sound, and water are used to accomplish the goal of increased function while minimizing pain. Both heat and cold provide analgesic effects. Heat is useful in both acute and chronic pain for analgesia, muscle relaxation, and enhancement of the stretchability of collagen. Cold may be more beneficial in acute pain for its ability to control edema; heat may exacerbate edema, if present. In general, use cold for the first 24 to 48 hours after an acute injury and heat thereafter.

Many forms of heat are available, including hot packs, shortwave and microwave diathermy, and ultrasound. Hydrotherapy provides heat but is much better prescribed as a debriding agent than a heating one. Such devices as moist air cabinets, paraffin baths, and fluidotherapy are indicated in some cases of arthritic pain.

The depth of penetration of heating modalities varies. Hot packs give superficial heat to the skin and subcutaneous tissue; microwave and shortwave diathermy provide deeper heat, warming some muscle layers. Ultrasound, working at the tissue-fluid interface, is the only heating modality that raises the intraarticular temperature of large joints significantly. Heating modalities are contraindicated in specific cases. See Table 2.5.

Table 2.5. Contraindications for Use of Heat

Insensate areas (risk of burns)
Acute infection, inflammation or edema
Compromised vascular supply
Tumors
Unknown underlying pathology

Electrical Modalities

Transcutaneous electrical nerve stimulation (TENS) modulates pain by applying electrical impulses to the skin. There are two basic types: high-frequency low-intensity TENS (conventional TENS), and low-frequency high-intensity TENS (electroacupuncture). Conventional TENS works because of the "gate" theory of pain. Presented simply, this involves incoming cutaneous sensory and proprioceptive impulses carried through larger myelinated nerve fibers, which inhibit pain impulses carried more slowly by unmyelinated nerve fibers at the level of the dorsal column of the spinal cord. The faster impulses arrive at the dorsal column first and "close the gate," forestalling propagation of the slower pain impulses.

The second type of TENS, high-voltage galvanic stimulation or electroacupuncture, uses a more pronounced jolt of electrical stimulation, which increases endogenous opioid substances in the brain. Electroacupuncture may be less useful in the treatment of some pain disorders because of the painful nature of the stimulus.

The advantage of TENS is that it is noninvasive. Several different electrodes and stimulator settings should be used before discontinuing it for failing to relieve pain. Individual response to TENS is the rule. Patients who respond to TENS may get prolonged relief from an implanted electrical stimulator. There are a few contraindications to TENS. To avoid vagal stimulation, it should not be placed over the anterolateral aspect of the neck. Theoretically, it may cause malfunction of cardiac pacemakers. Hypersensitivity to the electrodes (skin irritation) occasionally necessitates discontinuation but can be minimized if different electrodes are used.

Medications

Typically, other physicians will have prescribed patients numerous medications if they have had pain for any length of time. It is important to know which medications have been tried, which were effective, and how they were taken in order rationally to provide pharmacologic adjunct therapy in a rehabilitation program.

Narcotic analgesics are rarely indicated in the treatment of pain, other than in emergency or very acute situations. However, some patients may be dependent on or frankly addicted to narcotic analgesic medications. Do *not* prescribe pain medications on an as needed (PRN) basis; this reinforces pain behavior. Patients should take medication on a schedule, regardless of the level of pain. If they feel they do not need the prescribed amount of medication, they should reduce the dose. If they feel they need more pain relief, they should be instructed to try nonpharmacologic techniques first. Failing these, new therapy should be planned with their physician.

Nonsteroidal antiinflammatory drugs (NSAIDs) such as ibuprofen have both analgesic and antiinflammatory properties. Although there is significant variability between agents, usually the antiinflammatory effect is obtained at two to four times the analgesic dose. Generally, those NSAIDs with a longer half-life allow better patient compliance but do not afford as quick an analgesic effect after the dose is taken. The COX-2 antagonists may have a better side effect profile than other NSAIDs and offer the convenience of once-a-day dosing. Other side effects of NSAIDs include fluid retention and, rarely, renal or liver problems.

Muscle relaxants such as cyclobenzaprine (Flexeril), metaxalone (Skelaxin), methocarbamol (Robaxin), and carisoprodol (Soma) may be indicated for the short-term (10-day) treatment of acute muscle spasm. Drowsiness associated with these agents makes them potentially dangerous for certain patients such as machinery operators, whose mental alertness is required for safety. They should not be taken with alcohol.

Amitriptyline (Elavil) is a tricyclic antidepressant with excellent analgesic properties, probably based on CNS modulation of the serotonergic pathways. It can be effective for pain relief in doses much lower than those used for depression. Usually 25 to 100 mg at bedtime is sufficient for analgesia. The side effects include drowsiness, which is limited by use at bedtime, and anticholinergic effects.

The antiseizure medications gabapentin (Neurontin), topiramate (Topamax), valproic acid (Depakote), and carbamazepine (Tegretol) probably control pain through their membrane stabilizing effects. These medications are effective primarily in neuropathic pain syndromes. Monitor for side effects with any medication.

Other Treatments

Other treatment methods are listed in Table 2.6. Exercise is an important adjunct therapy. Finding the ideal combination of

Table 2.6.   Other Treatment Methods

What	Why	How	Limitations
Trigger point injections	Spreading out muscle fibers can relieve pain	Palpate an isolated painful point in muscle with pain referral; inject with 1–2 cc of 0.5% Procaine or 1% Xylocaine without epinephrine Normal saline works, but does not produce immediate effect Use ultrasound immediately afterward	Trigger points may recur, fibrosis of muscle
Spray and stretch techniques	Counterirritant effect similar to TENS and topical agents (liniments)	Use fluoromethane or other vapocoolant spray	Works best for large muscles (trapezius)
Massage	Decreases muscle tension	Various techniques	Labor-intensive, best for short-term, acute problems
Manipulation	Realignment of abnormal musculoskeletal positioning	Apply short-arm lever techniques appropriately	Remains controversial
Functional electrical stimulation (FES)	Used with surface EMG biofeedback, retrains/ strengthens muscles	Use of electrical current strengthens muscle	Burns, skin sensitivity

EMG, electromyographic; TENS, transcutaneous electrical nerve stimulation.

rest and exercise is a challenging concept for patients and practitioners alike. When acute inflammation of the muscle or joint is present, rest is necessary to allow healing to occur. However, muscle weakness and joint contracture can take place very rapidly when there is complete immobility. The key is PROM up to, but not past, the point of pain. The power required to range the joint may be provided by a therapist or by the patient after proper training. Causing pain during the ROM of the joint will only restart the vicious cycle of pain, immobility, contracture, and more pain.

Isometric exercise may be initiated even in the presence of acute joint inflammation. When combined with surface electromyographic (EMG) biofeedback techniques, isometric contraction and relaxation of the muscle can be coordinated easily.

Therapeutic exercise of a subacute joint begins with gentle PROM up to, but not past, the point of pain after application of a suitable heating modality, such as hot packs and ultrasound. This maximizes ROM and minimizes pain. As inflammation subsides, the patient becomes more active in the isotonic use of muscles around the joint. Therapy ultimately concentrates more on strengthening through resistive exercise. The timing of this program is highly variable, because it depends on the patient's tolerance and requires close follow-up by the therapist and the doctor.

It is difficult, if not impossible, to strengthen painful muscles. To develop a muscle training response requires forces applied to the muscle and other tissues that will not be tolerated by a patient in pain; no progress will be made. Refer to Fig. 2-3 for stages of recovery from acute pain.

Specific details regarding evaluation and treatment of back, neck, and fibromyalgic pain are listed in Tables 2.7, 2.8, and 2.9, respectively.

COMPLICATIONS

Many patients are sensitive about the psychologic overlay associated with pain. Allow the patient to gain some confidence in your ability to control acute pain using physical techniques. Then, educate about the usefulness of long-term lifestyle adjustment in the management of pain. Psychologic support may help the patient

Stage 1		Stage 2		Stage 3		
Pain relief through modalities	→	Regain normal resting muscle length through ROM and flexibility exercises	→	Gradual muscle strengthening	→	Recovery

Fig. 2-3. Stages of recovery from acute pain.

Table 2.7.   Back Pain—Evaluation and Treatment

History
Trauma—mechanism of injury
Past history, prior episodes, surgery
Locking, pop, snap, inability to straighten up
Radiating pain or numbness in the legs
Weakness, bladder or bowel dysfunction
Prior exercise/fitness level

Physical
Observation—skin markings, posture, pain behaviors
Range of motion—flexion, extension, lateral bending, rotation
Palpation—muscle, facet joint and spinous process tenderness
Manual muscle testing—quadriceps (L4); extensor hallicus
   longus (L5); gastrocnemius (S1)
Sensory—L4–S1, dermatomes
DTRs—ankle jerk (S1); knee jerk (L4)
Straight leg raise—sitting versus supine
Other tests—hips, sacroiliac joints

Differential diagnosis of acute back pain
Sprain—ligamentous, strain—muscle
Disc disease—degenerative, herniation, inflammatory
Arthritis
Spondylosis, spinal stenosis, spondylolysis, spondylolisthesis
Facet joint arthropathy, subluxation
Arachnoiditis, iatrogenic—"failed back syndrome"
Neurogenic, vascular—aortic aneurysm
Viscerogenic, gynecologic
Osteoporosis—fracture, dislocation, subluxation
Psychogenic—malingering
Malignancy—multiple myeloma, metastasis
Infectious—AIDS, TB, abscess

Treatment
Acute—rest, analgesia, superficial heat
Subacute—mobilization, PT (modalities, ROM, stretching,
   gradual exercise), education, posture, +/– bracing

AIDS, acquired immunodeficiency syndrome; PT, physical therapy; ROM,
range of motion; TB, tuberculosis.

tolerate pain that cannot be controlled medically. Never promise to
eliminate all pain!

Secondary gain, both monetary and emotional, can be a perva-
sive and often totally subconscious motivating factor in continuing
pain behaviors. Secondary gain must be eliminated before the patient can recover.

If not treated aggressively and effectively, acute pain may
progress to a chronic pain syndrome. Recognize psychosocial/
behavioral issues early to plan comprehensive pain management.

Table 2.8.   Neck Pain—Evaluation and Treatment

History
Trauma—mechanism of injury
Locking, crepitation, noise, spasm
Headache, dizziness
Jaw pain
Arm symptoms—numbness, weakness, leg symptoms
Past history, episodes
Dysphagia—severe spondylosis
Stress-related factors
Posture-related factors—computer terminal, phone

Physical
Observation
Range of motion, crepitation
Manual muscle testing upper extremities—deltoid C5, biceps
   C5–6, triceps C6–7, wrist extensors C6–7, intrinsics C8
Sensory—C4–T1 dermatomes
DTRs—biceps C5–6, triceps C7–8

Differential diagnosis of neck pain
Sprain—ligamentous, strain—muscle
Disc disease—degenerative, herniation, inflammatory
Arthritis
Spondylosis, spinal stenosis
Facet joint arthropathy, subluxation
Arachnoiditis, iatrogenic—"failed neck syndrome"
Neurogenic
Osteoporosis—fracture, dislocation, subluxation
Psychogenic—malingering
Malignancy—multiple myeloma, metastasis
Infectious—AIDS, TB, abscess
Torticollis, antecollis, retrocollis, other movement disorder

Treatment
Acute—rest, analgesia, superficial heat
Subacute—mobilization, PT (modalities, ROM, stretching,
   gradual exercise traction), education, posture, +/– bracing

PT, physical therapy; ROM, range of motion.

Table 2.9.   Fibromyalgia (and Myofascial Pain)—Evaluation and Treatment

History
Pain
Muscle stiffness
Tightness
Burning
Waxing and waning
Varies in location/intensity
Stress related
Sleep disorder
Headaches
Soft neurologic symptoms—numbness, weakness—in a nondermatomal pattern

Tolerance for exercise
Usually low
Generalized fatigue
Nutrition
Other medical stressors
Psychosocial stressors
Anxiety
Depression
Autonomic symptoms—sweating, irritable bowel

Physical
Trigger points—latent, active—in characteristic locations
Normal neurologic examination
Postural abnormalities—check head to toe—evaluate for leg-length discrepancy

Differential diagnosis (rule these out before making diagnosis of primary fibromyalgia)
Intrinsic muscle disease—myositis, myalgias (viral infections, etc.), infections, trichinella
Rheumatologic disease
Hypothyroidism[a]
Anemia[a]
Mitral valve prolapse[a]

Treatment
Patient counseling—diagnostic and therapeutic reassurance, avoidance of aggravating factors, frequent follow-up
Physical modalities—stretching, flexibility, exercises, attention to posture, position, local anesthetic sprays or injection, aerobic conditioning, muscle massage, stretching, ultrasound
Medications—amitriptyline (Elavil) and cyclobenzaprine (Flexeril) of significant benefit in controlled trials; start with 10 mg of either at bedtime and increase to 25–50 mg depending on response and toxic effects; NSAIDs and simple analgesics may be used in combination with above, but of no demonstrable efficacy; prednisone and narcotics should not be used

---

NSAIDs, nonsteroidal antiinflammatory drugs.
[a] May be a contributing factor.

SUGGESTED READINGS

Brown SE, Atchison JW, Gnatz SM et al. Pain rehabilitation. 2. Documentation of acute, subacute, and chronic pain. *Arch Phys Med Rehabil* 1998;79(Suppl 1):S54–S59.

Caillet R. *Soft tissue pain disability.* Philadelphia: FA Davis, 1977.

Caillet R. *Low back pain syndrome,* 5th ed. Philadelphia: FA Davis, 1995.

Gnatz SM. Temporomandibular joint disorders. In: Grabois M, Garrison, SJ, eds. *Physical medicine and rehabilitation: the complete approach.* Cambridge, MA: Blackwell Science, 2000.

Gnatz SM, Brown SE, Atchison JW et al. Pain rehabilitation. 5. Pain assessment and management of common disorders. *Arch Phys Med Rehabil* 1998;79(Suppl 1):S74–S76.

Gnatz SM, Childers MK. Acute pain. In: Grabois, M, Garrison, SJ, eds. *Physical medicine and rehabilitation: the complete approach.* Cambridge, MA: Blackwell Science, 2000.

Simons DG, Travell JG. *Myofascial pain and dysfunction, the trigger point manual,* 2nd ed. Baltimore: Williams & Wilkins, 1999.

Taub NS, Worsowicz, GM, Gnatz SM et al. Pain rehabilitation. 1. Definitions and diagnosis of pain. *Arch Phys Med Rehabil* 1998; 79(Suppl 1):S49–S53.

Wall PD. The gate control theory of pain mechanisms. A re-examination and re-statement. *Brain* 1978;101:1–18.

Wall PD, Melzack R, eds. *Textbook of pain,* 3rd ed. Edinburgh: Churchill Livingston, 1994.

Yunis MB. Diagnosis, etiology, and management of fibromyalgia syndrome: an update. *Compr Ther* 1988;14:8–20.

3

Amputations

Jay V. Subbarao and Gary S. Clark

GENERAL INFORMATION

This chapter focuses on the basic physiatric approaches to the most commonly occurring amputations: transtibial amputation (TTA) [formerly known as below knee amputation (BKA)], transfemoral amputation (TFA) [formerly known as above knee amputation (AKA)], transradial amputation (TRA) [previously termed below elbow (BE) amputation], and transhumeral amputation (THA) [previously referred to as above elbow (AE) amputation].

DEFINITIONS

An amputation is the removal of a limb or other appendage or outgrowth of the body. Disarticulation involves amputation through a joint. The portion of the limb that remains after amputation is known as the residual limb. (We encourage you to use the term *residual limb* in place of the pejorative term *stump* and also to refer to "a patient/person with amputation" rather than "an amputee.") A prosthesis is the manufactured device that allows the person with an amputation to regain function (e.g., for TTA/TFA, weight transmission during ambulation). Postamputation, phantom sensation is experienced by essentially 100% of individuals and is usually described as the sensation of the amputated limb still being present. Although this is a "normal" phenomenon after an amputation and not typically painful, a proportion of individuals develop phantom limb pain, which is a chronic pain syndrome involving the amputated limb and requires comprehensive care.

INCIDENCE/ETIOLOGY

Currently there are an estimated 1.5 million individuals in the United States with major limb loss, with more than 120,000 new amputations each year. There are a variety of causes for amputation, including dysvascular diseases, trauma, infection, malignancy, and congenital anomalies. Lower limb amputations account for 90% of all amputations, with 75% of these resulting from peripheral vascular disease and 20% from trauma.

Dysvascular disease can result in amputation from acute arterial insufficiency with gangrene or chronic nonhealing ulcers associated with poor blood supply with accompanying infection of skin (cellulitis) or bone (osteomyelitis). Risk of dysvascular amputation increases significantly when associated with diabetes (at least fourfold) and with aging. Men are at higher risk than women, and African American men and women are at much higher risk (two- to fourfold) than age- and gender-matched whites. In addition, there is a significant correlation of peripheral vascular disease with cardiovascular (myocardial infarction) and cerebrovascular (stroke) disease. Figure 3-1 shows common factors leading to amputation.

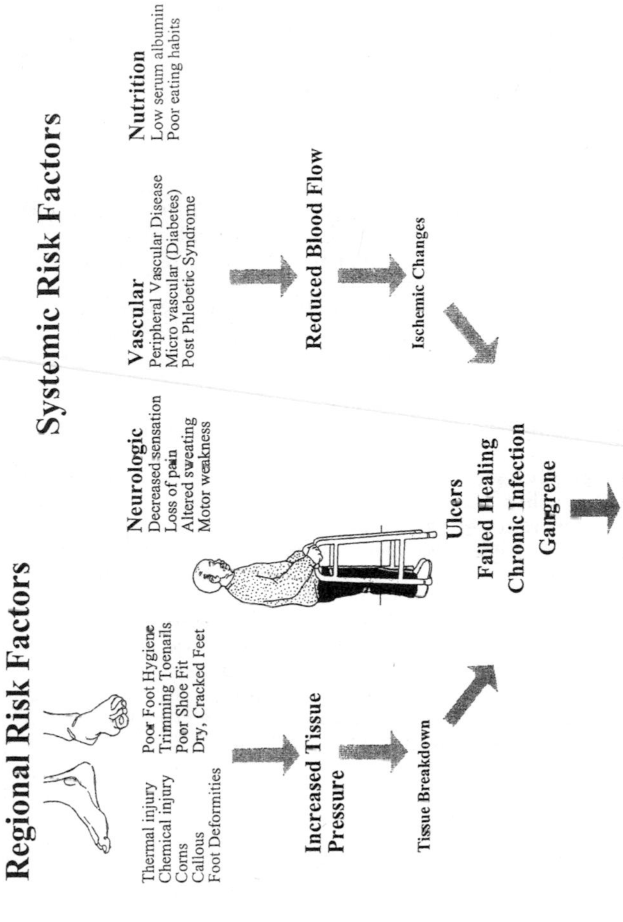

Regional Risk Factors

Systemic Risk Factors

Thermal injury   Poor Foot Hygiene
Chemical injury   Trimming Toenails
Corns   Poor Shoe Fit
Callous   Dry, Cracked Feet
Foot Deformities

Neurologic
Decreased sensation
Loss of pain
Altered sweating
Motor weakness

Vascular
Peripheral Vascular Disease
Micro vascular (Diabetes)
Post Phlebetic Syndrome

Nutrition
Low serum albumin
Poor eating habits

Increased Tissue Pressure

Tissue Breakdown

Reduced Blood Flow

Ischemic Changes

Ulcers
Failed Healing
Chronic Infection
Gangrene

Amputation

Fig. 3-1. Factors leading to amputations.

Trauma is the next most common cause for lower extremity amputation and the leading cause (75%) of upper extremity amputation. Motor vehicle accidents and work-related injuries, such as machine trauma, electrical or chemical burns, along with higher risk recreational activities account for most of these amputations. Among individuals 10 to 20 years of age, tumors are the most common cause of amputation. Congenital limb deficiency occurs in approximately 26 of 100,000 live births and is nearly twice as common in the upper limb 3 in the lower limb.

Overall, rates of dysvascular amputation continue to rise, whereas rates for amputation because of trauma and malignancy are declining. Rates of congenital limb deficiency remain stable.

PATIENT ASSESSMENT/EVALUATION

General Considerations

Assessing individuals with amputation involves much more than just choosing substitutes for lost body parts. The general health of the patient must be assessed, with particular attention to the cardiopulmonary, musculoskeletal, and neurologic systems (including cognitive function and vision). If there are general health limitations, these may adversely affect the patient's progress in the rehabilitation program and ability to achieve his or her highest functional level. A good understanding of the components and patterns of normal gait is essential for understanding the prosthetic gait patterns and gait deviations.

To assess possible mobility limitations, observe the patient performing a transfer, such as moving from bed to wheelchair without a prosthesis. If the patient can perform this activity independently, meaning, with or without an assistive device such as a walker, but without physical assistance, he or she is more likely to function well with a prosthetic device.

The higher energy requirements of ambulation after amputation as measured by oxygen consumption underscores the importance of an efficient cardiopulmonary status, because this can limit the distance and speed at which the patient can walk. A person with unilateral TFA, ambulating with a walker or crutches without a prosthesis, consumes approximately 65% more energy than a healthy individual with normal gait. Even after prosthetic fitting and training, significantly more energy is required for ambulation compared with normal gait (Table 3.1).

Table 3.1.   Energy Requirements for Various Levels of Amputation (Using Prostheses)

Amputation Level	Energy Increase (% Above Normal)
Unilateral, transtibial	10–20%
Bilateral, transtibial	20–40%
Unilateral, transfemoral	60–70%
Bilateral, transfemoral	>200%

Assessing the patient's cognitive status is relevant as well, because there are a variety of new tasks to learn after amputation. Examples include putting on (donning) and removing (doffing) the prosthesis, learning how to inspect the limb for injury, and cleaning and caring for the device. She or he should be aware of safety precautions to avoid injury. The patient's social support system is also important, because the family and/or caregiver may need to assist in compensating for physical, cognitive, or environmental limitations.

It is important to consider the underlying cause of the amputation. If amputation is a result of peripheral vascular disease, the opposite limb must be assessed for similar problems. If the amputation was related to cancer, there may be metastatic disease. For obvious reasons, other comorbid conditions that may contribute to functional loss should be documented, such as blindness, severe arthritis with joint deformity or limitation of motion, stroke with hemiparesis or ataxia, or end-stage renal disease with fluid fluctuations.

Residual Limb Evaluation

Finally, it is important to focus attention on the residual limb. Regardless of the site of amputation, there are a number of standard assessments that are important to record for the residual limb, as follows:

- *Length of residual limb* (measured to bone end and skin end, which often differ) from a fixed proximal skeletal landmark, such as from the medial joint line of the knee for TTA. A very short residual limb may be difficult to fit with a prosthesis, whereas a very long residual limb may preclude use of a prosthesis.
- *State of healing of the incision or scar and mobility* of the scar and surrounding soft tissue. If the scar becomes adherent to underlying bone, it is susceptible to break down from movement within the prosthetic socket during ambulation.
- *Soft tissue coverage* of the residual limb, particularly of distal bone. Too little soft tissue results in excessive distal bony prominence, which can be painful in a prosthesis and is more likely to break down; too much soft tissue distally can interfere with proper fit and function of the prosthesis.
- *Skin integrity* of the residual limb. Skin breakdown generally precludes wearing the prosthesis until the skin is intact.
- *Sensation* in the residual limb. A patient with impaired light touch and/or pinprick sensation is vulnerable to unrecognized skin irritation and breakdown.
- *Overall shape* of the residual limb. Ideally cylindrical or slightly conical for best prosthetic fit and function.
- *Full range of motion (ROM)*, both passive and active, in the joints of the residual limb. Joint contractures are the most common complication for individuals after amputation and complicate prosthetic fitting and function.
- *Joint ligamentous stability*. A prosthesis increases stress on proximal joints in the residual limb and the opposite extremity, and lax joint ligaments can result in instability and pain.

- *Strength* of the remaining musculature of the limb. Proximal or opposite limb or upper extremity weakness can render the patient unstable during ambulation.

Accurate assessment of these characteristics facilitates appropriate prosthetic fitting and, ultimately, maximizes level of function. This also serves to design a rehabilitation program, to effectively reverse or prevent secondary complications that limit function and reduce comfort. Although the role of the opposite limb differs for upper versus lower extremity amputations, it is crucial in both situations to assess the extremity for skin integrity, joint ROM and stability, sensation, and strength. Abnormalities in one or more characteristics will further limit functional potential.

REHABILITATION

Ideally, rehabilitation management begins before the actual amputation. The patient can be counseled regarding the therapeutic benefits of amputation, such as reduction in pain, elimination of infection, and restoration of functional independence. Patient education should include what to expect during postoperative care, the timing and sequence of different phases of rehabilitation, demonstration of a typical prosthesis, and discussion of realistic functional goals. The exercise program needed after the amputation can be explained and even initiated if the amputation is an elective one. A peer visitor program can be of great help if it can be arranged before or soon after the amputation, so that the patient can get first hand information from someone who has already been through the process.

Preprosthetic Training

If training is not initiated before the surgery, it should be started as soon as possible postoperatively. The goals at this stage are to achieve functional independence in self-care and mobility without a prosthesis, as well as to prepare the patient and his or her residual limb for prosthetic use. This includes learning to "ace-wrap" the residual limb with the figure-of-eight technique to maximize edema control, aid healing, and shape the residual limb. As the residual limb heals, compression and shaping can be continued by transitioning to an appropriately sized elastic shrinker sock. This is accomplished by exercising to build strength and endurance, with training in transfer techniques, wheelchair level of mobility, and, if appropriate, short-distance ambulation (hopping) with a walker. This is an important skill, because there will always be times when the patient will need to be able to walk without a prosthesis, such as at night, during prosthetic repairs, or in the event of skin breakdown that temporarily precludes wearing the prosthesis.

Other areas of focus include attention to general medical status, monitoring wound healing, and training the patient and family as appropriate in residual limb care. Some surgeons prefer application of a rigid cast dressing immediately after surgery and change it in 7 to 10 days.

Training also involves close inspection of the residual limb and opposite limb for skin status, ROM and stretching exercises, proper positioning of the residual limb to decrease risk of contractures, for example, no pillow under the knee, to lesser flexion at the knee joints, and gentle massage of the distal residual limb to avoid scar adherence and provide tactile input and desensitization from pain. Necessary adaptive equipment such as long-handled reacher and gait assistive devices or walkers to facilitate function are issued, with appropriate training. Patient and family education comprise the final component of the preprosthetic program.

Prosthetic Fitting

Although most patients undergoing amputation will clearly qualify for being fitted and trained to use a prosthesis, there are some situations in which a prosthesis may be *relatively* contraindicated (Table 3.2). It is important to emphasize that there are no absolute contraindications for prosthetic prescription, including age. For patients with severe cardiac disease or hemiparesis, it may be appropriate to consider a "cosmetic" prosthesis, which would provide the patient a more complete body image and facilitate socialization. In such cases, patients are typically mobile at a wheelchair level and do not use the prosthesis to transfer or walk.

The exact timing for prosthetic fitting depends on several factors but is usually in the range of 4 to 6 weeks. Key factors are a well-healed suture line and minimal edema of the residual limb. The remaining skin over the residual limb must also be intact, with stable size and shape of the residual limb. Patients with diabetic peripheral vascular disease or with residual wound infections typically require longer intervals for healing. The remaining residual limb assessment factors previously reviewed such as ROM, strength, and joint stability affect the design of the prosthesis and the patient's functional prognosis. A well-structured preprosthetic program facilitates early prosthetic fitting.

Table 3.2.   Relative Contraindications for Lower Extremity Prosthetic Prescription

- Severe cognitive deficits interfering with learning and safety awareness
- Severe cardiopulmonary limitations (Cardiac Functional Class IV)
- Neurologic disorders with residual deficits in balance, coordination, vision, or strength
- Severe and intractable pain in the residual limb aggravated by contact with prosthesis
- Active alcohol or substance abuse interfering with learning and safety
- Chronic or recurrent skin breakdown, particularly if related to infection
- Significant (>30°) flexion contracture of hip or knee, nonresponsive to ROM/stretching

ROM, range of motion.
DEVELOPED BY: HINES PACT PROGRAM

Most prostheses are custom fitted and fabricated and are made with total contact sockets. The socket is created by applying a plaster cast to the residual limb to create a "negative mold." The cast is removed and filled with a plastic material to form a "positive" replica of the limb, which serves as the model on which the synthetic prosthetic socket is molded. Prosthetic fabrication is aided by technologic advancements, thus improving the accuracy of socket fit and reduction in the fabrication time. Prostheses are either preparatory or definitive. A *preparatory prosthesis* (sometimes referred to as a temporary prosthesis) uses the same prosthetic principles for fit and function as the definitive prosthesis. The primary difference lies in using the preparatory socket to assist in the maturation (primarily shrinkage) of the residual limb, which usually occurs over 3 to 4 months. During this interval, decreasing residual limb size (because of edema absorption and pressure atrophy of soft tissue) is accommodated to maintain proper socket fit, by using one or more prosthetic socks of varying thickness (measured as one ply, three ply, or five ply). Once the residual limb has stabilized in size, depending on the patient's functional level, a *definitive prosthesis* (also referred to as the permanent prosthesis) can be prescribed. If there is excessive residual limb shrinkage to the point that the preparatory prosthesis does not fit well (i.e., too loose even with multiple prosthetic socks) with further shrinkage anticipated, a replacement socket for the preparatory prosthesis may need to be fabricated. Another potential advantage of using a preparatory prosthesis is the ability to use fairly basic prosthetic components for simplified initial gait training, with the option of upgrading to more advanced components in the definitive prosthesis based on the patient's level of function and needs.

If a definitive prosthesis is ordered as the initial (sole) device, it is typically fabricated only after the residual limb has matured completely characterized by completed shrinkage and shaping during the preprosthetic program. For these patients, the preprosthetic program is much longer, which delays prosthetic fitting and training. The risk of psychologic rejection of prosthesis is increased with delayed prosthetic fitting, as is the risk of phantom pain. Many third-party payers will fund only one termed definitive prosthesis for policyholders. A potential strategy in this situation might be to prescribe a definitive prosthesis up front, with a plan to fabricate a replacement socket rather than a whole new prosthesis, after stabilization of residual limb size.

Prescription Writing

To appropriately prescribe a prosthesis, it is important to become familiar with the materials available for use in its fabrication and how these will perform the weight-bearing or weight-transmitting functions of the prosthesis. In addition, knowledge of the indications, advantages, and disadvantages of the prosthetic components and designs is crucial to tailor the device to best (and most cost effectively) meet the patient's needs. The selection of components depends on individual patient characteristics, level of amputation, size and shape of the residual limb, tolerance for pressure from the prosthesis, and activity level. While writing a prosthetic prescription, it is important to also consider comorbid conditions and to incorporate the patient's goals and choices as well as ability to learn the use and management of the prosthesis. A typical prosthetic prescription includes the socket design, prosthetic joint(s) as appropriate, type of construction either endoskeletal or exoskeletal, the mechanism for suspension, and terminal device.

Socket design involves the interface between the residual limb and the prosthesis and is critical to proper functioning and comfort of the prosthesis. Considerable research has gone into developing and refining the most effective designs and materials to achieve this goal. There are one or more typical socket designs for each level of amputation, which are discussed subsequently. Each design takes advantage of "pressure tolerant" tissues for primary weight bearing or support, while incorporating pressure relief strategies for "pressure sensitive" areas. Weight bearing directly at the end of the residual limb occurs in Syme amputation only.

Prosthetic joints apply biomechanical engineering principles and research to try to simulate the function, if not the anatomy, of the amputated limb. Although there have been dramatic improvements in design and function of prosthetic joints and their control systems, these will never fully replace anatomic joints. This is true primarily because of loss of kinesthetic and proprioceptive sensation with prosthetic components (so the patient after amputation must use other senses, such as vision, to compensate), and because prosthetic designs cannot reproduce active antigravity muscle contraction (e.g., to extend the knee after TTA).

Endoskeletal construction involves a metal tube or pipe connecting the socket to the terminal device as the primary weight support mechanism, usually with a soft foam outer (cosmetic) covering. *Exoskeletal* designs feature a rigid plastic exterior shell extending from the socket to the terminal device and are very durable. Endoskeletal prostheses are lighter and more cosmetic but are typically more expensive for upkeep, because the foam cover is easily torn and requires frequent replacement. The alignment of the endoskeletal prosthesis may be easily adjusted by the prosthetist, whereas the exoskeletal prosthesis is a fixed device that cannot be adjusted once fabricated. Either design can be custom fabricated to match the shape and skin color of the opposite limb.

Suspension refers to keeping the prosthesis attached to the residual limb. For patients with lower extremity amputation, the primary concern is having the prosthesis remain securely attached during swing phase with the prosthesis. However, other activities, such as sitting and standing, can present challenges in maintaining position and alignment of the prosthesis on the residual limb.

The *terminal device* is the prosthetic equivalent of a hand or foot. Upper extremity terminal devices attempt to simulate the dexterity and grip capabilities of the human hand. Lower extremity terminal devices try to replicate foot and ankle functions of adapting to terrain, weight bearing, and push-off during ambulation.

Prosthetic Training

Once the patient receives the prosthesis, he or she will need additional training to learn how to appropriately function with the device. This typically involves occupational therapy with primary emphasis for training patients after upper extremity amputation and self-care activities in the persons with lower extremity amputation. Physical therapy trains patients after lower extremity amputation. Initially the patient learns how to correctly don and doff the prosthesis, with instructions to progressively increase wearing tolerance (how long he or she is able to comfortably wear the prosthesis, with no evidence of skin irritation or breakdown). The next step for individuals after lower extremity amputation is to gradually increase weight-bearing tolerance (duration of time the individual is able to stand and/or walk with the prosthesis, again without skin irritation or breakdown). The importance of frequent skin inspection is stressed, particularly over common areas of shearing or pressure.

Continuing therapy is needed to correctly learn how to use the prosthesis. Learning the correct sequence of maneuvers to position, stabilize, and operate the terminal device is the goal for individuals after upper extremity amputation. For patients who have had a lower extremity amputation, the focus is on developing a smooth, symmetric gait pattern for maximal energy efficiency and cosmetic appearance. Additional therapy efforts address continuing improvements in strength (particularly in key muscle groups) and endurance, as well as instruction in principles of energy conservation to avoid fatigue. The patient must also learn proper care and cleaning of the prosthesis.

Volpicelli has described seven ambulation levels to categorize the degree of mobility achieved by individuals after amputation (Table 3.3). Another method of quantifying ambulation after amputation involves characterizing patients as "community ambulators" (able to walk functional distances outside the house), "household ambulators" (only able to walk independently inside their house), or "therapeutic ambulators" (can only walk with the physical assistance of others; ambulation is therapeutic from a psychologic and/or physiologic standpoint).

Complications

Although more common when first learning to use a prosthesis, complications may occur at any time. The most frequent problems

---

Table 3.3.   Ambulation Levels of Lower Extremity Amputees

VI	Unlimited community ambulation
V	Limited community ambulation
IV	Unlimited household ambulation
III	Limited household ambulation
II	Supervised household ambulation
I	Wheelchair ambulation
0	Bedridden

From Volpicelli LJ, Chambers RB, Wagner FW Jr. Ambulation levels of bilateral lower extremity amputees: analysis of one hundred and three cases. *JBJS* 1983;65A:599, with permission.

involve residual limb *skin*. Incision dehiscence can occur from premature prosthetic fitting or from trauma to the residual limb (e.g., from a fall). An improperly fitting prosthesis may cause irritation, abrasion, or even ulceration of the skin at pressure areas in the socket. Adherent skin in the region of the incision may result in skin breakdown from the shear forces caused by pistoning up and down in the socket with ambulation. Bony prominences without a corresponding area of relief in the socket may result in focal skin damage. Also at risk for irritation are areas of previous skin grafting and vascular bypass incisions and grafts. Contact dermatitis can be caused by allergy to lotion, soap, or even prosthetic materials. Brawny edema, induration, and discoloration of the skin of the distal limb in a circular shape may indicate a "choke syndrome." This occurs when the residual limb becomes larger, typically from excessive weight gain or from wearing an excessive number of socks, and no longer fits into the total contact socket. The resulting gap between the skin of the distal limb and the distal socket wall creates pressure, causing fluid to accumulate and fill the potential space. This can lead to extensive skin breakdown but can be corrected by shrinking the residual limb (using an Ace wrap or shrinker sock) or socket modification to restore total contact. Local skin problems such as furuncles, folliculitis, or epidermoid cysts may also occur and prevent comfortable prosthetic function. The patient should be instructed to keep the skin clean by washing the residual limb (as well as the prosthetic socket and inserts) thoroughly at least twice a day (followed by patting the skin dry, and several minutes of air drying), in addition to frequent close inspection.

Patients with skin breakdown of their opposite ("good") leg present a special management challenge. One philosophy is to minimize use of the prosthesis for ambulation, even to the point of maintaining bedrest, to facilitate healing of the opposite extremity. On the other hand, individuals after bilateral lower extremity amputations are far more likely to be successful prosthetic ambulators if they have been trained with a prosthesis before the opposite leg was amputated. The related strategy is to aggressively train the patient to ambulate with the current prosthesis, so that when he or she progresses to amputation on the opposite side, the likelihood of ambulating with bilateral prostheses is maximized.

Bony outgrowths of the distal ends of amputated bones are more common in the upper limbs, in electrical injuries, and in children and may impair prosthetic fitting. *Joint* contractures as well as joint instability or arthritis can also limit prosthetic function. *Comorbidity* can significantly affect the level of function after amputation, particularly severe cardiac disease or neurologic impairments (e.g., weakness, incoordination, loss of balance, visual loss, cognitive deficits). It should be noted that overall 5-year survival rates after amputation are 75% for patients without diabetes, but only 39% with diabetes.

Psychoemotional issues can also impede an individual reaching his or her full functional potential. Examples include a patient who considers the amputation "a failure" of treatment, with subsequent denial of the amputation, rejection of the prosthesis, or severe depression with poor motivation. Rarely, a patient may be too fearful of falling to learn to use a prosthesis. Patients who adapt poorly to the limb loss are reported to complain of phantom pain with increasing intensity and frequency.

Pain may severely limit successful prosthetic use. The differential diagnosis of possible causes for pain involving the residual limb can be extensive. Patients may present with residual limb pain or even pain in the phantom limb, which is typically aching or cramping in nature. Performing ROM exercises along with massaging or tapping the residual limb may relieve the pain. The limb may contain a painful neuroma, diagnosed by palpation of a tender mass in the region of a peripheral nerve, with radiating pain in the distribution of the nerve when percussed. All nerves develop neuromas (a bulging at the nerve end) to some degree when severed. However, large neuromas, or those in critical locations where they are subjected to pressure or shear stress, may be painful and interfere with prosthetic gait. Treatment approaches include local injection with steroid, ultrasound, or rarely surgical excision and/or revision of the amputation.

Painful residual limbs may result from factors not directly related to the amputation or prosthesis. A lumbar herniated nucleus pulposus (HNP) may cause pain to radiate down the residual limb. Several of the usual clues used to diagnose this condition may be missing, including lower lumbosacral dermatomes for assessing sensation, distal muscles for assessing strength, or the patellar or Achilles tendons for assessing reflexes. Compounding the problem is the prosthetic gait pattern, which may predispose to HNP because of increased stress across the lumbar spine.

Although traditionally described as rare, the incidence of "phantom pain syndrome" is variably documented as ranging from 5% to 50% or more. This chronic and usually severe pain syndrome is characterized by pain that appears to originate in the amputated portion ("phantom") of the limb. This is postulated to be due to signals arising from the nerves proximal to the amputation site that previously carried sensation from the amputated portion. The exact neuropathologic basis of the normal phantom sensation versus the pathologic phantom pain is not well understood. Phantom sensation is a self-limiting process involving the sensation of the amputated limb still being present, although often altered in shape or length (telescoping). Although phantom sensation may involve tingling or other nonnoxious experiences, it does not require pain medications but instead patient education and reassurance. The presence of persistent pain generators (such as chronic infection or severe ischemia) before the amputation or delayed prosthetic fitting may increase the risk of phantom pain syndrome. Phantom pain does not respond to typical acute pain interventions such as narcotics but may be controlled by agents used to treat chronic neurogenic pain syndromes. Potentially effective medications include tricyclic antidepressants (such as amitriptyline or doxepin), antiarrhythmic agents (such as mexiletine), or membrane-stabilizing agents (such as phenytoin or carbamazepine). Topical capsaicin, which depletes Substance P, has been used successfully in some cases. Physical treatments such as desensitization massage or transcutaneous electrical nerve stimulation (TENS) may be taught by a therapist and used by the patient at home to control pain. Therapeutic heat or cold typically is of limited or temporary benefit, although contrast baths (alternating hot and cold water) may be more effective.

Follow-Up

Once the patient has been fitted and trained with a prosthesis, the functional outcome is usually good. Unless there is an underlying disease process or complication, the residual limb should adapt to prosthetic use such that the patient is typically able to wear and use it nearly the entire day. The patient should be followed at periodic intervals, initially monthly, then at increasing intervals for the first year after fitting. The focus during these return visits is on evaluating prosthetic fit and function, residual limb status, and the prosthetic gait pattern. The opposite limb should also be checked including vascular supply and sensation, skin breakdown, because of the high risk of losing the opposite extremity (up to 20% of patients with diabetic peripheral vascular disease may need a contralateral limb amputation within 2 years). Proper foot care and close monitoring of local and systemic factors have reduced the amputation rates.

After the patient reaches a stable state with the prosthesis, he or she must be seen by the physiatrist only if and when complications arise. The prosthetist generally continues to follow the patient regularly for minor adjustments and is the first level of intervention when problems occur. If this is unsuccessful in resolving the problem, the patient should be seen for a more comprehensive team evaluation, because any major change or replacement of the prosthesis requires a prosthetic prescription from the physician. The prosthesis will wear out over time or may malfunction. The socket, certain joint components, or the entire prosthesis may need to be replaced. The average prosthesis usually lasts 3 to 5 years, even with very heavy use. However, a prosthesis may last more than 10 years and still be functional for a less vigorous individual. Children during the growth period require frequent prosthetic modifications and/or replacement.

As with all aspects of rehabilitation, it is important to remember that the patient is the one who ultimately determines the definition of successful prosthetic use. Not all persons wear their prostheses during all waking hours or even every day. Success is achieved if the individual has reached his or her maximal functional potential or, alternatively, a level of function that he or she deems acceptable.

REHABILITATION BY SPECIFIC AMPUTATION SITES: The following are examples of the rehabilitation management of patients with amputation at different levels

Transtibial Amputations (TTA)

General Considerations

Although cardiopulmonary status is usually not a major issue at this level, general medical status should still be considered. Assessment of the patient's ability to transfer, or ambulate without a prosthesis, gives a general idea of overall fitness. Cognitive status is important because the patient will need to learn to properly don the prosthesis and master a different gait pattern.

Residual Limb Assessment

Tibial length ideally should be 5 to 7 inches or approximately one third of the original tibial length. The fibula should be no longer than the tibia and ideally should be about 1 inch shorter.

The residual limb is measured from the medial joint line of the knee rather than the tibial tuberosity. A bone length of less than 2 in. provides such a short lever arm that special prosthetic fabrication techniques may be needed. Residual tibial length of more than 8 in. makes standard fitting difficult. Extremely long residual limbs in TTAs have poor muscle coverage, because the distal one third of the lower leg is covered mostly by tendons, which predisposes to skin breakdown. In addition, the lever arm of the limb is longer, resulting in greater force on the distal skin during gait and compounding the breakdown problem. Usually the gastrocnemius muscle is brought anteriorly over the end of the tibia and surgically secured. The surgeon usually bevels the end of the tibia to remove the sharp edge of the transected bone. However, the most common site of skin breakdown in the transtibial limb is still at the anterior distal end, where the prosthesis rubs on the distal tibia. There must also be good skin integrity over the patellar tendon and anterior flares of the tibia because these are the major weight-bearing areas in the socket. The limb should be a slightly tapered cylinder, nontender, and pliable distally, rather than firm and unyielding. There should be minimal edema.

The scar(s) may be aligned in any direction but should not adhere to the underlying tissues. Adherent tissue creates more shear force on the skin inside the socket and may lead to more frequent skin breakdown during ambulation. Soft tissue integrity is particularly important at the end of the bone. Assess knee ROM; active full extension is necessary for good prosthetic function. There should be at least 70 degrees of active knee flexion. Hip extension should be full. Strength in all muscle groups about the knee and hip should be measured as good (4/5 on manual muscle testing) or as normal (5/5). Assess for tenderness, locking, or ligamentous laxity of the knee joint on both sides.

Preprosthetic Training

Training consists of shaping and maturing the limb for prosthetic application, as well as addressing joint mobility and strength in the entire residual limb. A specific exercise prescription must be written for active ROM for both the knee and the hip, with prolonged and gradual stretching if there is a contracture of either joint. Strengthening exercises should include the knee extensors and flexors as well as the major hip muscle groups and upper extremity muscles strengthened to facilitate the use of assistive devices for gait.

There are several appropriate methods for shaping and maturing of the limb. The method used by the physiatrist depends in part on the surgeon's preference. The most rapid method for preparing the limb for a prosthesis is the immediate fit rigid dressing. With this method, the residual limb is placed in a plaster cast to midthigh level in the operating room. This rigid dressing controls postoperative edema, thereby speeding up healing and shortening the preprosthetic phase. It also provides protection for the residual limb from trauma (such as hitting it against the side rail). Although the plaster cast can be windowed or temporarily removed to enable close examination of the limb, it must be closed promptly (within 30 to 45 minutes) to avoid accumulation of edema. The rigid dressing is generally left in place for 7 to

14 days and then replaced with another rigid dressing or with a preparatory prosthetic socket with a pylon that allows partial weight bearing on the residual limb. Patients with severe vascular dysfunction or infection (e.g., osteomyelitis) are not good candidates for rigid dressings because of the inability to closely monitor wound healing.

When the immediate fit rigid dressing method is not used, elastic wrapping should be used to control edema beginning immediately after surgery. An elastic bandage such as an Ace wrap should be applied from the distal thigh level, in a figure-of-eight method with greater pressure distally than proximally. This method is shown in Fig. 3-2. A 4- or 6-in. wide Ace wrap is routinely used for TTA depending on the size of the limb. The wrap is initiated proximally (step 1) and brought around the distal corner of the limb (step 2). The wrap is then brought proximally again (step 3) and wrapped around the remaining corner of the distal end (step 4); this sequence is repeated until complete residual limb coverage is attained. Circumferential wrapping must be avoided, because it will act as a tourniquet and trap edema distally, actually exacerbating the problem. The wrap should be applied snugly without causing pain. It should be reapplied each time it loosens, potentially every 3 to 4 hours. If the knee is at risk for a flexion contracture, a posterior plaster midthigh length splint can be used to maintain extension. Progressively firmer elastic wrapping should be applied as the suture line heals, even if sutures or staples are still in place. Wrapping must continue at all times, until full maturation of the limb, whenever the prosthesis

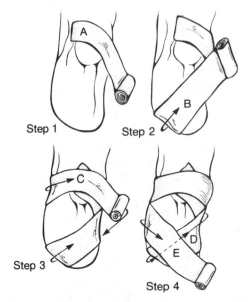

Fig. 3-2. Figure-of-eight method of transtibial amputation (TTA) residual limb wrapping.

is not worn. The patient must learn to apply this independently, so he or she can rewrap the limb whenever the wrap loosens. TuboGrip, a tube-shaped elastic wrap, may be substituted for the conventional elastic bandage. If adequate shrinkage is not obtained before measuring the patient for the prosthesis, then the prosthesis will force the edema out of the limb, rendering the socket too large. This may cause loosening and instability of the prosthesis during gait, pain in residual limb, or skin breakdown and require replacement of the prosthetic socket or potentially, surgical revision of the limb.

Special care should be taken with the suture line. Because there are several layers of tissue that are closed over the cut end of bone, the scar, including skin and all subcutaneous layers, is prone to adhere to the bone. Scar mobilization, which involves gentle massage of the skin around the suture line, should be prescribed to reduce adherence to underlying tissue and bone. This should be initiated as soon as tolerated and be performed more aggressively once the sutures are out. The patient should learn to perform scar mobilization independently.

Prosthetic Fitting

The socket commonly used in a TTA prosthesis is called a patellar tendon bearing (PTB) prosthesis. In this total contact socket, the body weight is borne on the patellar tendon, the anterior proximal tibial condyles medially and laterally, and the remaining soft tissues of the proximal anterior muscular compartment of the leg. These areas tolerate pressure well, as opposed to the anterior tibia and the distal tibial end, which are pressure intolerant. Figure 3-3 depicts areas of pressure-tolerant versus pressure-sensitive tissue for a TTA residual limb.

The socket is typically lined with a soft material, called a soft insert, to provide extra skin protection and patient comfort. A distal end pad may be prescribed to cushion the bottom of the socket if the hard socket wall is not well tolerated. A PE-LITE liner is a popular interface, is hygienic, and is easy to maintain. Patients generally don one or more woolen socks (one, three or five ply thickness) depending on the degree of shrinkage, then don the PE-LITE insert, and finally don the prosthesis. If the skin is very fragile or sensitive a nylon sleeve or sheath can be pulled over the residual limb before wearing the woolen socks, to reduce friction. Another increasingly popular socket design involves use of a silicone gel sleeve to better distribute weight bearing, minimize shear force, and provide cushioning for improved comfort.

The weight is transferred from the socket to the foot via either an exoskeletal or endoskeletal system as previously discussed. The prosthesis is fastened to the limb by a suspension system. The usual PTB suspension system consists of a supracondylar cuff suspension. A small leather cuff attached to the proximal edge of the socket medially and laterally encircles the distal thigh just above the femoral condyles and is secured by a buckle. An alternative suspension system is the PTB-SC, or PTSP (patellar tendon bearing/supra patellar) suspension. This system has a PTB socket with proximal extensions medially and laterally above the femoral condyles. The socket has removable pads (or a soft insert with built in pads) that, when slid into place, narrow

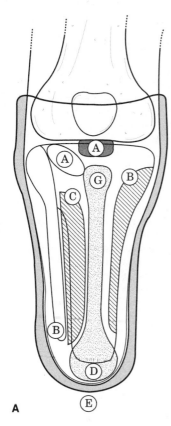

PATELLAR-TENDON-BEARING
BELOW KNEE PROSTHESIS
ANTERIOR ASPECT

Areas of Weight Bearing
A. Patellar tendon
B. Flare of medial tibial condyle
   and anteriomedial aspect
   of shaft of tibia
C. Anterolateral aspect of stump
   (pre-tibial group)
D. Portion of shaft of fibula
E. Gentle end-bearing if tolerated

Areas of Relief
A. Anterior and lateral edges of
   lateral tibial condyle
B. Head and distal end of fibula
C. Crest of tibia
D. Anterior, distal end of tibia
E. Distal end of stump if end-
   bearing is not tolerated

Height Anterior
A. Bisects patella

Height Lateral
A. 1/2 to 1 inch higher than
   anteriorly

Fig. 3-3. Model of pressure-tolerant and pressure-sensitive areas of transtibial amputation (TTA) residual limb.

the upper margin of the socket above the condyles to provide suspension, keeping the prosthesis firmly attached to the limb during the swing phase of gait. Newer suspension techniques take advantage of the intimate fit of silicone gel sockets to provide suction suspension; the gel liner is attached to the prosthetic socket via a pin on the distal surface which inserts into a locking port in the distal socket. This is commonly called ICEROS (Icelandic roll on suction socket).

The typical terminal device used as the ankle and foot mechanism is a solid-ankle/cushioned-heel (SACH) foot. Although the SACH foot has no moving parts, the compressible foam cushion heel mimics ankle plantar flexion at heel strike, allowing for a smoother gait. It is the lightest, least expensive, and most durable terminal device and requires the least maintenance. If the patient is very active, an energy-storing terminal device such as the Seattle Foot or Flex Foot may be more appropriate. These devices contain

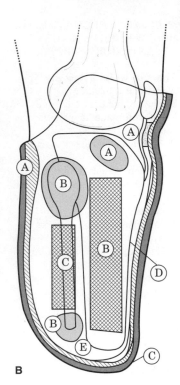

PATELLAR-TENDON-BEARING BELOW KNEE PROSTHESIS LATERAL ASPECT

Areas of Weight Bearing
A. Patellar tendon
B. Anterolateral aspect of stump (pre-tibial group)
C. Mid-portion of shaft of fibula
D. Posterior neurovascular bundle area
E. End-bearing if tolerated

Areas of Relief
A. Anterior and lateral edges of lateral tibial condyle
B. Head and distal end of fibula
C. Anterior, distal end of tibia
D. Crest of tibia
E. Distal end of stump if end-bearing is not tolerated

Height Anterior
A. Bisects patella

Height Lateral
A. 1/2 to 1 inch higher than anteriorly

Height Posterior
A. 1/2 inch higher than tibial plateau or center of patellar-tendon bar

B

Fig. 3-3. *continued*

a strong, flexible shank that bends at heel strike, storing energy. The foot recoils at toe-off, generating a force that mimics plantar flexion and gives a push-off that more closely replicates normal gait. A typical TTA prosthetic prescription is delineated in Table 3.4.

Prosthetic Training

Gait training in physical therapy with the TTA prosthesis should be initiated as soon as the device is fitted. The average length of training for a patient with TTA is 2 weeks. Gait training is initiated using parallel bars to instruct on "loading" on the prosthetic side and to train in proper heel-to-toe gait pattern. When the patient is ready, he or she is usually advanced to a cane

Table 3.4. Sample Prosthetic Prescription (Transtibial Amputation)

Right TTA prosthesis
PTB total contact socket
Silicone gel liner with locking pin suspension
Endoskeletal construction with cosmetic cover
SACH foot

PTB, patellar tendon bearing; SACH, solid-ankle/cushioned-heel; TTA, transtibial amputation.

or walker. The use of crutches with the prosthesis is generally avoided, because poor gait patterns tend to develop. The residual limb skin should be checked frequently by the therapist and patient for evidence of irritation or breakdown. If present, prosthetic adjustment may be necessary, and the patient should not wear the prosthesis until any skin lesions are healed and necessary prosthetic modifications are completed.

Transfemoral Amputation (TFA)

General Considerations

Cardiopulmonary status is of greater significance after TFA, because the TFA patient needs approximately 65% more energy (as measured by oxygen consumption) during prosthetic gait than that used in normal bipedal gait. Cognitive status is also a greater concern because the TFA prosthesis is more difficult to don than a TTA prosthesis, and the gait pattern is much more complicated because of the need to learn prosthetic knee control.

Residual limb length should ideally be more than 10 in. or in the middle third of the femur. This length is measured from the proximal edge of the greater trochanter. Femoral length of less than 8 in. makes it difficult to control the limb in the prosthetic socket. The positioning of the scar is not critical for fitting, but the scar should not adhere to any underlying tissue or be deeply invaginated. Ideally the bone should be covered with full-thickness soft tissue. Carefully inspect the skin in the groin and ischial areas for open areas or lesions. Sensation is usually intact unless areas of skin grafting are present. The limb should be a tapered cylinder. If excess tissue is present over the adductor tendons, the residual limb will be difficult to fit into the prosthesis, causing a painful pinching of the adductor roll between the top edge of the prosthesis and the ischium. The skin in the region of the groin tends to be glandular, and excreted material may become impacted in the glands, leading to skin lesions such as furuncles or abscesses. This should first be treated with education about frequent and effective hygiene and, if the problem persists, should be treated with an antibiotic solution such as Cleocin-T, a topical antibiotic particularly effective against anaerobic bacteria. Sweating may be a problem inside the socket and may be controlled by Dry-Sol, a potent antiperspirant.

Hip ROM, a critical measurement, is very difficult to assess accurately after TFA. The shorter and larger the limb, the more difficult hip ROM is to measure. TFA results in the unopposed pull of muscles inserting into the greater and lesser trochanters. The unopposed pull of these residual muscles, specifically the gluteus and iliopsoas muscles, places the femur in a flexed, abducted, and externally rotated position. This often results in significant hip flexion contractures and is further aggravated by patients who tend to remain in sitting or side-lying positions with the hip flexed. With a short or bulky limb, the femur may be flexed, abducted, or externally rotated inside the residual limb, even when the limb appears to be in a neutral position. The limb may appear to have full ROM, although the hip joint may have significant contractures that will impair prosthetic gait.

Hip extension can be accurately assessed by the Thomas test. The patient is placed in a supine position on an unyielding surface while the examiner fully flexes the contralateral hip. The patient is instructed to hold the thigh against the chest, thus controlling the rotation of the pelvis to allow accurate measurement of hip extension. Full flexion of the contralateral hip should be confirmed by checking that lumbar lordosis is completely flattened. This ensures full posterior rotation of the pelvis, securing the angle of the pelvis in relation to the examination table. Then the residual limb is placed in internal rotation and adduction. Only then can the extension of the hip of the residual limb be accurately assessed. A patient may have up to a 60-degree hip flexion contracture and still appear to have full hip extension if the Thomas test is not used, because anterior pelvic rotation, femoral external rotation, and femoral abduction allow the femur to lie flat on the examination table, mimicking full hip extension. A true hip flexion contracture greater than 10 degrees is enough to seriously impair ability to ambulate with a prosthesis.

Strength in the hip must also be accurately measured. The two hip muscle groups needed by a patient with TFA during gait are the abductors and the extensors. Half of normal hip extension is provided by the hamstrings, which are severed during the surgical procedure. Therefore, the degree of weakness must be carefully measured. The hip abductor muscles can accurately be measured with the hip in extension and internal rotation. With any degree of hip flexion or external rotation, the examiner will actually be measuring the strength of the hip flexors, because the action of these muscles will substitute for weak abductors.

Preprosthetic Training

Active hip ROM and stretching exercises are crucial. Lying prone is an ideal method of providing static stretch to the hip flexors, although it may be difficult for older patients or those with moderate contractures to tolerate. Progressive stretching may be accomplished by adding pillows under the distal residual limb with the patient in prone position. Strengthening exercises are indicated for the key hip muscle groups, the extensors and abductors.

Residual limb shaping and maturing should also start immediately by wrapping with an elastic bandage, usually with a 6-inch wide Ace wrap. The postoperative wound dressings should be discarded as rapidly as possible to ensure more rapid shaping. For the patient who cannot effectively wrap the residual limb, an elastic prosthetic shrinker sock may be substituted. It has the advantage of being easier to don and the disadvantage of being a fixed size. As the residual limb shrinks, the shrinker sock's compression diminishes, whereas Ace wrapping provides a custom fit with each application. It is vital that the Ace wrap or the shrinker include the entire residual limb, with special care that the medial part of the limb is wrapped proximally to the adductor tubercle, to avoid an adductor roll. The figure-of-eight wrapping method used is shown in Fig. 3-4. The process is similar to that used on TTA residual limbs. To adequately secure the compressive dressing high in the groin, especially with short residual limbs, the elastic Ace wrap must go around the waist, or alternatively a belting device must be used with the shrinker sock. In the first 2 weeks, the Ace wrap should be reapplied at least three times a day to accommodate volume changes.

Prosthetic Fitting

Prosthetic materials used for the socket and weight-transmitting portions of the TFA prosthesis are the same as for the TTA prosthesis. However, because the weight-transmitting portion is longer in the TFA prosthesis, the lighter weight of the endoskeletal system is of greater benefit than in a TTA prosthesis.

TFA sockets are of two types: the traditional quadrilateral socket and the newer CAT-CAM (contoured adducted trochanteric-controlled alignment method) or narrow mediolateral (ML) socket. Currently, the narrow ML socket is more commonly prescribed. Both of these sockets are total contact sockets. In the quadrilateral socket, weight bearing occurs on the ischial tuberosity, with the patient effectively "sitting" on the brim of the socket. Limb position within the socket is maintained by pressure from the anterior wall of the socket against the pressure tolerant anterior thigh, which keeps the ischial tuberosity in position on the posterior brim. Thus, the empty socket has a rectangular shape when viewed from above, with the narrow dimension in the anterior-posterior plane.

In contrast to the quadrilateral socket, weight bearing on a narrow ML socket is on the lateral aspect of the femur, in the area just below the greater trochanter. This is accomplished by compressing the limb in the socket medially. From above this socket is oval in appearance, narrower in the mediolateral plane, and is custom molded to the residual limb along the entire length of the socket.

Suspension in TFA prostheses is provided by the socket or by a belt around the waist. The socket suspension is called a suction socket, which is achieved by total contact and is made airtight with a one-way valve placed distally. When the limb is inserted into the socket, all the air is forced out through the valve. The prosthesis tends to pull away from the limb during the swing phase of gait, but negative pressure between the limb and the socket keeps the prosthesis from sliding off. However, this socket is difficult to apply and even small volume changes in the limb may create difficulties in donning the prosthesis. If the socket is not applied properly, an air leak may occur and suction is lost, allowing the prosthesis to slide distally and impairing stability. The

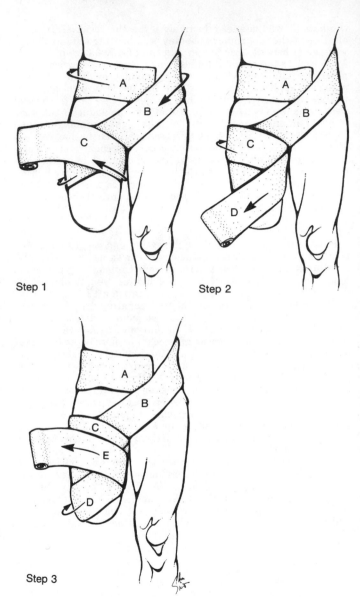

Fig. 3-4. Figure-of-eight method for transfemoral amputation (TFA) residual limb wrapping.

most common suspension belt is a Silesian belt, which is a webbed strap attached to the lateral brim of the socket. It fits around the opposite iliac crest, thereby holding the socket in place and minimizing rotation of the socket. In a young individual, a suction socket is the optimal choice. In the older or less vigorous person, a semisuction socket, or a looser fitting suction socket with prosthetic socks in conjunction with a Silesian belt, may be ordered. Similarly to TTA prostheses, a TFA residual limb can be fitted with a gel liner with a distal pin that inserts into a locking port in the prosthetic socket to provide suction suspension.

The knee joint is chosen in accordance with the patient's activity level and ability to maintain balance. A person with good balance and an average activity level is typically best served by a polycentric constant friction knee. If balance is a concern, a safety knee can be prescribed. The safety knee joint swings freely with a constant friction resistance as long as a vertical load is not applied. If vertical force is applied within 15 degrees of extension, the knee locks in place. If the person begins to stumble and fall, the knee locks even when flexed, allowing weight bearing. Thus, the person has time to regain balance. During the training phase, and in some cases on a permanent basis, an external knee locking mechanism may be used to achieve better stability. For a very active person, a hydraulic knee mechanism can be considered. The fluid in a hydraulic knee allows the knee to move at various speeds depending on the force applied. This allows an individual to walk at varying speeds, a major advantage over the constant friction knee. Technological advances and research resulted in C-Leg which stabilizes the knee in various degrees of flexion, thus facilitating circulation on uneven surfaces.

The foot and ankle device typically used in TFA prostheses is a single-axis foot. This terminal device has an ankle joint that moves freely in a plantar- and dorsiflexion plane, limited only by rubber bumpers. Thus, plantar flexion occurs immediately on heel strike, placing the prosthetic foot flat on the floor quickly and making the stance phase more stable on the prosthetic limb.

Upper Extremity Amputations

General Considerations

Cardiopulmonary and overall medical status are of lesser importance in the decision to fit a patient with upper extremity amputation with a prosthesis because energy expenditure is not a major issue. However, accurate assessment of the patient's cognitive status is extremely important because new skills of donning the prosthesis and manipulating the terminal device must be learned. A patient with blindness may require additional training because the terminal device has no kinesthetic or proprioceptive sensation.

Residual Limb Assessment

In the acute treatment phase, when considering limb length the general rule is to save all that is possible. Soft tissue coverage of bones is necessary whenever possible, especially at the distal aspect. The limb shape should mimic that of the normal limb; it should not be distally edematous or bulbous. The soft tissue and skin should move easily, without adhering to underlying structures. Scars should be well healed and not painful. The presence of exostoses or bone spurs should be determined.

Preprosthetic Training

Active ROM for each remaining joint should be implemented immediately after amputation. Special attention to the shoulder joint is crucial to preserve full painless range in the glenohumeral joint, especially external rotation. Begin wrapping the residual limb immediately after surgery. Static stretching may be needed. All remaining major muscle groups should be strengthened. Principles described for lower limb amputations also apply here. There may be multiple surgical scars, which are likely to adhere to underlying bone. Begin scar mobilization as soon as any adherence is noted, as well as routinely when the incisions are fully healed.

The hand of the unaffected limb in a person with unilateral upper extremity amputation will almost certainly become dominant regardless of prior handedness. The occupational therapy prescription should include orders to instruct the patient in performing activities of daily living (ADLs) with one-handed techniques, as well as assisting in switching hand dominance if the previously dominant hand is absent. The upper extremity prosthesis is often used as an assist in bilateral hand activities. Patients with bilateral amputations, and some with unilateral amputation, use the limb for lifting and other heavy manual activities.

Prosthetic Fitting

Prosthetic replacements are controlled and operated by either body-powered or myoelectric technology. In most cases, the body-powered prosthesis is ordered, at least as the initial device, because it is significantly lighter and easier to learn to use (and much less expensive). Usually an exoskeletal system with a total contact socket is prescribed. The suspension system in the body-powered prosthesis also serves as the cabling system to transmit body movement into function of the terminal device. Traction on the operating cable, via biscapular adduction, opens the terminal device, and strong rubber bands close the device for grasping. The most common type of suspension used is a Northwestern Ring Figure-of-Eight, shown in Fig. 3-5.

The wrist joint replacement unit does not usually function as a true wrist, but rather has a "quick disconnect" receptacle that allows a variety of terminal devices to be interchanged. Alternatively, a constant friction wrist unit may be ordered that allows prepositioned wrist flexion and extension and that is lighter. The elbow joint in an transhumeral prosthesis usually consists of an internally locking elbow with a turntable. The elbow is switched between locked and unlocked positions by placing traction on a second "switching" cable, usually operated by shoulder depression. When the elbow is locked, traction on the operating cable opens the terminal device. When the elbow is unlocked, traction on the operating cable flexes the forearm segment of the prosthesis. The forearm is extended by force of gravity. The turntable allows the forearm to be moved passively toward and away from the body, mimicking internal and external rotation of the humerus. When a prosthetic shoulder joint is required following a shoulder disarticulation, a constant friction hinge, which may be passively positioned, is ordered.

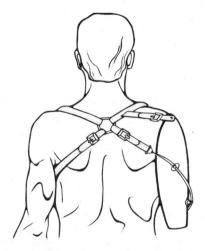

Fig. 3-5. Posterior view, Northwestern 0-ring figure-of-eight suspension device for transhumeral amputation (THA) prosthesis.

The terminal device is the most important part of an upper extremity prosthesis and may be either a hook or a hand. The hook is a functional device, whereas the hand, whether designed as a functional unit or solely for cosmetic effect, is not as functional. This is because the hook allows the individual to visualize what he or she is manipulating, whereas the prosthetic hand has limited function because of the fingers blocking the patient's view. There are at least 50 different hook terminal devices, the most common being the Dorrance 5X for TRA amputation and a Dorrance 5XA for limbs amputated above the elbow. Both types use a cover made of rubber, which is easily torn or marred. There are also pediatric hook sizes.

Myoelectric Prostheses

A myoelectric prosthesis uses small electric motors to power movement of the terminal device. The myoelectric prosthetic hand closely resembles a human hand and is usually positioned in a "three-jaw chuck" grip, in which the stationary thumb opposes the mobile index and middle fingers in a pinching movement. This movement is controlled by the wearer via surface electromyographic (EMG) electrodes that sense the activity of selected muscles in the residual limb, usually the wrist extensors. Activation of this muscle group triggers activation of the motor, which is incorporated into the prosthetic wall. A battery pack is also incorporated into the prosthesis and requires daily charging. A myoelectric prosthesis may use a harness similar to a body-powered prosthesis or may simply be slid over the residual forearm and be suspended from the epicondyles. As an alternative to the myoelectric hand, a myoelectric hook terminal device may be installed and may be slightly more functional, although less cosmetic. A myoelectric elbow joint is also available, although the large forearm segment is difficult to move with the small motors available. Major disadvantages of myoelectric devices at this time include their extremely high cost, considerable weight, and need for frequent adjustment and repairs. Also, the myoelectric hand uses a rubber cosmetic cover glove that is easily torn or stained and is expensive to replace.

Prosthetic Training

Training in the use of an upper extremity prosthesis is performed by an occupational therapist. The patient typically will attend daily therapy sessions for the first 2 weeks, tapering to three times a week, for a total of 20 to 25 training sessions. The patient should learn how to place the terminal device where desired and how to open and close it. Independence in ADLs is the primary goal of therapy. Patients with upper extremity amputations frequently reject their prostheses unless the prosthesis substantially improves their functional level.

Pediatric Amputations and Children with Limb Deficiencies

Children with congenital amputations or limb deficiencies are prone to exostosis or bony overgrowth, an additional complication not usually seen in adults. The child's skeletal system retains the ability to grow, leading to the development of new bony prominences at the ends of long bones after amputation that outgrow the covering skin and soft tissue. This may lead to skin breakdown and infection and may require surgical correction.

Prosthetic fitting in the child should follow developmental guidelines. Upper extremity prosthetics may be provided when the child begins to sit, about age 6 months ("fit to sit"). Lower extremity prostheses may be provided when the child begins to stand and walk, age 9 to 14 months ("fit to stand"). The pediatric patient requires close follow-up during the growth period to ensure that the prosthetic device used is appropriate. Children and their parents require close monitoring and counseling to adapt to limb loss and they should be encouraged to be involved in age-appropriate social and recreational activities.

SUGGESTED READINGS

Atkins DJ, Meier RH, eds. *Comprehensive management of the upper-limb amputee.* New York: Springer-Verlag, 1989.

Bryant PR, Pandian G. Acquired limb deficiencies in children and young adults. *Arch Phys Med Rehabil* 2001;82(3 Suppl 1):S3–S9.

Colwell MO, Spires MC, Wontotcik L et al. Lower-extremity prosthetics and rehabilitation. In: Grabois M, Garrison SJ, Hart KA et al, eds. *Physical medicine and rehabilitation: the complete approach.* Malden, MA: Blackwell Science, 2000:583–607.

Gonzalez IG, Myers SJ, Edelstein JE et al. *Downey & Darling's physiological basis of rehabilitation medicine,* 3rd ed. Boston: Butterworth Heinemann, 2001:427.

Huang ME, Levy CE, Webster JB. Prosthetic components, prescriptions, and indications. *Arch Phys Med Rehabil* 2001;82(3 Suppl 1): S17–S24.

Inman VT, Ralston HJ, Todd J. *Human walking.* Baltimore: Williams & Wilkins, 1981.

Leonard JA, Meier RH III. Upper and lower extremity prosthetics. In: DeLisa JA, Gans BM, eds. *Rehabilitation medicine: principles and practice,* 3rd ed. Philadelphia: Lippincott-Raven, 1998:669–698.

McAnelly RD, Faulkner VW. Lower limb prostheses. In: Braddom RL, ed. *Physical medicine & rehabilitation.* Philadelphia: WB Saunders, 1996:289–320.

Northwestern University Medical School Prosthetic-Orthotic Center. *Lower- and upper-limb prosthetics for physicians, surgeons, and therapists.* [course notebook] 1989.

Pandian G, Huang ME, Duffy DA. Perioperative management. *Arch Phys Med Rehabil* 2001;82(3, Suppl 1):S9–S16.

Sherman RA. Published treatments of phantom limb pain. *Am J Phys Med* 1980;59:232–244.

Wu Y, Krick H. Removable rigid dressing for below-knee amputees. *Clin Prosthet Orthot* 1987;11:33–44.

Arthritis

John J. Nicholas and C. George Kevorkian

There are many different types of arthritis, but rheumatoid arthritis (RA), osteoarthritis (OA), and the spondyloarthropathies, including ankylosing spondylitis (AS) are the main kinds managed by the physiatrist. The treatment of RA is the most complex, but the techniques and modalities appropriate to RA can be applied to nearly all other forms of arthritis.

RHEUMATOID ARTHRITIS

RA is a chronic polyarthritis and a diffuse, multisystem, connective tissue disease. The hallmarks of RA are a positive test for immunoglobulin M (IgM) rheumatoid factor (RF); bilateral, usually symmetrical joint inflammation; erosive changes noted radiographically; and persistent inflammatory synovitis of many joints, especially the hands.

Epidemiology

The prevalence of RA is approximately 1%, and increases with increasing age. Women are affected about three times as frequently as men, although this gender difference is reversed in older patients. RA has a worldwide distribution. A genetic predisposition exists, because first-degree relatives of persons with seropositive erosive disease are five to six times more likely to develop severe RA. A strong association with the major histocompatibility complex gene product, HLA-DR4, and a preponderance of whites and Japanese with classic or definite RA have been demonstrated.

Etiology and Pathology

Various theories have been advanced to explain RA, including infective agents, cellular hypersensitivity, genetic predisposition, and immune complex involvement. None has gained unequivocal acceptance.

A probable early event in the disease process is an antigen-antibody reaction at the synovial level with activation of complement. Acute pathologic findings include microvascular injury, edema of subsynovial tissues, and synovial lining cell proliferation and joint exudates.

Examination of the synovium reveals edema, villous synovial projections, and hypertrophy and hyperplasia of the synovial lining cells (both A and B type cells). Vascular changes such as capillary obstruction, neutrophil infiltration, areas of thrombosis, and perivascular hemorrhage are common. Mononuclear cells predominate in the subsynovial stroma. As inflammation continues, pannus, an inflammatory synovial tissue, is produced and ultimately invades the bone and cartilage and leads to cartilage and soft tissue damage.

Clinical Features

The onset of RA is usually gradual; however, 15% to 20% of patients present acutely. Symptoms of fatigue, anorexia, malaise, weight loss, weakness, and generalized "aches and pains" usually herald the onset of RA, which is initially polyarticular in approximately 75% of patients. The small joints of the hands and feet are affected early and other joints such as the knees, cervical spine, feet, and temporomandibular shoulders are commonly affected later. Morning stiffness of greater than 30 minutes duration, considered a result of synovial congestion, joint capsule thickening, and synovial fluid, is common.

Approximately 10% of patients have a mild, transient polyarthritis followed by a lasting remission and 10% have inexorable downward progression. The remaining 80% exhibit a characteristic waxing and waning of symptoms. The degree of articular severity and the presence of extraarticular manifestations may not correlate; however, both of these manifestations are more likely to be severe in patients with high titers of RF.

Patients rarely die of RA; death results from associated features such as vasculitis, cervical spine subluxation, complications of drug therapy, and infection. The course of the disease varies with the individual patient, but certain aspects indicate a less favorable outcome. These include insidious onset, youthful onset, being female and/or Caucasian, presence of rheumatoid nodules, high titers of RF and C-reactive protein, and markedly elevated sedimentation rate.

Numerous authors have proposed functional classifications for RA patients. Steinbrocker's practical criteria are listed in Table 4.1.

Table 4.1. Functional Criteria in Rheumatoid Arthritis (RA)

Grade	Definition	Remarks
I	Capable of all activities	—
II	Moderate restriction	Physical abilities adequate for normal activities, despite handicaps of discomfort or limited motion of one or more joints
III	Marked restriction	Activity limited to self-care and a few duties of a nonstrenuous occupation
IV	Bed and/or chair bound	Capable of little or no self-care

Adapted from Steinbrocker O, Traeger CH, Batterman RC. Therapeutic criteria in rheumatoid arthritis. *JAMA* 1949;140:659–662, with permission.

The term *symmetrical* used radiologically, refers to bilateral joint involvement, although not necessarily to the same degree. Bony ankylosis is rarely a feature. See Table 4.2.

Table 4.2.   Radiologic Features of Rheumatoid Arthritis (RA)

Early Changes	Late Changes
Soft tissue swelling	Uniform narrowing of joint (cartilage space)
Juxtaarticular osteoporosis	Bone destruction
Marginal erosions	Joint malalignment and subluxation

Management

Management of RA can serve as a general model for physiatric care of many of the arthritides. The comprehensive management of the RA patient involves prescription of appropriate medications as well as use of a variety of resources familiar to physiatrists. Aspirin, in doses of 3 to 6 g daily, is often the initial drug of choice. Levels should be monitored, and a level producing tinnitus obviously must be reduced. Doses below 3 g/day are usually only analgesic.

If aspirin is contraindicated, cannot be tolerated, or does not produce the desired therapeutic effect, a trial of nonsteroidal antiinflammatory drugs (NSAIDs) is indicated. If these agents fail to suppress the disease adequately, a variety of drugs such as gold, steroids, penicillamine, and antimalarials are available. In addition, there are a variety of newer very effective medications such as methotrexate, leflunomide, etanercept, and infliximab. Consultation with a rheumatologist is recommended at this level of disease management.

Physiatric Management

The physiatrist should become familiar with the wide array of resources available for treatment of arthritis patients and with his or her role as team leader and treatment coordinator.

The goals of arthritis rehabilitation are as follows:

- Maintain or improve range of motion: prevent deformities
- Limit disability
- Protect susceptible joints
- Decrease pain and stiffness
- Use joints and muscles efficiently and safely
- Improve strength in selected muscles and overall endurance
- Control weight and maintain appropriate nutrition

Optimal arthritis rehabilitation is characterized by a motivated, well-informed patient following a regimen prescribed and coordinated by a knowledgeable physician, administered by a well-trained therapist, and coordinated with other medical and surgical treat-

Table 4.3.   The Arthritis Rehabilitation Team

Physiatrist
Patient and family
Patient educator
Occupational therapist
Physical therapist
Pharmacist
Nurse
Psychologist/psychiatrist
Dietician
Social worker
Vocational counselor

ments. The regimen should include sufficient instructional treatments, an ongoing basic home program, and modification of the program as disease state changes. Poor rehabilitation outcomes can result from the omission of any of these elements (Table 4.3). The patient and family should be made aware that physical medicine and rehabilitation treatments do not cure arthritis, substitute for adequate rest, replace prescribed medications, or usually result in rapid improvement.

Agents used for arthritis rehabilitation include modalities, exercise, rest, splints, education, and/or other techniques.

Modalities

A variety of explanations have been advanced to explain the mechanisms of analgesia production by heat, such as local axon reflex, endorphin production stimulation, gating theories, and others. See Table 4.4. There is no first-line superficial heating apparatus of choice; patient acceptance is paramount. Deep heating modalities include shortwave, microwave, and ultrasound; these are rarely used but may benefit selected patients.

Table 4.4.   Heat Modalities

Rationale	Agents	Deep Heat
• Analgesic	• Infrared lamp	• Shortwave
• Sedative	• Baker	• Microwave
• Antispasmodic	• Contrast baths	• Ultrasound
• Metabolic	• Hydrocolator packs	
• Remote effects	• Fluidotherapy	
	• Whirlpool	
	• Hot tub bath	
	• Paraffin baths	
	• Electric blankets and heating pads	

Cold

Heat and cold have similar analgesic and antispasmodic effects. Their metabolic and remote effects are essentially opposite. Application of cold typically aggravates joint stiffness; therefore, cryotherapy should be used with caution, even though this modality is effective in treating acutely inflamed soft tissue injuries. See Table 4.5.

Table 4.5. Cryotherapy	
Rationale	Agents
• Analgesic	• Cold water
• Metabolic	• Ice packs
• Antispasmodic	• Ice massage
• Antispastic	• Slush
• Remote effects	• Evaporants

Hydrotherapy

The mechanical buoyancy of water immersion in a pool or tank helps to decrease stress on weight-bearing joints and allows for easier ambulation and exercise. See Table 4.6. Use of pressure gradient gloves may reduce finger swelling (Table 4.7). Other

Table 4.6. Hydrotherapy	
Rationale	Agents
• Sedative	• Whirlpool
• Mechanical	• Hubbard tank
• Sensory	• Wading tank
	• Therapeutic pool
	• Showers
	• Contrast baths

Table 4.7.   Other Therapeutic Agents
Local injections
TENS
Biofeedback
Acupuncture
Operant conditioning
Pressure gloves

TENS, transcutaneous electrical nerve stimulation.

Table 4.8.   Goals of Exercises

Preserve or improve ROM
Increase strength in selected muscles
Improve endurance
Improve coordination
Improve function
Relax tense muscles
Improve posture

ROM, range of motion.

techniques such as joint injections and acupuncture may benefit selected patients.

Exercise

Most arthritic patients cannot tolerate multiple muscle strengthening. Judicious selection of muscles to be strengthened is essential. The shoulder abductors, hip and knee extensors are often the most important muscles on which to focus. See Table 4.8 for exercise goals and Table 4.9 for types of exercises. Isometric exercises are preferred, at 10 repetitions or less, usually in selected muscles such as the hip extensors, quadriceps, and deltoid muscles.

Modify or temporarily discontinue any exercise or activity that apparently increases pain, stiffness, or swelling persisting for 24 hours or more. Although isometric exercises are preferred, low-resistance isotonic exercises may be safe, especially for those patients for whom isometric exercises are contraindicated, such as severe hypertensives. See Fig. 4-1. Exercise must be performed very carefully in the presence of marked joint destruction. Patients may even begin endurance training to tolerance under water or walking on smooth surfaces. The application of heat or cold by patient preference before exercise often facilitates this effort.

Table 4.9.   Classification of Exercises

Passive (maintains ROM)
Active assistive (increases ROM)
Active (maintains ROM, improves endurance)
Resistive (increases strength)
Stretching
Reeducation
Coordination
Relaxation
Postural
Deep breathing

ROM, range of motion.

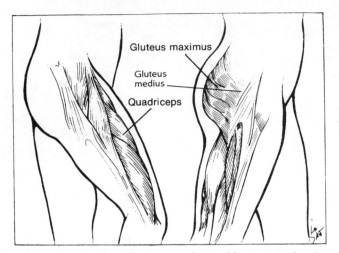

Fig. 4-1. Important muscles to strengthen and keep strong for sit to stand and stair-climbing activities.

Physicians and patients should know when range of motion begins to diminish. At this time stretching exercise should be taught. Stretching painful joints may seem hurtful but will diminish contractures in the long run. Patients must also be reminded not to substitute *work* for exercise. Exercise is a regularly and precisely limited performance with the goals of increasing strength and endurance. Work is no substitute for exercise.

Rest

Instruct the patient to get 10 hours of bed rest daily but not to become inactive. See Table 4.10 for the effects of rest.

Assistive Devices

Prescribe assistive devices liberally as needed for common activities. Utensils with built-up handles, modified pens and grip pencils, reachers, etc., as well as joint-sparing and energy conserving techniques should be taught by occupational therapists.

About one third of RA patients have some significant mobility difficulty. Mobility may be assisted with the use of canes with handle modification or platforms, crutches, walkers with platforms (volar armrests), and shoes with carefully prepared orthotist high toe boxes ugly shoes. Other transportation aids include stair gliders (elevators); wheelchairs, including electric models and scooters; and adapted vans and automobiles.

Education

Patient education should be ongoing, especially education about scientific, efficacious medical treatments as opposed to un-

Table 4.10. Effects of Rest

Beneficial	Harmful
Decreases pain	Psychologic effects
Decreases joint metabolism	Depression
	Anxiety
Decreases joint inflammation	Dependency
Useful adjuvant to anti-inflammatory medication	Muscle atrophy
	Deconditioning
May minimize cartilage and collagen destruction	Postural deconditioning
	Deep vein thrombosis
	Negative calcium and nitrogen balances
	Increased tendency to contracture formation

proved "quick-fix" miracle cures or complementary medications and treatments. Information about home, employment, and recreational adaptations to physical disabilities must be repeated as the patient ages and the disease progresses. Family members also benefit from continued exposure to this information. The local Arthritis Foundation is a source of educational materials as well as peer support groups and trained counselors. Medical social workers, home health services, and vocational rehabilitation also educate patients through evaluation and training. Psychologic support may be requested for personal, social, sexual, vocational, and family problems.

The Rheumatoid Hand

An understanding of the pathophysiology and kinesiology of the rheumatoid hand is essential for adequate treatment.

The wrist is affected early in most patients, often resulting in a flexion deformity. Radial deviation of the metacarpals commonly precedes and contributes to the more noticeable ulnar deviation at the metacarpophalangeal (MCP) joints. Normal anatomic factors exist that enhance ulnar deviation, including the following:

- The long finger flexors pull ulnarly during power grip
- The shape of the metacarpal heads (heads of IV and V are normally ulnarly directed; the radial condyle has a more prominent shoulder)
- The radial collateral ligament is longer and thinner than the ulnar and therefore more easily stretched
- Intrinsic muscle factors, particularly the ulnar insertions of the intrinsics that are more efficient than the radial; also, the abductor digiti minimi pulls ulnarly

Activities of daily living, such as opening car doors, unscrewing motions (counterclockwise), and power grip motions often favor

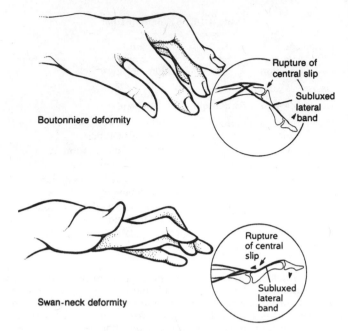

Fig. 4-2.   Mechanisms of common finger deformities.

ulnar forces. Common finger deformities include boutonniere (buttonhole), swan-neck, and thumb deformities. See Fig. 4-2.

Assessment of rheumatoid hand function is essential. Account for swelling, pain, tenderness, strength, and coordination. There is no correlation between hand function and joint range of motion or deformity.

The purpose of exercise for the RA hand is to preserve function and prevent deformities. The basic hand exercise prescription includes:

- Stretching of interossei [flexing distal interphalangeal (DIP) and proximal interphalangeal (PIP) while extending MCP joint]
- Active range of motion exercises for wrist, thumb, and fingers
- Reeducation and gentle manual resistance exercises for the weakened finger extensor muscles

Exercises such as squeezing a rubber ball or sponge are contraindicated, because they primarily involve the lumbricales and finger flexors, already mechanically dominant forces in RA. These exercises increase the development of muscle imbalance and hand deformities. Use only active range of motion (AROM) or gentle active assistive range of motion (AAROM) exercises; avoid passive range of motion (PROM).

Splints

Splinting should enforce the beneficial effects of rest and result in symptomatic decrease of inflammation, especially in the acute disease. The major goals are to:

- Relieve pain
- Maintain position of function
- Discourage abuse of affected joints
- Assist function, both presurgically and postsurgically

Splint immobilization should help in reducing synovitis and resulting pain. Splints likely do not prevent deformities from occurring or correct deformities already present. Presurgical and postsurgical splints are highly individualized, often intricate, and are not used by the typical RA patient.

Resting wrist splints are the most practical and useful. These should almost always be prescribed to patients in the acute stage. If both hands are involved, the patient should alternate use daily. In the acute stage, resting splints should provide a 10- to 20 degree-wrist cock-up, to keep the wrist aligned properly, supply some radially directed force to the fingers to offset ulnar deviation, and to provide support under the heads of the proximal phalanges to prevent volar subluxation and keep the MCP joints extended. The resting splint should keep the hand in a predominantly neutral position. Functional splints provide some support to an isolated joint while allowing use of the hand. Dynamic splints use springs or rubber bands in an attempt to improve alignment or range of motion.

It is likely that knee contractures can be prevented or improved by wearing posterior shell extensor splints; but this of course will not occur if the splint is usually placed on a shelf in the bureau drawer.

Treatment of the Foot in RA

Most RA patients have foot deformities. Gait analysis of such patients commonly reveals a slower gait velocity, decreased step length, and excessive foot pronation. A prolonged double support phase is common; initial ground contact is with the medial border of the pronated foot rather than the lateral. Treatment consists of footwear modifications, use of modalities, and exercises. Specific shoe design is shown in Table 4.11. Common problems and interventions are presented in Table 4.12.

Table 4.11. Shoe Design Elements

Extra-depth shoe
High, wide toe box
Force-absorbing sole orthotics
Steel shank (from heel to MTP joint)
Firm heel counter
Tie lacing with multiple lace holes (for wide pressure distribution)
Velcro tongue closures

MTP, metatarsophalangeal.

**Table 4.12.   Common Rheumatoid Arthritis
(RA) Foot Problems and Interventions**

Problem	Intervention
Forefoot	
Metatarsalgia (including involvement of first metatarsal phalangeal joint)	Metatarsal bar Rocker bottom to shoe Metatarsal pad insert Plastazote insert Inner sole wedge
Hallux valgus Hammertoes	Extra-depth shoe with wide toe box
Midfoot	
Midtarsal joint pain	Use of tennis shoes Adhesive arch strapping Steel shank
Hind foot	
Painful subtalar joints and painful heel	Crepe sole Padded heel insert UCBL orthosis Plastic heel cup Arch supports Steroid injections PTB weightbearing brace

PTB, patellar tendon bearing; UCBL, University of California Berkeley
Laboratory

A variety of custom-molded shoes are available and may be
necessary in treating a severely deformed foot. If pain and disability become intractable, a final solution may be the use of a
tendon patellar weightbearing brace to unload the ankle.

Use caution in making modifications to a shoe; it often becomes
heavier and, therefore, may not be practical for the patient. See
Table 4.13.

Instruct the panel to perform heel cord stretching, AROM of the
ankle and subtalar joints, and flexion and extension of the toes
daily. Foot whirlpools may provide analgesia and can be used at
home.

OSTEOARTHRITIS

Definition

OA, also known as degenerative joint disease, is the most common joint disease and is considered to be the leading cause
of disability in older adults. OA is characterized pathologically
by the progressive deterioration and ultimate loss of articular
cartilage with reactive changes at the joint margins and in the
subchondral bone.

Table 4.13.   Shoe Modifications

Heel pads, cups
UCBL insert (especially for plantar fasciitis)
Plastazote insert
Metatarsal bars and/or inserts
Medial heel wedge/Thomas heel (for pronation)
Lateral shoe wedge

UCBL, University of California Berkeley Laboratory

Epidemiology

The prevalence of OA markedly increases with increasing age. OA is classified as either idiopathic (primary) or secondary (attributable to an obvious underlying cause).

Age, gender, vocation and avocation, race, and heredity all may play a role in the clinical manifestations of OA. In the elderly populations, OA is more common in the thumb and other finger joints in women; hip OA is more common in men. The clinical patterns of joint involvement often relate to prior vocation or avocation. For example, OA is common in the ankles of ballet dancers, although this is an uncommon site in the overall population. Native Americans are more likely to develop OA than whites; the exact role of obesity as a primary etiologic factor is still uncertain except in obese women's knees.

Clinical Features

Clinical manifestations of OA include development of joint pain, stiffness, enlargement, and associated limitation of movement. Typically, only one or a few joints are involved. Early in the disease, pain results from joint use and is relieved by rest. With progression of the disease, pain at rest may become common, as well as pain brought on by minimal movement. Enlargement may result from increased synovial fluid or bony proliferation. Joints commonly involved include DIP and PIP joints, base of thumb, hip, knee, and spine. Shoulder and elbow are involved more rarely.

Treatment

The conservative treatment of OA involves medications, reduction of joint load, and rehabilitative therapy. Drug therapy is essentially symptomatic, and analgesics such as aspirin and acetaminophen should be used. NSAIDs should be prescribed if severe joint inflammation is present or if a trial of analgesics has failed. Systemic glucocorticoids are usually not indicated, but intraarticular or periarticular injections, for example the anserine bursa, may provide symptomatic relief.

Methods to relieve joint loading include:

- Correction of postural abnormalities
- Orthotics, braces
- Well-padded shoes, such as running shoes
- Use of canes or walkers
- Judicious rest, although not prolonged immobilization
- Weight loss

Rehabilitative therapy includes splints to stabilize the MCP joint of the thumb; isometric exercises, especially to the knee extensors and hip extensors; and heat and cold modalities to joints. Recently developed knee braces can correct varus or valgus deformities to unload the tibial condyles in unicompartmental OA of the knee. Simple knee sleeves also will relieve knee pain in mild cases.

ANKYLOSING SPONDYLITIS AND OTHER SPONDYLOARTHROPATHIES

AS is the prototype disease of a group of interrelated seronegative spondyloarthropathies. Disorders include Reiter's disease, certain forms of psoriatic arthritis, juvenile chronic polyarthropathy, acute anterior uveitis, reactive arthritis, and the enteropathic arthritides. These disorders are not considered rheumatoid variants. Common features of the spondyloarthropathies include:

- Seronegativity for IgM RF
- Association with sacroiliitis/AS
- Presence of enthesopathy (inflammation/ossification at the site of ligamentous insertion into bone)
- Association with the histocompatibility antigen, HLA-B27
- Tendency to familial clustering as well as overlap (two or more spondyloarthropathies in the same family)
- Association with certain co-diseases such as psoriasis, chronic inflammatory bowel diseases, urethritis, and acute anterior uveitis

AS is reviewed as a typical representative of this group.

Definition

The term AS is not necessarily ideal for this disease, as only a minority of patients progress to a bent, fused, flexed spine. Moll defined AS as a chronic disorder of the spine and sacroiliac (SI) joints, in which inflammatory lesions are associated with progressive stiffening of the spine and radiologic calcification of spinal ligaments.

Among the most widely accepted criteria for diagnosis of AS are those developed in Rome (1961) and New York (1966). The most common way to satisfy the criteria is radiologic evidence of grade III or IV bilateral sacroiliitis together with a history of pain and/or limitation of motion. The presence or absence of the HLA-B27 antigen does not alone confirm the diagnosis. This disease is almost always diagnosed by means of a radiologic examination confirming sacroiliitis. Therefore, a patient with symptomatic bilateral sacroiliitis, although lacking the HLA-B27 antigen, likely still has AS.

Epidemiology

The prevalence in whites is approximately 1%. The sex ratio for sacroiliitis is almost identical, but males are much more likely to have clinical spinal disease. Thus, the male to female ratio is 3:1 to 5:1. The geographical distribution of AS is similar to that of the HLA-B27 antigen and is, therefore, rare in African and American blacks and Japanese. The disease usually presents between 15 to 35 years of age.

Clinical Features

Common symptoms include the gradual onset of low back pain, usually worse in the morning, and morning stiffness is common. Activity usually decreases the discomfort. Typical musculoskeletal clinical features are shown in Fig. 4-3. In established cases, spinal mobility and chest expansion are reduced. Progressive postural changes, such as forward stoop, are associated with tightness of heel cords, hamstrings, flexors, and pectorals. Other conditions associated with AS include ulcerative colitis, psoriasis, urethritis, iritis, aortic incompetence, and cardiac conduction defects. See Fig. 4-4.

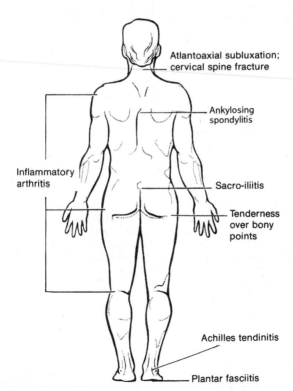

Fig. 4-3. **Musculoskeletal clinical features of ankylosing spondylitis.**

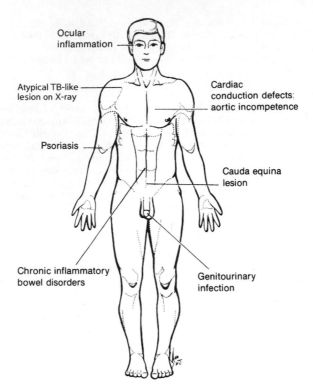

Ocular inflammation

Atypical TB-like lesion on X-ray

Psoriasis

Cardiac conduction defects: aortic incompetence

Cauda equina lesion

Chronic inflammatory bowel disorders

Genitourinary infection

Fig. 4-4.   Nonmusculoskeletal clinical features of spondyloarthropathies.

Radiology

Radiologic features include sacroiliitis—changes vary from blurring of the joint margin to sclerosis and eventual SI joint fusion spinal changes—syndesmophyte formation; in severe cases, the classical fused-bamboo spine; ossifying discitis; intervertebral fusion; and fractures. Other abnormalities are erosion and ankylosing of peripheral joints (particularly hip), ischial tuberosity whiskering, and periosteal elevations. For severe hip conditions, total hip arthroplasty is usually preferred to other forms of hip surgery. Postoperatively there is an increased incidence of heterotopic ossification.

Laboratory

RF is almost always negative; the HLA-B27 antigen is positive in at least 95% of cases with spondylitis. Erythrocyte sedimentation rate and alkaline phosphatase are usually elevated at some stage of the disease.

Management

Comprehensive physiatric management includes use of medication, physical therapy, and patient education.

NSAIDs are the initial drugs of choice and a rheumatologist should be consulted if NSAIDs do not suffice.

Physical Therapy

The objectives of physical therapy are to maintain normal spinal column position, strengthen spinal muscles, increase breathing capacity, maintain joint mobility, and relieve symptoms. Exercises include deep breathing, back extension and strengthening; and stretching of pectorals, hip flexors, hamstrings, and heel cords. Modalities may be employed as needed. (Spinal extension exercises and push-ups may help extend the spine.)

Patient Education

An education program includes a description of the disease and its course, with a rationale of needed exercises and development of posture consciousness. The need for adequate rest should be stressed and the use of proper sleeping surfaces, including a firm mattress with few, if any, pillows. The patient must always be vigilant to correct the tendency toward spinal flexion that occurs on a daily basis.

Outcome

The prognosis of AS is usually better than that of RA, in that only a minority of patients ultimately develop a significant disabling spinal deformity. Progressive disease is less common in women.

SUGGESTED READINGS

Biundo JJ, Rush PJ. Rehabilitation of patients with rheumatic diseases. In: Kelly WN, Harris ED, Ruddy S et al, eds. *Textbook of rheumatology,* 6th ed. Philadelphia: WB Saunders, 2001:763–775.

Convery FR, Minteer MA, Amiel D et al. Polyarticular disability: a functional assessment. *Arch Phys Med Rehabil* 1977;58:494–499.

Hicks JE, Gerber LF. Rehabilitation of the patient with arthritis and connective tissue disease. In: DeLisa JA, Gans B, eds. *Principles and practice of rehabilitation medicine,* 3rd ed. Philadelphia: JB Lippincott, 1998:1047–1081.

Klippel JH. Arthritis Foundation. *Primer on the rheumatic diseases.* Atlanta, GA: Arthritis Foundation, 2001.

Kremer JM. Rational use of new and existing disease-modifying agents in rheumatoid arthritis. American College of Physicians-American Society of Internal Medicine. *Ann Intern Med* 2001; 134:695–706.

McGuire T, Kumar VN. Rehabilitation management of the rheumatoid foot. *Orthop Rev* 1987;16:83–88.

Nicholas JJ. Physical modalities in rheumatological rehabilitation. *Arch Phys Med Rehabil* 1994;75:994–1001.

Nicholas JJ. Exercise prescription for the arthritic patient. In: Shankar K, ed. *Exercise prescription.* Philadelphia: Hanley & Belfus, 1999:277–296.

Nicholas JJ. Rehabilitation of patients with rheumatological disorders. In: Braddom RL, ed. *Physical medicine and rehabilitation,* 2nd ed. Philadelphia: WB Saunders, 2000:743–761.

Nicholas JJ, Aliga N. Rehabilitation following arthroplasty. In: Grabois M, Garrison SJ, Hart K, et al, eds. *Physical medicine and rehabilitation, the complete approach.* Malden, MA: Blackwell Science, 2000:1551–1564.

Steinbrocker O, Traeger CH, Batterman RC. Therapeutic criteria in rheumatoid arthritis. *JAMA* 1949;140:659–662.

Swanson AB, Swanson GD. Pathogenesis and pathomechanics of rheumatoid deformities in the hand and wrist. *Orthop Clin of North Am* 1973;4:1039–1056.

Swezey RL. *Arthritis: rational therapy and rehabilitation.* Philadelphia: WB Saunders, 1978.

5

Burns

Karen Kowalske and Phala Helm

Burn injuries affect more than 2 million individuals annually. Approximately 100,000 burn patients are hospitalized each year with most requiring some type of rehabilitation intervention. The most common age groups injured are age 17 to 25 years (75% to 85% male) burned by flammable liquid and ages 2 to 4 years burned by hot water. The most common area of the body burned is the upper extremity (70%), and the next most common area is the head and neck. The predominant cause for a major burn is flame (55% to 60%), followed by scalds (10% to 15%), electrical (5% to 10%), flash fires (5% to 10%), and grease (6%). Other causes include contact with hot objects, tar, chemical, and ultraviolet (UV) light. Most burn centers nationwide now also take care of frostbite and skin disorders such as toxic epidermal necrolysis and necrotizing fasciitis.

More than 60% of burn injuries occur at home or other private dwellings, whereas 20% of injuries occur at the place of work. Seven percent of injuries occur in a conveyance (auto, plane, etc.). This is important because patients injured in a conveyance are more likely to require amputation and extensive rehabilitation.

Rehabilitation of the burn patient begins within the first 24 hours after injury and may last for up to 2 years depending on the size of the burn and complications that occur. The rehabilitation phase of care uses a team approach to address the needs of the patient. The patient is taught that recovery depends primarily on the patient's commitment to hard work and sometimes painful exercise programs.

ASSESSMENT

Care of the burn patient begins with the assessment of the depth of burn, the overall total body surface area (TBSA) involved, and the severity. These factors, combined with the patient's age and associated injuries are important for determining the treatment plan as well as the morbidity and mortality associated with the injury. The amount of tissue injured by a burn depends on the duration and intensity of thermal exposure and the systemic responses to the heat damage. The characteristics of the skin also contribute to the depth of the burn. In children, the rete pegs are not well developed and in older adults they are atrophied; therefore, the depth of burn when compared with normal skin is increased in these age groups.

Understanding the depth of burn is based on an understanding of the anatomy and physiology of the body's largest organ. Skin serves many purposes that when interrupted cause significant impairment (Table 5.1). Understanding of the layers of the skin is essential to determining the classification of burn depth and understanding the potential complications following this type of injury (Fig. 5-1 and Table 5.2).

Table 5.1.   Functions of the Skin

Protects against infection
Prevents loss of body fluids
Controls body temperature
Functions as an excretory organ
Functions as a sensory organ
Produces vitamin D
Determines identity (e.g., cosmetic)

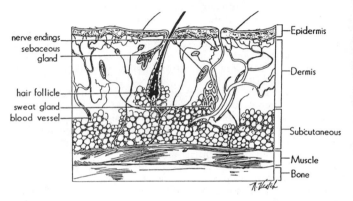

Fig. 5-1.   Anatomy of the skin.

Table 5.2.   Depth of Burns

Depth of burn is measured by degree
1st degree (superficial)—epidermis injured, characterized by ery-
    thema and mild pain
2nd degree—(superficial partial thickness) entire epidermis and
    portions of dermis are destroyed. Blisters form. It is a wet-
    appearing, painful wound.
Deep 2nd degree—(deep partial thickness) extends more into
    dermis. Usually no blisters and wound is red in some areas
    and white in deeper parts. Painful.
3rd degree—(full thickness) entire epidermis and dermis are de-
    stroyed. Appears waxy white or leathery brown or black. Lack
    of pain due to destroyed nerve endings.
4th degree—(deep full thickness) involves muscle, tendon, and
    bone. Appears charred. May require flap or amputation. May
    have pain in the surrounding tissues.

SIZE OF BURN

The total body surface area (TBSA) is often estimated by using the "rule of nines." Developed by Pulaski and Tennison, the rule of nines attributes 9% to each of several body areas with 1% for the perineum (see Fig. 5-2). It is easy to use but does not allow for differences in proportion of head and lower extremities in infants and children as compared with adults. A more accurate estimation of the TBSA burned is the Lund and Browder method (Fig. 5-3). Another easy but less accurate measure is to use the patient's palm as a measure of approximately 1% TBSA.

It is essential that all patients with major burns be transported to a regional burn center emergently for appropriate resuscitation and timely treatment. Most patients with moderate burns would also benefit from burn center treatment. Most minor burns may not require specialized treatment (Table 5.3).

TREATMENT

Initial management of a burn injury is directed at decreasing the potential for further tissue damage. Rapid removal of burned clothing is essential because burned clothing can retain heat for extended periods. Cooling the burn wound can help neutralize retained heat and decrease pain if applied within seconds to minutes postburn. Cooling has disadvantages because it can increase body heat loss thus decreasing body temperature. The best indication for cooling is in superficial second degree burns less than 15% TBSA for heat neutralization and pain control. Never use ice for cooling because of decrease in cutaneous blood flow resulting in tissue neurosis.

Following major burn injury, there are massive fluid and protein shifts in the burn tissue as a result of increased vascular permeability. The largest shift of fluid occurs in the first several hours postburn and can cause burn shock if the fluid is not replaced. Evaporative loss results in heat loss and a caloric drain on

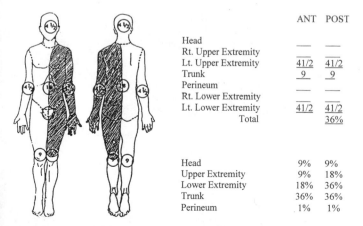

	ANT	POST
Head	—	—
Rt. Upper Extremity	—	—
Lt. Upper Extremity	4 1/2	4 1/2
Trunk	9	9
Perineum	—	—
Rt. Lower Extremity	—	—
Lt. Lower Extremity	4 1/2	4 1/2
Total		36%

	ANT	POST
Head	9%	9%
Upper Extremity	9%	18%
Lower Extremity	18%	36%
Trunk	36%	36%
Perineum	1%	1%

Fig. 5-2. Estimation of size of burns by rule of nines.

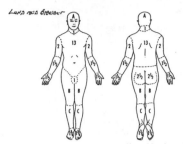

Relative Percentage of Areas Affected by Growth

	Age in Years					
	0	1	5	10	15	Adult
A - ½ of head	9½	8½	6½	5½	4½	3½
B - ½ of one thigh	2¾	3¼	4	4¼	4½	4¾
C - ½ of one leg	2½	2½	2¾	3	3¼	3½

Fig. 5-3. Lund and Browder. Relative percentage of areas affected by growth.

Table 5.3. Classification by Burn Severity

Minor burn
15% TBSA, 1st and 2nd degree burn in an adult
10% TBSA, 1st and 2nd degree burn in a child
2% TBSA, 3rd degree burn in child or adult, not involving eyes, ears, face, or genitalia

Moderate burn
15–25% TBSA, 2nd degree burn in an adult
10–20% TBSA, 2nd degree burn in a child
1–10% TBSA, 3rd degree burn in child or adult, not involving eyes, ears, face, or genitalia

Major burn
25% TBSA, 2nd degree burn in an adult
20% TBSA, 2nd degree burn in a child
All 3rd degree burns greater than 10% TBSA
All inhalation injuries

TBSA, total body surface area.

the patient. Bacterial contamination of the burn wound can occur immediately because of impaired defenses including loss of skin barrier, impaired local blood flow, and impaired systemic immune response.

Fluid Resuscitation

Immediate fluid resuscitation is essential following major burn injury. A shift of body fluids to the involved areas can cause intravascular hypovolemia and massive edema of both injured and uninjured tissues. If treatment is inadequate, acute renal failure and death can occur. Several formulas are available for calculating the fluid needs but serve only as guidelines. The fluids should contain sodium and resuscitation should be completed within the first 48 hours. Individual adjustments are critical for maintaining urine output.

Escharotomy/Fasciotomy

Escharotomy is an incision through the burned tissues to relieve increased tissue pressure. Massive edema in extremities that are burned circumferentially can cause neurovascular compromise. Early assessment of blood flow is essential. This is evaluated by physical examination, arterial Doppler, and tissue pressures. If tissue pressures are greater than 40 mm Hg or if pulses are diminished, escharotomy is indicated. Escharotomies are sometimes required on the chest wall if thick eschar limits chest expansion. With very deep burns such as those from an electrical cause, fasciotomies may be necessary to relieve increased compartment pressures.

Wound Care

Topical antimicrobial agents are the mainstays of wound care following burn injury. Initially, the wound is cleaned with mild soap and water. Most burn programs across the country have discontinued "tanking" in which the patient is submerged in water. With this technique, it is difficult to maintain body temperature, wound cross contamination can occur, and it may worsen hyponatremia. Instead, a spray technique is used. Next, nonviable tissue is removed with blunt or sharp techniques, and the topical agent is applied. Many antimicrobials are effective in decreasing burn wound sepsis. Silver sulfadiazine (Silvadene) is the most widely used because it soothes exposed nerve endings and has few side effects. Sulfamylon is often used on ears because of its increased depth of penetration. For small wounds, any of the antibiotic ointments can be used.

Biologic dressings act as a skin substitute and provide temporary coverage for the burn wound. These can be obtained from human cadavers (allograft) or from pigs (heterograft or xenograft). These are primarily used as an immediate coverage for clean midpartial-thickness wounds. The dressing becomes adherent and does not require daily dressing changes. It decreases fluid loss, relieves pain, and encourages the growth of granulation tissue. The dressing should gradually separate as the underlying wound heals. If it remains adherent for more than 10 days, silver sulfadiazine can be used to remove it. If it is left on too long it can become incorporated into the underlying tissues.

Allograft can also be used following excision as a "test" graft. If the allograft remains adherent, then it is likely that the bed is ready for autografting.

Synthetic dressings can be used to cover open wounds until they heal or can be autografted. The ideal characteristics of a synthetic dressing are for it to be inexpensive, readily available, non-allergenic, permeable, and easily removable. One product that meets these criteria is Biobrane. It has a bilaminar structure with silicone on the outside and nylon bonded to the bottom and covered with collagen. It is an excellent cover but must be stretched and held in place most often with staples or Steri-Strips. Therefore, it is most often applied in the operating room. Xeroform is a sulfur-impregnated gauze. It can be used moist as a nonstick dressing or can be allowed to dry out and adhere like a biologic dressing.

Debridement

Removal of devitalized tissue facilitates healing. With dressing removal, adherent tissue can be removed. Topical agents and any loose devitalized tissue can be removed with a coarse gauze or brush. Adherent devitalized tissue can be removed sharply with a scalpel or scissors. Enzymatic agents can be used in small areas that are being treated conservatively. For larger areas, surgical debridement is required. The two primary techniques for surgical debridement are tangential excision and fascial excision. Fascial excision removes the burn tissue and occasionally some level of viable tissue. Fascia provides an excellent wound base for grafting and decreases surgical blood loss particularly on the chest. The downside of fascial excision is the loss of subcutaneous fat that then creates a significant long-term cosmetic deformity. Tangential excision shaves thin layers of burn eschar sequentially until viable tissue is apparent. To control the increased blood loss with this technique, tourniquets can be used. This technique requires an experienced surgeon to determine the level of tissue viability. Early excision and grafting following major burn injury has decreased morbidity, mortality, and length of hospitalization.

Skin Grafting

With the exception of small wounds, all full-thickness burns and some slow-healing deep partial-thickness burns require skin grafting. Autografting takes skin from one part of the body, usually the anterior thigh, and moves it to the area of injury. Most wounds are covered with a split-thickness graft, which creates a partial-thickness wound in the area of the donor site. This skin can then be meshed and expanded to provide additional coverage of the wound. Meshed graft has better wound adherence but greater cosmetic deformity. The greater the mesh the greater the wound coverage but cosmetic deformity is increased because the area between the mesh heals by secondary intention. Sheet grafts require more skin to cover a set area and have a better cosmetic appearance but separate if a hematoma forms under the graft. Sheet grafts are always used on the face and can be used on the dorsal hands if the overall burn area is small. Following grafting, the wound is immobilized for 3 to 5 days. Once the bulky dressings are removed, gentle exercise can resume. It should be noted that split-thickness skin grafts have no dermal appendages and, therefore, do not have normal shear tolerance. Integra is a new artificial dermis that can be used to treat large burns. This product is placed surgically on a clean granulation bed. One to 2 weeks later, the outer coating is removed and an epidermal autograft is placed. This has an advantage that the donor site is less deep but treatment requires two surgical procedures. Cultured skin can be grown from a small biopsy. It is one cell layer thick and expensive. Therefore, it is used only for the largest of burns. Cultured skin is fragile and has a tendency to contract over time and, therefore, may require surgical release or regrafting.

Positioning

The general principle for positioning following burn injury is to put the injured area in a position of stretch without compromising the underlying neurovascular bundle. For small burns, local positioning for maximum stretch can be used. For large burns, entire body positioning is critical (Table 5.4). It is also important to alternate positions to avoid contractures. Sustained stretch in both directions is used to maintain full range of motion. Careful attention should be paid to tissue integrity to avoid splitting the skin.

Splinting

Splinting is an essential component of acute and long-term burn care. Following initial fluid resuscitation, patients can develop profound edema, particularly in the hands. These patients should be splinted with the wrist in 10 degrees of extension, 60 degrees metacarpal phalangeal (MP) flexion, and full extension of the proximal interphalangeal (PIP) and distal interphalangeal (DIP) joints. Splinting is also used after wound healing to prevent and treat contractures. These splints are placed so that the scar band is on maximal stretch. For patients who are critically ill, the ankles should be positioned in neutral to avoid plantar flexion contractures. For contractures unresponsive to splinting, serial casting can be used.

COMPLICATIONS

A variety of physical and psychologic complications result from burns, as listed in Table 5.5.

Nonhealing Wounds

Nonhealing wounds complicate the rehabilitation course because they may limit the ability to cast or splint and the ability to apply pressure garments. Often, nonhealing wounds are colonized by methicillin-resistant *Staphylococcus aureus*. Local care with Bactroban or drying agents may facilitate wound closure. Careful attention must be paid to avoid any shearing forces across the skin. Wounds open for many years are at risk for Marjolin's ulcer, a malignant form of skin cancer.

Exposed Tendons

If there is a deep full-thickness burn on the dorsal aspect of the hand or if the extensor tendons are exposed, range of motion should be modified to provide tendon glide only. This technique is stretching for MP flexion while maintaining PIP and DIP extension, flexing the PIP with MP and DIP extension, and stretching

Table 5.4.   Positioning to Prevent Deformity

Area Burned	Resulting Deformity	Position of Prevention
Neck Anterior aspect or circumferential	Flexion contracture of neck	No pillow under head
Neck Posterior aspect (only)	Extensor contracture of neck	Prone—pillow under upper chest to flex cervical spine. Supine—small pillow under neck
Axilla Anterior	Adduction and internal rotation	Shoulder joint in abduction (80 degrees to 90 degrees) and external rotation
Posterior	Adduction and external rotation	Shoulder in forward flexion and 80 degrees to 90 degrees abduction
Pectoral region	Shoulder protraction	No pillow. Shoulders abducted and externally rotated
Chest or abdomen	Kyphosis	As above and hips neutral (NOT flexed)
Lateral trunk	Scoliosis	Supine, affected arm abducted
Elbow Anterior surface or circumferential	Flexion and pronation	Arm extended and supinated
Wrist Total or volar surface	Flexion	Splint in 15 degrees extension
Dorsal surface	Extension	Splint in 15 degrees flexion
Hip (includes inguinal and perineal burns)	Internal rotation, flexion and adduction, possible joint subluxation if contracture severe	Neutral rotation and abduction and maintain extension by prone position or pillow under buttocks

continued

Table 5.4. *Continued*

Area Burned	Resulting Deformity	Position of Prevention
Knee (popliteal surface or circumferential)	Flexion	Maintain extension, using posterior splints or suspend heels with plastic heel protecting boots NO PILLOWS under knees while supine or under ankles while prone
Ankle	Plantar flexion if foot dorsiflexor muscles are weak or their tendons are divided	90 degrees dorsiflexion with splint if possible rather than footboard

the DIP with PIP and MP in extension. This avoids placing the entire tendon on stretch, which could cause tendon rupture. Patients are immobilized in slight MP flexion with full PIP and DIP extension when not in therapy. When splints are removed for wound care, the patient and wound technician should be instructed to avoid fisting, which could rupture the tendon. If tendon rupture does occur, the finger should be immediately immobilized in PIP and DIP extension for a minimum of 5 weeks to facilitate tendon reattachment.

Exposed Bone

Skin graft will not stick over exposed bone or tendon. Therefore, these areas must heal by secondary intention. The pinprick technique can be used to facilitate granulation. This technique involves stimulated the surrounding tissue with a sterile needle to the point of bleeding. These cells differentiate into granulation cells, thus providing a bed for epithelialization. For large areas of exposed bone, burr holes can be drilled to the marrow, allowing for stem cell migration with subsequent granulation tissue formation.

Scarring

The burn wound, unless immediately excised and grafted, begins its secondary healing. The wound may be covered with eschar, which is made up of nonviable tissue, coagulated protein, and residue from topical antibiotics. Regeneration of the skin (epithelialization) begins when epithelial cells at the wound edge divide and proliferate as do the epithelial cells from the base of the hair follicles and sweat glands. After epithelialization, peripheral nerves regenerate and may be associated with pain and itching.

Table 5.5.   Burn Sequelae

Defect	Cause
Hypopigmentation, hyperpigmentation	Melanin abnormality and donor site choice
Sensory impairment	Sensory nerve fibers fail to penetrate thick scar tissue
	Damaged in full-thickness burns
Abnormal skin lubrication	Loss of sebaceous glands due to depth of burn
	Unable to penetrate heavy scar
Abnormal sweating, heat intolerance	Loss of sweat glands due to depth of burn
Cold intolerance	Abnormal vasomotor response
Pruritis	Dry skin from lack of lubrication
Fragile skin	Loss of normal elasticity; thin
Ingrown hairs, pustules	Hair cannot penetrate thick scar and becomes infected
Permanent tanning	If exposed to direct sunlight before 12–18 months post-born
Marjolin's ulcer	Chronic recurring ulcers
Callused feet (Fig. 5.24)	Deep excision of feet
	Skin adherence to bone
	Bony abnormality
Comesis	Permanent scarring
	Flattened facies
	Body part amputated
Joint pain	Repeated minor trauma to hands and knees
	Joint pinning
Psychologic, social	All of the above
Fatigability	
Lack of endurance	

Depending on the depth, healing is usually complete in 14 to 21 days. The wound that remains open for more than 3 weeks develops dense scar tissue called hypertrophic scar. Hypertrophic scar is differentiated from keloid because it does not expand out of the area of the original injury. These scars are thick, hyperemic, pruritic, and often painful. Hypertrophy of scars peaks between 3 and 6 months and partially resolve between 12 and 18 months. The disappearance of hyperemia is a good indication that the scar is mature. Although the long-term utility of pressure garments has been called into question, most burn centers continue to use custom pressure garments on areas of hypertrophic scarring. Because graft skin retains a normal collagen matrix, it is less likely to hypertrophy and may not require pressure garment treatment. Significant scarring in grafted areas is seen when the graft is highly meshed and widely expanded. Other things that help decrease scarring are custom face masks, moisturizing, scar massage, silicone, and steroid injections. For scarring on the face or alopecia, tissue expansion of the normal skin followed by scar excision and rotational flap can be used to restore a more normal skin appearance.

Contractures

Contractures are a common complication following major burn injury, affecting 30% to 50% of patients. If the patient develops a contracture, treatment focuses on stretching. This may be combined with paraffin. For patients with a burn injury, paraffin is used at 118°F. This is a lower temperature than that used in other populations and is necessary to avoid burning the newly healed skin. If the paraffin is too warm, it can be placed in a bowl and allowed to cool before application. The paraffin can be applied by hand or with a brush and is then covered with cellophane. The patient is then placed in a position of maximum stretch and held there for 20 minutes. The paraffin warms and moistens the tissues, which allows for an easier stretch. If paraffin is not used, the skin should be well moisturized with lotion before stretching. If full range of motion cannot be obtained with passive range of motion, the patient can be treated with splinting or casting. Splints are easy to make and apply. They are good for mild contractures or for maintaining range of motion. They are also easily removed and, therefore, not a good choice for noncompliant patients, especially small children. Serial casting can be used with significant contractures. The cast keeps the skin stretch at near maximum range for 3 to 7 days, followed by removal, stretching, and recasting in an improved range. Casts must be well padded to avoid tissue shear. If a scar band is very narrow or unresponsive to conservative treatment, surgical release will be necessary.

Neuropathy

Neuropathy is a common complication of severe burn injury. Careful evaluation reveals two patterns. First is a generalized peripheral polyneuropathy. This pattern is similar to critical illness neuropathy. It occurs in older adults and in the sickest of patients. Mononeuropathies or mononeuropathy multiplex occur in patients with an electrical burn and in other patients with very deep burns. Inappropriate positioning, elevated tourniquet time or pressure, or direct pressure on the nerve may contribute to these neuropathies. The most common neuropathies seen after burn injury are peroneal, ulnar, and median. Peroneal neuropathies can occur by direct heat injury or by prolonged positioning in the frog-leg position with hip flexion and external rotation, knee flexion, and ankle plantar flexion with inversion. This position puts the peroneal nerve on maximum stretch and predisposes it to ischemia at the fibular head. The ulnar nerve can be compromised by direct pressure or by positioning with elbow flexion and forearm pronation. This position narrows the diameter of the ulnar groove and predisposes to injury. The median nerve can be compromised at the carpal tunnel. This is usually associated with significant hand edema. Early carpal tunnel release may be indicated to relieve this pressure.

Reflex Sympathetic Dystrophy (RSD)

RSD or complex regional pain syndrome type 1 is a rare complication of burn injury occurring in less than 1% of patients. It primarily occurs in the hand, and less often in the foot, and usually presents with significant edema and pain out of proportion to the tissue injury. It is seen more often in partial-thickness burns and in patients reluctant to perform range of motion exercises from the time of initial injury. It is worse with immobilization and usually responds to oral steroids combined with aggressive range of motion.

Central Neurologic Complications

Central neurologic complications following burn injury are rare. Traumatic brain injuries can be seen with falls after an electrical injury or with car or motorcycle crashes. Anoxia is seen following cardiac arrest with electrical injuries or with severe inhalational injures. Strokes can occur soon after injury in those patients with underlying vascular disease. Late neurologic complications are extremely rare but can occur months to years after a high-voltage electrical injury. These present with a pattern consistent with a stroke or spinal cord injury without any other clear cause.

Heterotopic Ossification (HO)

HO occurs in 1% to 4% of patients following major burn injury. It most commonly occurs in the elbows and less often in the shoulders, knees, and hips of patients who have been very ill with large TBSA burns. The underlying cause of this condition is still unclear. Although medication intervention has been attempted, it usually does not affect formation. Early resection followed by continuous passive range of motion (CPM) may be successful in some patients.

Amputations

Amputations are necessary following deep full-thickness or fourth-degree burns that involve muscle and bone. This depth of burn is seen with high-voltage electrical injuries and when patients are trapped in a closed space such as an automobile or a house. Care is taken to maximize extremity length. Careful prosthetic fitting is essential to avoid skin breakdown over the stump, which is often covered with grafted tissue. A silicone sleeve can be used to maintain moisture and decrease shear forces across the stump. Long-term monitoring for subsequent bony overgrowth is essential.

PREVENTION

As healthcare providers, it is essential that we are aware of the basics of burn prevention (Table 5.6). Simple measures such as a working smoke detector can decrease the incidence and severity of injury.

CONCLUSION

Patients who survive a major burn injury require extensive rehabilitation intervention for prevention and treatment of contractures, deconditioning, neuropathy, scarring, and other more

Table 5.6. Burn Prevention for Common Conditions That Can Result in Burns

1. Scald burns from bathing—set hot water temperature at 124°F
2. Radiator burns—do not remove cap on a hot radiator
3. Automobile failure to start—do not *prime* carburetor
4. Grease fire in kitchen—do not carry burning grease outside, smother burning grease with soda or flour
5. Scald burns from hot liquid on range—turn all pot handles inward so child cannot reach
6. Burning candles—do not reach over. Do not wear loose clothing close to burning candles. Place in protective container
7. Burning trash—do not throw combustible liquids on trash to start the fire. Keep garden hose in area where trash is burned
8. Barbeque pit fires—do not start fire with combustible liquids
9. Lawn mower fires—wait until mower is cool before adding gas
10. Hot irons—keep children out of areas with hot irons
11. House fires—do not smoke in bed. Check smoke detector battery frequently. Do not use combustible cleaning solutions in area around hot water heater
12. Vaporizers—do not use hot water vaporizers close to child's bed
13. Electric blankets can catch fire
14. Methamphetamine lab explosions—you know the answer
15. Insensate extremities—do not soak in hot water, do not walk on hot cement, do not warm feet with heating pad or next to a radiator

unusual complications. The rehabilitation team must work closely with the surgical team to time interventions. With comprehensive treatment, most burn patients do well. Return to work rate is high and overall life satisfaction is good. This information is useful to help patients through what is one of the most painful injuries imaginable.

SUGGESTED READINGS

Demling RH, LaLonde C. *Burn trauma*. New York: Thieme Medical Publishers, 1989.

Fisher SV, Helm PA. *Comprehensive rehabilitation of burns*. Baltimore: Williams & Wilkins, 1984.

Helm PA, Fisher SV, Cromes GF. Rehabilitation of the patient with burns. In: DeLisa JA, ed. *Rehabilitation medicine: principles and practice*. Philadelphia: JB Lippincott, 1998:1575–1597.

Richard RL, Staley MJ. *Burn care and rehabilitation: principles and practice*. Philadelphia: FA Davis, 1994.

Cancer Rehabilitation

David X. Cifu and Theresa Gillis

OVERVIEW

Currently 1 million people in the United States are under active treatment for cancer; 1.5 million are considered cured. The lifetime probability for developing cancer is one in three. More than 600,000 people per year are diagnosed with cancer. Fifty percent of all cancers occur in persons older than 65 years. A variety of factors, including type of cancer, therapeutic interventions, variable periods of bedrest, and the comorbidity often seen in older adults, combine to produce significant long-term or permanent functional loss as a result of cancer. Timely cancer rehabilitation can return the individual to functional independence, thereby improving quality of life.

FUNCTIONAL ASSESSMENT

The functional status of a cancer patient can be correlated with the outcome of the underlying disease. The Karnofsky Performance Status Scale, the most widely used measure of the functional status of cancer patients, allows a consistent means of categorization. Match rehabilitation goals to the patient's functional level. See Table 6.1.

TREATMENT

The regimens used to maintain function include mobilization, activity, nutrition, social support systems, and pain control. This overall program is used in combination with specific interventions based on the organ systems affected. Cancer rehabilitation concentrates initially on early discharge from the acute care setting. Continued rehabilitation occurs in the home environment. The intensity of the rehabilitation effort and the clinical setting depend on the type, site, and extent of involvement of the cancer.

Mobilization

Use daily bedside physical therapy to teach independence in bed mobility, through such activities as rolling from side to side and moving from a supine to a sitting position, as well as transfer skills, such as bed to chair. Nurses reinforce these learned activities.

Progressively increase the patient's time out of bed. Use a sitting program for patients who have difficulty with sitting secondary to orthostatic disturbances or skin breakdown. Assess skin integrity before and after sitting to prevent breakdown. Patients are to be out of bed, in a chair, throughout the day, as much as tolerated.

Activity

Encourage patients to do as much for themselves as possible, such as dressing, grooming, and feeding, as well as to use their

Table 6.1. Karnofsky Performance Status Scale

General Category	Index	Specific Criteria
Able to carry on normal activity, no special care needed	100	Normal, no complaints, no evidence of disease
	90	Able to carry on normal activity, minor signs or symptoms of disease
	80	Normal activity with effort, some signs or symptoms of disease
Unable to work, able to live at home and care for most personal needs, varying amount of assistance needed	70	Cares for self, unable to carry on normal activity or to do work
	60	Requires occasional assistance from others but able to care for most needs
	50	Requires considerable assistance from others and frequent medical care
Unable to care for self, requires institutional hospital care or equivalent, disease may be rapidly progressing	40	Disabled, requires special care and assistance
	30	Severely disabled, hospitalization indicated; death not imminent
	20	Very sick, hospitalization necessary; active supportive treatment necessary
	10	Moribund
	0	Dead

From Mor V, Laliberle L, Morris JN et al. The Karnofsky Performance Status Scale: an examination of its reliability and validity in a research setting. *Cancer* 1984;53:2002–2007, with permission.

own strength for mobility, either ambulating or propelling a wheelchair. Provide reachers, gait devices, and other aids to allow independent function. Physical appearance is important; encourage the use of wigs, makeup, and other aspects of cosmesis such as prosthetic facial features and limbs and modified clothing.

Formulate an individualized program for stretching, positioning, self range of motion, strengthening, and conditioning, in addition to regular physical and occupational therapy. Educate family and friends in ways to encourage and support independent activities.

When the patient achieves enough functional independence to be discharged, teach a specific home program of exercises to promote continued improvement. Consider a home safety evaluation. Schedule periodic evaluations and home or outpatient physical and occupational therapies, if needed. Consider the patient's expected functional outcome when ordering expensive equipment; devices may not be useful if the patient soon experiences a physical decline.

Social Support

The use of a multidisciplinary team approach (including an oncologist, a physiatrist, appropriate therapist(s), a social worker, a psychologist, an oncology nurse, a dietitian, and, the patient) is necessary to attempt to address all concerns. Select facilities such as the acute care hospital, the hospice, and the home with supportive care, through awareness of availability and the patient's care needs and wishes. Involve family members and friends, as appropriate, to achieve a smooth transition from one environment to another and to maintain adequate patient care.

Nutrition

Encourage good nutrition. Offer foods pleasant in appearance, smell, and taste. Anorexia, changes in ability to smell and taste, oropharyngeal and esophageal lesions and infections, and problems with digestion and absorption are common.

Maintain independent feeding and, if possible, independent preparation of food, by promoting mobilization and activity. Preserve the patient's autonomy as much as possible. Supplement the diet liberally as soon as possible with foods high in calories and protein to maintain strength and endurance. Obtain assistance from dietitians and nutritionists. Use enteral feeding or intravenous hyperalimentation only as a last resort to support nutritional needs. The oral route is the most physiologic approach.

Pain Management

Pain is present in 40% of people with intermediate-stage cancer and in 60% to 80% of people with advanced-stage cancer. Cancer pain, as categorized by Foley, allows for a systematic treatment regimen (see Table 6.2).

First, ascertain the type of cancer pain present. Categorize the patient using this pain classification. Treatment of the underlying cancer is the first line of therapy. Surgery, radiotherapy, and chemotherapy directed at the tumor may all result in decreased pain.

Table 6.2. Foley's Cancer Pain Classification

I	Patients with acute cancer-related pain associated with diagnosis of cancer or associated with therapy
II	Patients with chronic cancer-related pain associated with cancer progression or therapy
III	Patients with preexisting chronic pain and cancer pain
IV	Patients with a history of drug addiction and cancer-related pain
V	Patients dying with cancer-related pain

From Foley KM. Cancer pain syndromes. *J Pain Symptom Manag* 1987; 2(2):S13–S17, with permission.

Next, use nonnarcotic pain relievers such as aspirin, acetaminophen, and nonsteroidal antiinflammatory drugs in combination with physical modalities such as vibration, transcutaneous electrical nerve stimulation (TENS), massage, and heat or cold. Encourage continued mobilization and activity. Avoid physical modalities using heat over an area of known tumor involvement.

As the next line of treatment, prescribe an oral opioid, in combination with a nonnarcotic pain reliever depending on the degree of pain and the clinical situation. In cases of acute pain syndromes, as well as in terminal patients, use narcotic medications more rapidly and liberally.

When appropriate opioid preparations are ineffective, consider invasive neurosurgical and anesthetic procedures performed by experienced personnel as useful adjuvants for pain control.

In addition to pharmacologic intervention, use behavioral approaches such as relaxation training, distraction, guided imagery, hypnosis, and behavioral training.

COMPLICATIONS

Bony Metastases

Obtain bone scans and x-ray films when there is evidence of bony involvement such as fracture, bone pain, or specific tumor type, to define the extent of the problem. Although local immobilization (e.g., using a sling or a halo-vest) or radiation therapy may forestall fractures, surgical correction, specifically intramedullary rodding, is necessary to promote weight bearing and continued activity. In addition, surgical intervention is indicated prophylactically in all cases in which greater than 50% of the bone cortex is destroyed or in lesions greater than 3 cm in diameter.

Orthopedically repair pathologic fractures by pinning, rodding, or replacing rather than casting or otherwise immobilizing, to allow early mobilization and weight bearing.

Treat pain from metastases with local immobilization, medications, physical modalities, radiation therapy, and/or chemotherapy (hormonal manipulation). If the pain is intractable, surgical intervention is indicated.

Amputation

With the advent of limb salvage procedures, amputation secondary to cancer has become less frequent, particularly in children. Rehabilitation following limb salvage is similar to that of joint replacement patients; however, expect a longer period of immobilization and/or nonweight bearing. In addition, more extensive bracing and assistive devices may be required.

Fit the patient with a conventional prosthesis as soon as possible, following basic principles of amputee rehabilitation. (See Chapter 3.)

Observe for common problems, including poor skin healing, as a result of radiation and chemotherapy, weight fluctuations, and generalized deconditioning.

Neurologic Involvement

Rehabilitate the patient with primary or metastatic spinal cord cancer using principles of spinal cord injury rehabilitation. (See Chapter 17.)

Primary and metastatic brain tumors may present with headache, focal neurologic deficit, seizures, or diffuse encephalopathy. Following acute treatment such as surgery, radiation therapy, and corticosteroid administration, employ stroke rehabilitation techniques. (See Chapter 19.)

Abnormalities of the neuromuscular system, both focal, such as Pancoast tumor and compression neuropathy, and systemic, such as peripheral neuropathy, may be the result of cancer or may be treatment related. Diagnose and treat these problems, using rehabilitative strategies for neuromuscular diseases. (See Chapters 11 and 14.)

BREAST CANCER

Advances in breast surgery have eliminated many of the complications associated with radical mastectomy such as edema, pain, immobility, and poor cosmesis. Educate the patient about appropriate positioning, range of motion, pain control, and activities.

The patient will be immobilized at the shoulder at the time of surgery. On the fourth postoperative day, begin active motion of the affected elbow, wrist, and hand, as well as the unaffected upper limb. Initiate motion of the affected shoulder in the supine position at day 5 to 7. Progress to upright activities when the sutures are removed at 2 weeks. At that time, add activities of daily living (ADLs) and strengthening for the patient's home program. Most patients require compression with an elastic bandage, followed by use of a custom-fitting gradient pressure garment for management of edema. In the rare patient who develops lymphedema despite appropriate interventions, use pneumatic intermittent compression and/or compression garments, such as a custom glove and sleeve.

SUGGESTED READINGS

Dietz JH. Rehabilitation of the cancer patient. *Med Clin North Am* 1969;53:607–624.

Foley KM. Cancer pain syndromes. *J Pain Symptom Manag* 1987; 2:S13–S17.

Hirsh D, Grabois M, Decker N. Rehabilitation of the cancer patient. In: DeLisa JA, ed. *Rehabilitation medicine: principles and practice.* Philadelphia: JB Lippincott, 1988:660–670.

Laban M. Rehabilitation of patients with cancer. In: Kottke FJ, Stillwell GK, Lehmann JF, eds. *Krusen's handbook of physical medicine and rehabilitation,* 4th ed. Philadelphia: WB Saunders, 1990:1102–1111.

Portnoy RK. Practical aspects of pain control in the patient with cancer. *Cancer J Clin* 1988;38:327–351.

Recommendations for Cancer Prevention. *Department of Cancer prevention and control manual.* Houston, TX: The University of Texas MD Anderson Cancer Center, 1989.

7

Cardiovascular Conditioning Exercise and Cardiac Rehabilitation

Donna M. Bloodworth

Virtually all persons can participate in exercise except those individuals in the throes of acute disease or trauma. Cardiovascular conditioning exercise, performed at a moderate to high intensity, maintains and improves cardiac health in persons with no heart disease. Examples of moderate exercise are walking at a brisk pace of 3 to 4 miles per hour. In persons who have cardiac risk factors but no symptoms of cardiac disease, exercise treadmill testing determines the intensity of cardiovascular conditioning exercise that the person may safely perform. Persons who have suffered cardiac events perform cardiovascular conditioning exercise at low intensity and with telemetry monitoring, as part of cardiac rehabilitation program, which also involves other lifestyle changes to modify risk factors. For persons with cardiac risk factors and persons with cardiac disease, participation in regular exercise at the appropriate intensity lowers future risk of cardiac illness.

DEFINITIONS

The *ACSM's Guidelines for Exercise Testing and Prescription* define *physical activity* as body movement caused by skeletal muscle contraction that increases energy expenditure. *Physical exercise* is a structured form of physical activity that occurs regularly so as to develop or maintain fitness. *Cardiovascular fitness,* or *peak exercise capacity,* as Dennis explains, is the maximal ability of the cardiovascular system to deliver oxygen to exercising skeletal muscle and then the maximal ability of the exercising muscle to extract oxygen from the blood. Regular cardiovascular conditioning exercise improves peak exercise capacity.

The general public thinks of cardiovascular conditioning exercise as *aerobic exercise* or *endurance exercise* (Table 7.1). Biking, swimming, jogging, and cross-country skiing are examples. *Cardiovascular conditioning exercise,* or aerobic exercise, involves prolonged periods of rapid alternating use of large muscle groups, which causes an increase in heart rate (HR). The amount that HR increases indicates the intensity of the exercise. Exercise enthusiasts describe endurance exercise as a "high reps, low resistance" activity. Variations on endurance exercise include exercise for weight loss, which is sustained for a longer duration to expend calories (according to Rippe and Hess), and exercise to increase bone density, in which the duration of exercise and the type (i.e., weight bearing) matters but not the intensity. The concept of aerobic exercise differs from *strengthening exercise,* also called *resistance exercise* or weight lifting. Strengthening exercise involves moving a heavy resistance or weight through the arc of motion of a muscle to build muscle bulk and strength. Exercise enthusiasts

Table 7.1. Types of Exercise and Their Prescription

Exercise Type	Examples	Prescription
Endurance, healthy person under 45 yrs	Biking, jogging, swimming, cross country skiing	20 to 30 minutes, 3 to 5 times per week to a heart rate of 70 to 85% maximum; high reps, low resistance
Strengthening	Free-weight lifting, fixed axis weight machines	5 to 10 repetitions of maximal tolerated weight or lifting to fatigue of a lesser amount of weight; low reps, high resistance
Weight loss	Biking, jogging, swimming, cross country skiing	30 to 60 minutes, 5 per week; or sufficient to expend 1,500 to 2,000 calories per week; endurance type
Increase bone density	Walking briskly, stair climbing, running, weight bearing exercise	30 minutes, 5 times per week; heart rate not important; must be weight bearing

reps, repetitions

describe this activity as "low reps, high resistance." This chapter presents these examples to underscore that the variables of exercise including resistance, repetitions, duration, intensity, and frequency can be manipulated to effect different physiologic results on the participant.

Physical exercise stresses or exerts the cardiovascular system; therefore, physicians and exercise physiologists define and stratify exercise participants in terms of cardiac risk factors (Table 7.2). For the purposes of exercise participation, an individual is defined by cardiac risk and falls into one of four categories:

1. Younger individuals with no cardiac symptoms and one or no risk factors for cardiac disease
2. Men older than 45 years, women older than 55 years, or any age person with two or more cardiac risk factors
3. Any individual with signs or symptoms of cardiopulmonary disease or a known cardiac event
4. Any individual with acute cardiac, pulmonary, metabolic, infectious, or traumatic disease

Exercise is contraindicated in persons with acute cardiac, pulmonary, metabolic, or infectious disease or trauma (Table 7.3). Healthy men younger than 45 years and women younger than 55 years may participate in exercise of moderate to vigorous intensity without prerequisite exercise treadmill testing. Men older

Table 7.2.   Risk Factors for Coronary Artery Disease

Family history of MI, revascularizing surgery or sudden death
  before age 55 years
Cigarette smoking within the last 6 months
Hypertension (systolic BP over 140 mm Hg, or diastolic BP over
  90 mm Hg on two occasions)
Elevated total serum cholesterol greater than 200 mg/dL, over
  elevated LDL cholesterol over 130 mg/dL
Impaired fasting glucose (over 110 mg/dL on two occasions)
Obesity (body mass index over 30 kg/m^2)
Sedentary lifestyle

BP, blood pressure; LDL, low density lipoprotein; MI, myocardial infarction.

than 45 years, women older than 55 years, and a person of any
age with two or more risk factors for cardiac disease should complete a maximal exercise treadmill test (ETT) before embarking
on a moderate to vigorous intensity exercise program. Persons
with signs or symptoms of cardiac disease or subacute cardiac
events should complete a symptom-limited ETT before beginning
monitored, low-intensity exercise. The initial exercises for a cardiac patient include ankle pumps and mobilization to a chair and
later slow, short-distance walking. Table 7.4 summarizes recommendations for evaluation and recommended activity level among
these groups.
   Persons with signs or symptoms of cardiac disease or subacute
cardiac events are candidates for cardiac rehabilitation programs.
Cardiovascular conditioning exercise is only a component of cardiac rehabilitation. Pollock and Wilmore define *cardiac rehabilitation* as a process of restoring physical, psychologic, and social

**Table 7.3.   Contraindications to
Exercise and Exercise Stress Testing**

Unstable angina, or recent myocardial infarction
Severe resting hypertension
Symptomatic, orthostatic or exercise-induced hypotension
Second- or third-degree heart block
Severe atrial or ventricular arrhythmias
Acute febrile or medical illness or instability such as pneumonia,
  GI bleed, or DVT
Cardiogenic shock or uncompensated heart failure
Pericarditis
Critical aortic stenosis

DVT, deep venous thrombosis; GI, gastrointestinal.

Table 7.4. Indications for Exercise Treadmill Testing (ETT) and Exercise Intensity Based on Cardiac Risk Stratification

Patient Stratification	ETT Indicated	Exercise Intensity
Male <45 yr; female <55 yr; one or no risk factors	No	Moderate or vigorous
Male >45 yr; female >55 yr; two or more risk factors	Maximal ETT	70 to 85% of maximal attained heart rate
Subacute cardiac event, or symptoms of cardiac disease	Symptom limited ETT	Low
Acute disease or trauma	Not applicable	None; contraindicated

function to optimal levels in those individuals who have had prior manifestations of coronary artery disease (CAD). Until the 1950s and 1960s, physicians recommended 6 weeks of bedrest after myocardial infarction (MI); however, this practice came under question and literature in these decades began to support the early mobilization of a cardiac patient to a chair and participation in progressive endurance exercises after the infarction healed. The *ACSM's Guidelines for Exercise Testing and Prescription* describe modern components of cardiac rehabilitation including exercise training; risk factor modification through diet, medication, and exercise; medical follow-up; and psychosocial and vocational counseling.

Endurance, or *cardiovascular conditioning activity* is only one of many forms of physical exercise. Endurance exercise involves repetitious movement at low resistance so as to drive HR and induce a cardiovascular conditioning effect. Physicians' prescribing cardiac exercise must stratify or define patients according to risk for cardiac events so that appropriate exercise testing may occur if indicated and so that appropriate intensity may be prescribed. For persons with heart disease, cardiac rehabilitation is a multifaceted program, of which endurance exercise is a component.

ANATOMY AND PHYSIOLOGY

Consider the human organism to be a cardio-pulmonary-muscular system designed to do work, that is, to move mass over distance. The anatomic and physiologic integrity of the heart, lungs, and muscles affect the physical fitness of organism and the ability to perform sustained work. Obviously, but beyond the scope of this review, disease or impairment of any of these organs, for example valvular heart disease, chronic obstructive pulmonary

Oxygen uptake = (Cardiac output in liters/minute)   x   (Arterial O_2 – venous O_2)
Maximal Oxygen uptake* = Maximal cardiac output   x   (Arterial O_2 – venous O_2

Fig. 7-1.   Oxygen uptake: Fick equation.

disease, or muscular dystrophy, decreases the organism's ability to perform sustained work.

The maximal ability of the individual to do work reflects his or her cardiovascular fitness: The gold standard of measurement of cardiovascular fitness is maximal oxygen consumption or VO_2 max. Maximal oxygen consumption is defined as the level of exercise achieved by an individual at the point when fatigue or symptoms prevent further exercise. Oxygen consumption is not a convenient method of determining fitness because of the specialized equipment required to measure oxygen use. Therefore, more practical and clinically useful means of evaluating cardiovascular fitness is necessary.

Oxygen consumption (VO_2) consists of HR, stroke volume (SV) of the heart, and the ability of the end organ, or muscle, to extract oxygen from the arterial blood before it is dumped into the venous system (CaO_2 – CvO_2). The mathematical relationship of these variables is the Fick equation (Fig. 7-1). Clinically, the HR and HR_{max}, or maximal HR, are used to evaluate how hard a person is working (in terms of that person's maximal cardiovascular ability). The maximal HR that an individual can obtain decreases physiologically with aging; the maximal HR can be approximated by subtracting age from 220 (Fig. 7-2). However, this estimation is only a rough guideline; the only objective way in which an individual's maximum HR can be determined is by exercise treadmill testing. Exercise testing on a treadmill, or with an arm ergometer for persons unable to walk, assists in determining the maximal HR that an individual can achieve. The individual's maximal HR provides some indication of cardiovascular fitness, or the maximal amount of internal work that can be done.

A second type of work to consider is the external work that is being accomplished. Some individuals have more efficient cardio-pulmonary-muscular systems than others and, therefore, can accomplish more external work at the same HR or oxygen consumption than the inefficient individual. However, an inefficient cardio-pulmonary-muscular work system can become more efficient. This is the goal of cardiovascular exercise; when efficiency improves as a result of cardiovascular conditioning exercise, a training effect is said to have occurred.

The Fick equation suggests the possible variables that might be made more efficient by a cardiac conditioning exercise program. Studies suggest that in normal subjects at maximal work levels, conditioning exercise increases VO_{2max} by increasing SV and by in-

Approximate maximal heart rate = 220 - age in years

Fig. 7-2.   Approximation of maximal heart rate based on age.

creasing end-organ extraction of oxygen, meaning increasing $(CaO_2 - CvO_2)$.

The muscle's extraction of oxygen from the blood is increased by increased size of capillary beds in the muscle and increased mitochondrial density. Maximal HR is physiologically set and decreases with age. Table 7.5 reviews the chronic effects of exercise on the heart, lungs, muscles, and vascular delivery system. The practical and clinical corollary to this increased efficiency is that, at submaximal external work levels after training effect has occurred, a lower HR, lower SV, and lower myocardial oxygen demand will be required to do the same amount of external work as compared with the untrained state.

After cardiac events, patients have additional reasons for loss of efficiency of the cardiovascular system. Dennis writes that several factors contribute to physical incapacity following cardiac events, including (a) treatments like medication and bedrest, (b) intravascular volume depletion, (c) left ventricular dysfunction, (d) residual myocardial ischemia, (e) age, (f) autonomic function, (g) skeletal muscle performance, (h) noncardiac medical diagnoses, (i) physical capacity before the event, and (j) symptoms during physical activity. Dennis explains that bedrest is the primary iatrogenic cause of physical deconditioning after myocardial event. Three hours of upright posture decreases the deconditioning effect of bedrest. Left ventricular dysfunction is the primary physiologic cause of physical deconditioning.

After cardiac transplant, the literature documents several changes that decrease exercise capacity. Schwaiblmair et al. noted decreased oxygen uptake and ventilation-perfusion mismatch. Interestingly, Richard et al. showed that chronotropic incompetence of the denervated heart did not significantly decrease exercise capacity. By contrast, Quigg et al. showed that chronotropic incompetence, especially for patients on calcium channel blockers, does lower peak oxygen consumption after exercise training. Lampert et al. wrote that, although the mitochondrial density of skeletal muscle increases significantly after the endurance training of transplant patient, the capillary-fiber density does not and may contribute to limiting exercise training effect. Despite these changes in the physiologic integrity of the heart, lungs, and muscles, Kobashigawa et al. wrote that heart transplant patients do respond to cardiovascular conditioning exercise and these patients' peak oxygen consumption improves with regular endurance exercise.

EPIDEMIOLOGY

Most patients in cardiac rehabilitation programs are recovering from the sequelae of CAD, as opposed to other cardiac pathology such as congenital, myopathic, or valvular disease. In the United States, CAD remains the number one cause of death, killing over 500,000 Americans annually. Thrombus formation in an atherosclerotic artery is found in most persons who die of transmural MI.

The United States' age-adjusted mortality rate for MI, however, is declining; in the 1950s this rate was 226 per 100,000, but by 1987, age-adjusted mortality for CAD had declined almost 50% to 124 per 100,000. Decline in mortality rate is attributed to advances in medical treatment and technology, including prehospital care, the wide availability of coronary care units, the

Table 7.5.   The Effects of Exercise and Other Factors on Maximal Oxygen Consumption (Maximal Cardiovascular Fitness)[a]

	Determinants of Maximal Values	Effects of Exercise in Normals	Effects of Exercise in Cardiac Patients
HR_{max}	Age, sinus node medications	None	May be lower due to medication or chronotropic effects of MI
SV_{max}	Heart size, conditioning effects	Increases	May decrease
$CaO_{2\,max}$	Pulmonary diffusion, ventilation and perfusion, anemia, inspired O_2 concentration	None; decreases if pulmonary disease	None; decreases if pulmonary disease
$CvO_{2\,max}$	Skeletal aerobic enzymes, fiber types, genetics, capillary bed	The greatest training effect is peripheral	The greatest training effect is peripheral
CaO_2^- CvO_2	O_2 extraction by muscle, sympathetic redistribution of blood to muscles	The greatest training effect is peripheral Increases	The greatest training effect is peripheral

[a]Adapted from Yanowitz FG, ed. *Coronary artery disease prevention.* New York: Marcel Dekker, 1992, with permission.

Table 7.6. CAD Risk Factor (RF), and Effects on CAD with Modification

Risk Factor	Modifiable	Decreases Risk of Cardiac Event and Death if Improved
Advanced age	No	—
Male gender	No	—
Family history	No	—
Sedentary lifestyle	Yes	Yes
Elevated lipids	Yes	Yes
Smoking	Yes	Yes
Hypertension	Yes	No; control reduces stroke risk
Diabetes	Yes	No
Type "A" personality	Yes	Possible

CAD, coronary artery disease.

use of thrombolytic agents, and improved diagnostic techniques and surgical interventions. However, a significant decline in the age-adjusted mortality rate of CAD has been attributed to patient-implemented lifestyle changes to reduce risk of cardiac disease.

Risk factors for atherosclerotic CAD (Table 7.2) include elevated serum cholesterol, cigarette smoking, hypertension, diabetes mellitus, advanced age, male gender, history of previous cardiac event or abnormal electrocardiogram (ECG), and a family history of CAD before the age of 50 years. The control of hypertension has not been shown to decrease cardiac risk, possibly because the medications used increase serum lipids. However, dietary and medical control of hyperlipidemia, smoking cessation, increased exercise, and modification of "Type A" behavior may also slow atherosclerotic disease progression or reduce disease recurrence or mortality (Table 7.6). Instruction in the prevention of the progression or recurrence of CAD through risk factor modification is a significant portion of the cardiac rehabilitation program.

EVALUATION

Before prescribing a cardiovascular conditioning exercise, the physician should interview the patient regarding the presence of cardiac risk factors (Table 7.2) or signs of cardiac disease. Some individuals should complete an ETT. These persons include men older than 45 years, women older than 55 years, any age person with two or more cardiac risk factors, and any individual with signs or symptoms of cardiopulmonary disease or a known cardiac event.

An *exercise treadmill test (ETT)* is a standardized, progressive, endurance evaluation, which the subject usually performs walking, jogging, or running on a treadmill. For persons with impaired leg function because of paralysis or arthritis, arm ergometer forms of the test also exist. Technicians place ECG electrodes on the test subject, who then mounts the treadmill and begins to walk; every 2 to 3 minutes the speed or inclination of the treadmill increases. The various speed and inclination combinations of the treadmill compare with approximate metabolic intensity, measured in MET. One *MET,* or *metabolic equivalent,* is the amount of oxygen consumed at rest, or 3.5 ml O_2/kg/min. The term MET is often used in exercise physiology. One MET describes energy required for the average person to sit quietly at rest, arms and trunk supported. Activities of increased workload are described in terms of this average metabolic rate. For example, self-care activities, on average, are at 3 MET workload and cause average people to require three times the O_2 consumption that they would use if resting quietly; slowly climbing stairs is a 5 to 7 MET activity and the average person will increase O_2 consumption five to seven times.

There are many published protocols of exercise treadmill testing. In general, exercise treadmill protocols increase the external workload, in regular increments of 1 to 3 MET depending on the protocol, in regular time intervals or every 2 to 3 minutes. MET, or workload, is increased by speeding up and/or elevating the treadmill. For example, a person undergoing a diagnostic maximal treadmill test may use a Bruce protocol that rapidly progresses to 3 MET activity and increases 2 to 2.5 MET in intensity every 2 minutes. On the other hand, a cardiac patient during a predischarge low-level symptom-limited test would probably undergo a modified Bruce or a Naughton protocol that starts at a level of 1.5 MET and even after 12 minutes only reaches an intensity of 4 MET.

There are at least three strategies for exercising a patient during an ETT. These strategies differ in intensity, rate of increase of intensity, and type of patient studied. The strategies include maximal ETT, submaximal ETT, and symptom-limited low-level ETT. It is probably safest for the resident physician and patient to clarify with the cardiologist or ETT lab physician which protocol and strategy will be used. It should be noted that all ETTs (maximal, submaximal, and low-level symptom-limited) should end if symptoms occur. This requirement necessitates that the attendant of an ETT is aware of and can recognize the criteria for ending an ETT. Table 7.7 compares features of maximal, submaximal, and symptom-limited, low-level stress tests; however, use of these terms is not universally accepted.

In the evaluation of patients who have sustained cardiac events, submaximal or symptom-limited, low-level tests might be used; each institution has its own protocol for testing. Be aware that there are different protocols and strategies of testing; clarify the test to be used and criteria for ending the test with the attending physician. Throughout any treadmill test, monitor ECG, patient appearance, blood pressure, HR, and symptomatology. Stop the test at patient request; if equipment fails; or for increasing angina, 2-mm horizontal or down-sloping ST depression or elevation, supraventricular or ventricular tachycardia, exercise-induced intraventricular conduction delays, exercise-induced hypotension, severe hypertension, bradycardia or significant heart block, or progressive ventricular ectopy.

Table 7.7. Submaximal and Symptom-Limited Exercise Treadmill Test (ETT)

	Maximal ETT	Submaximal ETT	Symptom-Limited ETT
Absolute endpoint	Symptoms of cardiovascular insufficiency or disease	Symptoms of cardiovascular insufficiency or disease	Symptoms of cardiovascular insufficiency or disease
Relative endpoint	Maximal obtained HR or age-predicted HR (some labs)	Predetermined % of age-predicted maximal HR (often 60%); or predetermined MET level (often 5 METS), or Borg scale	HR obtained at time of symptoms
Protocol	Bruce in 60% of labs	Variable, often low level	Low level: low MET initiation point and small increments of increase MET intensity (e.g., Naughton, Modified Bruce)
Special uses			Patient after cardiac event

HR, heart rate; MET, metabolic equivalent.

Contraindications to ETT are essentially the same as those of Phase 1 of a cardiac rehabilitation program and also include digitalis or other drug effect and presence of a fixed-rate pacemaker.

For cardiac patients performing a low-level stress test, poor prognosis is associated with inability to achieve 5 MET activity, malignant ventricular arrhythmias, exercise-induced hypotension, and significant ST segment elevation or depression.

TREATMENT

In practice, patients often ask doctors how they can get into shape. The physician first must query whether the patient is interested in weight loss, improved cardiovascular fitness, or strength increase; then, the physician queries what types of exercise the patient prefers so that physician can outline a prescription to achieve the patient's goals. For example, a 30-year-old, with no cardiac risk factors, wants to participate in a jogging program to improve cardiovascular fitness. This person does not require a preexercise treadmill test because of the age and lack of risk factors; the individual's maximal HR is 200 minus 30, or 190 beats per minute. To achieve improved cardiovascular fitness, that is, improved maximal cardiac output, the individual should jog intensely enough to increase HR to 133 to 160 beats per minute, three to five times per week for 20 to 30 minutes.

The amount of exercise necessary to induce a cardiovascular conditioning effect in a normal person is 30 minutes of aerobic exercise three to five times per week at an intensity of 70% of maximal HR. The 30 minutes of aerobic activity is always preceded by stretching warm-up and cool-down periods of 10 to 15 minutes each. In persons who are younger than 45 years with no cardiac risk, use the equation, (220 – age) to determine maximal HR and then take 70% of that number to determine target HR during exercise. However, perform a maximal ETT in men older than 45 years, women older than 55 years, or any person with two or more risk factors for CAD to determine objectively maximal heart; then take 60% to 70% of the objectively demonstrated maximal HR to determine target HR. A submaximal or symptom-limited stress test is necessary if a cardiac event has occurred.

Persons who have sustained a cardiac event are prescribed a different intensity of exercise. They also participate in 30 minutes of aerobic activity, preceded and followed by 15 minutes of stretching, but intensity is 60% of maximal HR obtained on a symptom-limited ETT.

Some patients with chronic stable angina will predictably have onset of pain at certain levels of exercise-induced HR and systolic blood pressure (SBP), called the double product (HR × SBP), or the rate-pressure product. These patients should exercise 10 beats per minute below their symptomatic HR to develop a training effect. As they become more conditioned, meaning fit, they will be able to do more external work, even though they never exceed their symptomatic HR.

A physician prescribing cardiovascular conditioning exercise specifies a duration of exercise, a target HR, and a number of times per week to perform the exercise. Depending on the patient's age, cardiac disease risk factors, or history of cardiac event, the physician increases or decreases the duration of exer-

Table 7.8. Diagnoses of Patients Who May Benefit from Cardiac Rehabilitation

Myocardial infarction
Status post CABG
Status post coronary angioplasty
Status post valve replacement
Status post valvuloplasty
Status post surgical correction of congenital cardiac defects
Status post cardiac transplantation
Compensated congestive heart failure
Chronic stable angina
Persons with increased risk for CAD, after medical clearance

CABG, coronary artery bypass graft; CAD, coronary artery disease.

cise and increases or decreases the target HR. High-risk individuals, or those with known cardiac or pulmonary disease, should complete a symptom-limited exercise treadmill before initiating an endurance exercise program; the maximal HR should be less than 60% and the duration of exercise 10 to 15 minutes. These persons (Table 7.8) may also participate in a cardiac rehabilitation program.

Cardiac rehabilitation usually has three distinct, successive phases (Table 7.9). The phases of cardiac rehabilitation, when successful, lead to a cardiac patient's functioning safely at maximal physiologic, psychosocial, and vocational ability through an independent, self-monitored program of aerobic exercise, stress management, sensible diet, and recommended medical follow-up.

Cardiac Rehabilitation: Phase 1

Phase 1, the inpatient acute phase of cardiac rehabilitation, is the initiation point and cornerstone for all other phases. Activity resumption and prescription; dietary changes and education; stress management techniques; and planning for vocational, family, and sexual needs begin in this stage.

Physicians should prescribe activity with appropriate precautions and monitor the patient's response to prescribed activity. The initial management of patients with acute ischemia is bedrest, with appropriate medical evaluation and treatment (Table 7.10). Patients ordered bedrest longer than 3 to 4 days are at risk for complications of immobility. To prescribe activity with appropriate precautions, examine the patient and review the chart for signs and symptoms that might contraindicate or limit activity (Table 7.11). Record these findings.

Begin activity when the patient is free of chest pain and early complications have been ruled out, usually at 36 hours to 4 days after admission. Approach activity cautiously if there are findings of moderate hypertension, moderate aortic stenosis, coexistent chronic medical disease, incisional drainage, sinus tachycardia, or ventricular aneurysm. Patients with uncomplicated cardiac events or first-degree heart block, sinus bradycardia, and infrequent

Table 7.9.   **Three Phases of a Cardiac Rehabilitation**

	Location	Initiation	Duration	Monitored	Activity/Intensity
Phase 1	Inpatient	2–4 days	Hospitalization	Yes	Progress to independent self-care and short-distance ambulation
Phase 2	Outpatient	3 weeks from onset	8–12 weeks	Yes	Progressive cardiac conditioning 1 hour 3 times per week (target heart rate based on submax ETT)
Phase 3	Community	After	Lifetime	No	Maintenance of cardiac conditioning 1 hour 3 times per week

ETT, exercise treadmill test.

Table 7.10. History and Exam Findings of Significance in the CAD Patient

Historical features
Continued angina
Perioperative or extended infarct
Post or concurrent history of CVA, COPD, renal and/or hepatic disease, systemic ASVD, arthritis, electrolyte imbalance, diabetes
Fixed-rate pacemaker
Medications that reduce heart rate response

Physical findings
Resting hypertension
Orthostatic or symptomatic hypotension
Uncompensated heart failure: rales, edema, jugular distension, hypoxia, tachypnea, S_3 gallop, sinus tachycardia over 120 beats/min
Fever; incisional drainage (CABG); PE, DVT
Focal neurologic signs
Ventricular fibrillation and tachycardia
Signs of PVD, arthritis, skin pressure
Tubes and drains that limit mobility (central, chest, surgical, etc.)

Diagnostic studies
CPK values
CPK-MB values
LDH values
Troponin levels
ECG
Chest x-ray (pneumonia, edema)
Telemetry strips for atrial fibrillation and flutter, degrees of heart block, PVC triplets, more than 6 PVCs/min
Echocardiogram for pericarditis or critical aortic stenosis

ASVD, atherosclerotic vascular disease; CABG, coronary artery bypass graft; COPD, chronic obstructive pulmonary disease; CPK, creatinine phosphokinase; CVA, cerebrovascular accident; DVT, deep venous thrombosis; ECG, electrocardiogram; LDH, lactate dehydrogenase; PVC, premature ventricular contraction; PVD, peripheral vascular disease.

premature ventricular contractions (PVCs) may generally proceed with Phase 1 activity. Appropriately prescribed and monitored early activity and ambulation is safe and does not increase risk of complications. The patient must be monitored during and after activity for signs and symptoms of activity-induced cardiovascular dysfunction (Table 7.11). Always stop activity if adverse symptoms occur.

Precautions written as part of the exercise prescription should reflect the physician's concern for activity-induced adverse cardiovascular effects. While in Phase 1, the patient should not participate in activity that raises the HR more than 20 beats per minute over the resting HR. In Phase 1, activities are performed

Table 7.11.   Signs and Symptoms of Activity-Induced Cardiovascular Dysfunction

Angina
Nausea
Dyspnea
Altered mental status
Activity-induced hypotension
Fatigue
Pallor
Cyanosis
Hypoxia
Activity-induced dysrhythmia

for 5 to 30 minutes, 2 to 3 times each day; coronary artery bypass graft (CABG) patients progress slightly faster than MI patients. A sample program of a multistep, graded-activity program for Phase 1 cardiac rehabilitation is in Table 7.12.

Goals that the patient should achieve by the time of discharge, meaning the end of Phase 1, include self-care and activities of daily living (ADLs) and household ambulation, except stair climbing. The patient should also understand and be able to take medications independently, adhere to prescribed diet, check pulse rate, and identify symptoms of recurrent disease. Occasionally, before discharge or at 3 weeks after the CAD event, the patient undergoes a submaximal, or in some cases, a symptom-limited ETT to determine the level of cardiovascular fitness, work capacity, or symptomatic HR for the purposes of Phase 2 exercise prescription.

Almost all ADLs can be performed at an energy cost of 4 MET or less. Stair climbing requires 5 to 6 MET. Patients unable to achieve normal ADLs without symptoms have severe impairment of the cardiovascular system by the New York Functional Classification System (Table 7.13).

If a cardiac patient only tolerated 4 MET of activity intensity on a Naughton ETT protocol, he or she would not be ready to perform the 5 to 7 MET activity of stair climbing.

Cardiac Rehabilitation: Phase 2

Once the patient is discharged from the hospital, the comprehensive cardiac rehabilitation program moves into higher gear. The goal of Phase 2 is to provide the patient with the information and experience that will permit him or her to pursue an independent cardiac conditioning and wellness program after graduating from the structured program. This phase usually begins within 2 weeks of discharge from the hospital, and sessions last 1 hour per day, three times per week for 8 to 12 weeks. Phase 2 usually takes place in a hospital or clinic. Requiring close physician supervision, this phase places emphasis on exercise and physical reconditioning; frequently, patients are monitored by telemetry during exercise.

As already discussed, initial exercise intensity is determined by results of a submaximal or symptom-limited, low-level ETT.

**Table 7.12. Sample Phase 1
Cardiac Rehabilitation Activity Outline**

Step	MET Workload	Location	Activities
1 (Initiated in ICU before PM&R consult)	1.5	Patient room	Ankle pumps, deep breathing and cough; P-AAROM all limbs; feed self
2 (Initiated in ICU before PM&R consult)	1.5	Patient room	Above; plus, transfer to bedside commode and chair; light grooming
3	1.5	Patient room	AROM, stretching, up in chair, bathing, slow paced ambulation
4	1.5 to 2.0	Nursing station	Supervised ambulation for 75 feet, dressing activity
5	1.5 to 3.0	Nursing station or gym	Ad lib ambulation on nursing station, 2 to 3 stairs, ADLs at sink; ambulation 100 to 300 feet, stationary bike (no resistance) for 3 minutes, warm-up activity
6	1.5 to 3.0	Gym	Ambulate 500 feet, 2 sets of steps or 8 stairs, 5 minutes stationary bike; teach to take pulse rate

ADLs, activities of daily living; AROM, active range of motion; ICU, intensive care unit; P-AAROM, passive and active assisted range of motion; PM&R, physical medicine and rehabilitation.

Intensity is increased on a weekly basis as symptoms and conditioning permit. There are many published protocols of activity, but a suggested activity outline is provided (Table 7.14). Contraindications to Phase 2 are essentially the same as those to ETT or Phase 1.

In general, the patient begins Phase 2 at an external intensity level of 5 MET and through aerobic conditioning progresses to 8 MET activity before discharge to Phase 3, after 8 to 12 weeks.

Education about diet, stress, medication, exercise, and symptomatology continue in Phase 2. Preparations to return to work, including job site evaluation or duty modification, are completed in this phase.

Table 7.13.   New York Heart Association Functional Classification System

Class	Limitation of Activity	METS	O_2 Consumption
I	No limits, no symptoms with ordinary activity	7 or more	24 cc/kg/min or more
II	Symptoms with ordinary activity; comfort at rest	5–6	17–21 cc/kg/min
III	Comfort at rest; symptoms with less than normal activity	3–4	10–14 cc/kg/min
IV	Discomfort with any activity; may have symptoms at rest	1–2	3.5–7 cc/kg/min

By discharge, the patient should be ready for the responsibilities of Phase 3, including a daily self-administered exercise program, carryover of lifestyle associated with low cardiac risk, and compliance with medications and medical follow-up. The patient should also have adequate knowledge of his or her disease and symptoms to pursue vocational, recreational, and sexual activities safely.

Cardiac Rehabilitation: Phase 3

Phase 3 of cardiac rehabilitation should be considered a permanent change in lifestyle and should continue throughout the person's life to minimize cardiac disease morbidity and mortality.

The cardiac transplantation group form a special population of cardiac rehabilitation patients. Before transplant, these patients have often been bedridden and are severely deconditioned by the symptoms of the disease. Prescription for exercise after transplant should be based on the results of a symptom-limited ETT. The patient is exercised at about 50% of the maximal HR achieved on symptom limited ETT, 4 to 5 days per week and starting at 15 minutes but progressing to 60 minutes.

Complications

There is risk associated with recreational exercise in healthy persons, exercise treadmill studies, and cardiac rehabilitation participation. The *ACSM's Guidelines for Exercise Testing and Prescription* refer to about one death for every 400,000 jogging hours. However, the rate of cardiac death for a sedentary lifestyle is seven times this rate. The rate of complications with ETT varies widely from 0.06% to 9%, including MIs and arrhythmias. For cardiac rehabilitation programs the rate of major cardiovascular complication, including death, is about one event per 60,000 participant hours.

Table 7.14. Suggested Activity Levels for Phase 2 Cardiac Rehabilitation

Level	Timing	Activities
1	3–4 weeks p/MI	8 minutes × 2 on stationary bike at 35% MET obtained on ETT (MET-ETT)
	monitored	8 minutes × 2 on arm ergometer at 30% MET obtained on ETT
		12 minutes at 50% MET-ETT on treadmill
2	4 weeks	8 minutes on bike at 45% MET-ETT × 2
		8 minutes on arm ergometer at 35% MET-ETT × 2
		12 minutes at 60% MET-ETT on treadmill
3	4–5 weeks	Same, except increase treadmill intensity to 70% of MET-ETT
4	5 weeks	Bike: 12 min at 45%
		Arm ergometer: 8 min × 2 at 45% MET-ETT
		Treadmill: 12 min at 75% MET-ETT
5	5–6 weeks	Bike: 15 min at 45% MET-ETT; otherwise, the same
6 Discontinue monitor if stable	6 weeks	Arm ergometer: 8 min × 2 at 45% MET-ETT
7	6–7 weeks after MI	Bike: 15 minutes at 3.7 METs
		Treadmill: 15 min at 75% MET-ETT
		Arm ergometer: 8 min × 2 at 4.5 METs
		Treadmill: 14 min at 3.9 METs
		Rowing machine: low resistance for 3–5 min
8	7 weeks	Bike: 15 min at 4.9 METs
		Arm ergometer: 8 min × 2 at 5.5 METs
		Treadmill: 20 min at 3.9 METs
9	9 weeks	Bike: same
		Arm ergometer: 8 min × 2 at 6.4 METs
		Treadmill: 22 min at 6 METs
10	11 weeks	Bike: 15 min at 6.1 METs
		Arm ergometer: same; treadmill 25 min at 6 METs
11	12 weeks	Bike: same; arm ergometer: 25 min at 6 METs
11	12 weeks	Bike: same; arm ergometer: same; treadmill 27.5 min at 6 METs
12	13 weeks	Bike: same; arm ergometer: same; treadmill 30 min at 6 METs

ETT, exercise treadmill test; METs, metabolic equivalents.

SUGGESTED READINGS

Dennis C. Rehabilitation of patients with coronary artery disease. In: Braunwald E., ed. *Heart disease: a textbook of cardiovascular medicine*, 5th ed. Philadelphia: WB Saunders, 1997:1392–1403.

Fardy PS, Yanowitz FG. *Cardiac rehabilitation*. Baltimore: Williams & Wilkins, 1995.

Franklin B, American College of Sports Medicine. *ACSM's guidelines for exercise testing and prescription*. Philadelphia: Lippincott Williams & Wilkins, 2000.

Kobashigawa JA, Leaf DA, Lee N et al. A controlled trial of exercise rehabilitation after heart transplantation. *N Engl J Med* 1999; 340:272–277.

Lampert E, Mettauer B, Hoppeler H et al. Skeletal muscle response to short endurance training in heart transplant recipients. *J Am Coll Cardiol* 1998;32:420–426.

Pollock ML, Schmidt DH. *Heart disease and rehabilitation*. New York: John Wiley and Sons, 1986.

Pollock ML, Wilmore JH. *Exercise in health and disease*. Philadelphia: WB Saunders, 1990.

Quigg R, Salyer J, Mohanty PK et al. Impaired exercise capacity late after cardiac transplantation: influence of chronotropic incompetence, hypertension, and calcium channel blockers. *Am Heart J* 1998; 136:465–473.

Richard R, Verdier JC, Duvallet A et al. Chronotropic competence in endurance trained heart transplantation recipients: heart rate is not a limiting factor for exercise capacity. *J Am Coll Cardiol* 1999; 33:192–197.

Rippe JM, Hess S. The role of physical activity in the prevention and management of obesity. *J Am Diet Assoc* 1998;98(10 Suppl 2): S31–38.

Schwaiblmair M, von Scheidt W, Uberfuhr P et al. Lung function and cardiopulmonary exercise performance after heart transplantation: influence of cardiac allograft vasculoplasty. *Chest* 1999;116:332–339.

Shephard RJ, Miller HS. *Exercise and the heart in health and disease*. New York: Marcel Dekker, 1999.

Yanowitz FG, ed. *Coronary artery disease prevention*. New York: Marcel Dekker, 1992.

8

Chronic Pain

Martin Grabois

Chronic pain is difficult and frustrating to control. Patients who experience it are often viewed as management problems and, therefore, as undesirable. Most physicians, including medical students, house officers, and practitioners, often lack understanding, have little training, and have even less interest in management of chronic pain. The aim of this chapter is to provide an understanding of chronic pain syndromes, a summary of evaluation techniques available, and treatment techniques used in its management. Hopefully, this increased knowledge will result in improved management of patients with chronic pain and chronic pain syndrome.

CHRONIC PAIN DEFINITION AND CHARACTERISTICS

Pain, in general, is an unpleasant sensory and emotional response to a stimulus associated with acute or potential tissue damage lasting less than 3 months. Acute pain is a normal symptom resulting from a noxious stimulus. It serves a useful biologic purpose by warning the organism of injury and causing the organism to seek help and guard the affected body part. It is usually time limited, and its intensity gradually decreases as the noxious stimulus is removed. Chronic pain syndrome is an abnormal condition in which pain is no longer a symptom of discreet tissues injury but in which pain and pain behavior become the primary disease and has specific characteristics (Table 8.1). Chronic pain syndrome is distinct from a chronically or intermittently painful disease state in which the patient experiences pain but manifests function and behavior appropriate to the degree of tissue injury. In chronic pain syndrome, subjective and behavioral manifestations of pain persist beyond objective evidence of tissue injury. Chronically painful conditions can lead to chronic pain syndrome but not all persons with chronically painful conditions manifest chronic pain behavior and disability. The difference between acute and chronic pain is further compared and contrasted in Table 8.2.

EPIDEMIOLOGY

Pain has become an increasing source of disability in the United States. It is noted that 16.5% of the adult population in the United States is disabled to some degree with half that number too disabled to work. Musculoskeletal disorders are noted to be the most frequent cause of disability and rank second in frequent causes of visits to physicians' offices and third in frequent causes of hospitalizations and surgical procedures. The total economic cost of all musculoskeletal conditions exceeds $65 billion annually. The Nuprin Report stated that 27% of the United States population suffers pain for greater than 101 days per year, resulting in staggering costs in days lost from work. We are now spending $70 billion a year on lost days for painful conditions or lost

---

Table 8.1. Characteristics of Chronic Pain

Persists long after healing should have occurred

Alteration of behavior and mood: depression, "pain behaviors," anger, moodiness, and anxiety

Limitation of activity: deconditioning, loss of strength, and flexibility

Vocational dysfunction and financial distress

Altered marital, family, and social relationship: stress, conflict, withdrawal, and dependency

Not always clear relationship to organic pathology

Litigation, disputes with insurance carriers or worker's compensation

Multiple nonproductive tests, surgeries, medical treatments, and therapies

Inappropriate or excessive use of medication and medical services

---

productivity, worker's compensation payments, and healthcare cost. Walsh and Dumitru suggested that our system of disability compensation in the United States increases frequency of certain types of disabilities and may delay recovery following occupational injuries. Chronic pain results when acute pain is not adequately evaluated and/or treated; when curative treatment or control is not available; or when pain-reinforcing complications such as secondary gains and social, economic, or psychosocial factors are prominent. Thus, in a small but significant number of acute pain patients, the pain continues and even intensifies in nature. The physical sensation of pain is complicated by physical factors such as inactivity, psychologic factors such as depression, and environmental factors such as compensation (Fig. 8-1). Chronic pain can be caused by ongoing pathologic processes (e.g., arthritis), chronic nervous system dysfunctions (e.g., phantom limb pain), or a combination of both processes. The evaluation of a chronic pain patient should focus on defining the pain sources as nociceptive, neuropathic, or neuropsychologic, while recognizing potential modifiers of the complaints. In an effort to optimize the care of patients with chronic pain, the International Association for the Study of Pain (IASP) Subcommittee on Taxonomy has developed a scheme for the coding of chronic pain syndromes. Codification of chronic pain presentations should enhance communication between treating physicians and provide direction of research efforts in this field. The pain diagnoses are separated into somatic, neuropathic, and psychologic causes. The IASP classification system further defines five axes based on (a) the anatomic region affected, (b) systemic cause, (c) temporal characteristics, (d) intensity, and (e) initiating cause. Each of these factors plays an important role in defining the treatment of pain. More recently, with the advent of managed care, approval for evaluation and treatment of patients with chronic pain in an interdiscipli-

Table 8.2. Differences Between Acute Pain and Chronic Pain

Chronic Pain	Acute Pain
Remote, ill-defined onset; duration unpredictable	Temporal features
Nonapparent	Recent, well-defined onset; expected to end in days or weeks
Intensity variable	Biologic function
Irritability or depression	Essential warning; impels rest and avoidance of further harm
May or may not give any indication	
	Variable
Recurrent (such as headache, sickle cell anemia), due to nonprogressive or slowly progressive diseases (such as hemophilia, inflammatory bowel disease, osteoarthritis, and many neuropathic pains) Pain determined by psychologic factors	Associated affect
	Anxiety common when severe or cause is unknown
	Associate pain-related
	Pain behaviors common (such as moaning, splinting, rubbing, etc.) when severe or cause is unknown
	Associated features
	May have signs of sympathetic vegetative signs, hyperactivity when severe such as lassitude, anorexia, weight loss, insomnia, loss of libido
	Types and examples
	Monophasic (such as postoperative, traumatic, due to progressive medical diseases) such as cancer and AIDS

nary or multidisciplinary chronic pain program has become more difficult.

PAIN MANAGEMENT CONCEPTS

The best management for chronic pain is prevention. This involves identifying contributing factors and addressing them in the early stages of the acute pain syndrome. As acute pain changes to subacute pain, these contributing factors usually become apparent. At this point a multidisciplinary team approach is often indicated, with comprehensive evaluation and use of appropriate medication, modalities, and gradual introduction of physical reconditioning activities. Identifiable psychosocial and environmental issues, although not usually prominent at this stage, if present must be recognized and managed. However, once these factors become prominent and last longer than 6 months the treatment strategy should be modified. When pain becomes chronic it in-

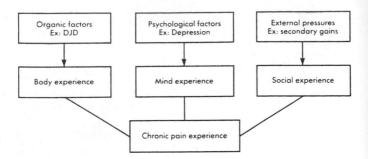

Fig. 8-1. Chronic pain: interaction of organic, psychologic, and social factors. (From Grabois M. Chronic pain. In: Goodgold, ed. *Rehabilitation medicine*. St. Louis: Mosby, 1988:664, with permission.)

creases in complexity, and the patient becomes more resistant to treatment. Concepts used in the treatment of acute pain such as inactivity, surgical intervention, narcotic medications, and physical modalities will not usually result in success. It is at this point that the concept of pain clinics or programs, which involve the interdisciplinary team for comprehensive evaluation and treatment, becomes appropriate and essential. Treatment goals at this time address improving the quality of life and functional capabilities of the individual with alleviation or modification of pain if possible and the remedy of factors that contribute to the perpetuation of the chronic pain syndrome. Winning strategies for pain clinics now seem to center around low price, customer satisfaction, demonstrated exceptional outcome, prestige, ease of access, and the development of practice parameter and/or clinical pathways. Having an appropriate utilization review program can control costs and still provide patients with good outcomes. Involvement in a vertically integrated healthcare network with access and referral mechanism for patients is very helpful in sustaining a multidisciplinary pain clinic.

PAIN CLINIC TEAM AND PATIENT SELECTION

Members of the multidisciplinary pain management team are listed in Table 8.3. The physician usually provides overall leadership and is the patient manager. Nonclinical administrative management often is under the supervision of a coordinator. In smaller programs, however, these positions may be combined. The physician is responsible for the initial evaluation and referral to the team. Members of the team who are consulted subsequently evaluate and assist in the selection of appropriate patients for treatment. Although evaluations are on a one-to-one basis, the team makes the decision to accept or reject a potential patient during a team interaction. Appropriate patients are those who demonstrate chronic pain, are motivated to participate, do not have significant complicating factors such as secondary gains, and accept the concepts and goals of the pain program (Table 8.4).

Table 8.3. The Pain Rehabilitation Team		
Clinical	Administrative	Consultants
Physiatrist/ patient manager	Program coordinator	Pharmacologist
Psychologist and/ or psychiatrist	Secretarial/ clerical staff	Dietitian
Physical therapist		Recreational therapist
Occupational therapist		Chaplain
Vocational counselor		Other physician specialists
Social worker		
Rehabilitation nurse		

ASSESSMENT AND EVALUATION

The evaluation includes examination of etiologic factors and a comprehensive pain evaluation, including a complete history, physical examination, quantification, functional evaluation, and psychosocial evaluation. Appropriate diagnostic tests are obtained but not repeated if previously performed. The evaluation should be as objective and quantitative as possible. It is essential to obtain and review the patient's pertinent medical records and review a pain questionnaire completed by the patient before examination (Fig. 8-2).

History

In taking a history, one should emphasize the following components in the clinical history:

1. Pain description: location, radiation characteristics, time sequence, what makes it worse or better, and patient's activity level

Table 8.4. Guidelines for Candidate Selection for the Pain Management Program
The candidate:
Has had chronic pain of more than 6 months' duration
Can comprehend the abstract principles of the pain management program
Is independently mobile (for attendance of appointments)
Is cooperative and willing to follow the principles of the pain management program
Has had appropriate evaluation techniques performed and/or reviewed
Has had appropriate surgical and conservative treatment for pain
Accepts concept of program

Complete the entire form by checking or circling answers.
Fill in blanks.   Use ink only.

NAME: _____   DATE: _____
ADDRESS: _____   AGE: _____
PHONE: _____   BIRTH DATE: _____
OCCUPATION: _____   MARITAL STATUS: _____
REFERRING PHYSICIAN: _____   LEVEL OF EDUCATION: _____

1. Onset of pain (Give specific date; if accident, describe.) _____

2. Surgery for pain (list below/none)

Procedure	Date	Surgeon

3. Location of pain:
   Indicate on the diagram the following:
   a. Entire painful area (xxxxx)
   b. Single most painful spot (*)
   c. Numbness (ooooo)
   d. Tingling area(s) (-----)

4. Does the pain move from one area to another? (yes/no)
   If yes, describe. _____

5. Pain scale:

0	1-2	3-4	5-6	7-8	9	10
No pain	Minimal	Mild	Moderate	Severe	Excruciating	Unbearable

   Using this scale, rate the pain:
   Now_____ Best times _____ Worst times _____

6. A. List all pain medications you now take.

Name	Amount	Frequency

   B. Do you drink alcohol for pain relief? (yes/no) _____
   Describe the type and amount: _____

Fig. 8-2.   Sample pain management program questionnaire.

7. A. Circle all physical and/or occupational therapies you have experienced for pain treatment:

Hot packs	Cold packs	Paraffin	Laser
Exercises	Massage	Fluidotherapy	TENS
Ultrasound	Whirlpool	Neuroprobe	Biofeedback
Other _____			

   B. Place a check mark by those that gave the most relief.

8. Using (X) for decreases, (O) for increases, indicate the effect of the following:
   ___ walking   ___ sleeping   ___ sexual activities   ___ alcohol
   ___ sitting   ___ fatigue   ___ bending   ___ medications
   ___ standing   ___ tension   ___ working   ___ bowel movements
   ___ reclining   ___ exercise   ___ house cleaning   ___ lifting

9. In a 24-hour period, indicate the hours you spend
   in pain ____;   reclining because of pain ____;
   reclining for other reasons ____;   sleeping ____.

10. Circle the numbers indicating pain limitations.

Activity	Normal	Mildly limited	Moderately limited	Severely limited
Walking	1	2	3	4
Running	1	2	3	4
Bending	1	2	3	4
Lifting	1	2	3	4
Sitting	1	2	3	4
Stair climbing	1	2	3	4
Resting	1	2	3	4
Sexual Activities	1	2	3	4
Working	1	2	3	4
Hobbies	1	2	3	4

11. Were pain not a problem, what would you like to do that you cannot do now? _____

12. When did you last work your regular job?   (date)
13. Is your case Workman's Compensation?   (yes/no)
14. Are you involved in a lawsuit because of the pain?   yes/no
    Describe: _____

Fig. 8-2. (continued).

2. Prior pain evaluations: physicians, hospitalizations, and diagnostic tests performed
3. Psychosocial/vocational evaluation: behavioral responses to pain, adjustments to impairment and disability, family and work history and dynamics
4. Past treatment: medical, surgical, and rehabilitative

Because rehabilitative pain management programs emphasize improving patient functioning rather than focus primarily on the relief of pain, functional evaluation, especially in activities of daily living (ADLs), household activities, vocational activities, and mobilization (sitting, standing, transferring, and ambulation), must be included in the comprehensive measurement of pain patients. Often the key question is how much a patient can do rather than how much it hurts.

Physical Examination

One should perform the initial comprehensive physical examination in a traditional manner with concentration on the musculoskeletal and neuromuscular systems and body mechanics. More thorough evaluation of other systems depends on the location of the pain (e.g., chest pain suggests cardiac evaluation).

Measurement of Pain and Its Effects

Although the measurement of induced acute pain is relatively easy and reproducible, the measurement of chronic pain is not. The measurement of chronic pain and its effect is in its infancy; there has been a proliferation of assessment instruments and methods that await further study, but none is universally accepted. Pain is a subjective phenomenon and it is not directly measurable. Hence, it is the effects of chronic pain that are measured. A combination of techniques is often needed to evaluate appropriately the chronic pain patient, including measures of self-reported pain, biomechanical, physiologic, psychologic/behavioral, functional, familial/social, and medical parameters. Some of these parameters are provided in Table 8.5, and Table 8.6 lists several accepted, published scales in use.

Diagnostic Tests

Diagnostic studies should be considered an extension of the clinical examination. It is inappropriate to repeat diagnostic studies previously performed satisfactorily, especially if there has been no significant change in the clinical examination. Studies should only be ordered if the diagnosis has not yet been established or if the results will change your treatment approach.

Classification of Patients

At the conclusion of the evaluation process it may be helpful to classify patients into categories based on their symptoms, objective findings, and psychosocial findings. This will have implications for the treatment approaches to be used. The Brena and Chapman Emory Pain Estimate Model attempts to achieve this concept. It has been modified with examples as shown in Table 8.7.

Table 8.5. Assessment Methods of the Effects of Chronic Pain

Subjective pain—whole body diagram[a]
Pain intensity rating scales[a]
Visual analogue scales[a]
General pain measurement (McGill Questionnaire)[a]
Biomechanical flexibility[a] (ROM measurements)
Endurance[a] (activity duration, such as walking; treadmill or ergometer testing)
Strength[a] (number of repetitions lifting a given weight; performance on Cybex or KinCom machine; static and dynamic body mechanics)
Physiologic—EMG muscle tension[a] (biofeedback)
Critical evoked potential
Autonomic responses
Oxygen consumption with exercise
Psychologic/behavioral—personality factors[a] [Minnesota Multiphasic Personality Inventory (MMPI)]
Mood (Beck Depression Inventory)
Frequency of "pain behaviors"
Stress management and coping skills[a]
"Meaning" of pain to patient/family[a]
Functional—basic ADL skills[a]
Housework
Yard work
"Up time" (activity diary)[a]: sitting, standing, walking, reclining, lying
Hobbies
Prevocational and/or vocational status
Familial/social—marital distress
Family distress
Social withdrawal
Contribution of family, social, and economic systems to maintaining pain behavior
Medical—patterns of medication usage[a]
Use of healthcare system
Effectiveness of therapies
Sleep patterns
Effects of other health problems

ADL, activity of daily living; EMG, electromyographic; ROM, range of motion.
[a]Measures used at Baylor College of Medicine.

Table 8.6.   Accepted Published Tests

Pain
McGill Pain Questionnaire[a]

Functional status
Sickness Impact Profile
Pain and Impairment Relationship Scale
Functional Assessment Screening Questionnaire

Psychologic status
Minnesota Multiphasic Personality Inventory (MMPI)
Back Depression Inventory

Several factors in single scale
Picaza Scale[a]
Hendler Screening Test for Chronic Back Pain Patients
Emory Pain Estimate Model

[a]Used at Baylor College of Medicine.

PAIN MANAGEMENT PROGRAMS

An example of an interdisciplinary comprehensive pain management program is outlined in Fig. 8-3. The program should be done in a day-hospital setting with weekly team conferences held to monitor progress, identify new problems, and modify the treatment plan as needed. Patients should be discharged from the program with 24-hours notice at any time if they are not benefiting from the program or cooperating with the program.

TREATMENT APPROACHES

By the time the patient with chronic pain is seen in a pain clinic, most traditional medical and surgical interventions have been attempted and have been unsuccessful. It is important not to repeat these treatments unless it is felt they have not been used properly or unless they may be beneficial when used in combination with other forms of treatment that could ultimately yield a better result. The cause of the chronic pain syndrome should be determined from a medical and psychosocial point of view and the location of "pain generator" should be noted. Attempts to decrease or eliminate the pain generator(s) are important and should be carried out first, followed by consideration of other treatment options. The goals in treating the patient with chronic pain are to modify medication, modulate the pain response, increase activity, restore physical functioning, and alleviate psychosocial and vocational dysfunction. Basically the techniques used should restore patient function to the highest level within the limits of the remaining pain or other physical limitations (Fig. 8-4). Treatment methods are usually employed in combination to achieve treatment goals. For example, remediation of sleep disturbance may require medication adjustment, psychologic techniques such as relaxation training or stress management, and an activity/physical restoration program. Treatment techniques should be integrated into a comprehensive treatment program and not used in isolation.

Table 8.7. Classification of the Patient with Chronic Nonmalignant Pain with Examples and Treatment Strategies

Class	Symptoms	Objective Findings	Psychosocial Components	Example	Treatment Strategies
IA	High	High correlation	High	Rheumatoid arthritis	Behavior modification approach with emphasis on medication and physical modalities
IB	High	High correlation	Low	Rheumatoid arthritis	Medication and modalities approach
IIA	High	Low correlation	High	Musculoskeletal/low back pain	Behavioral modification approach
IIB	High	Low correlation	Low	Musculoskeletal/low back pain	Physical modalities and exercise

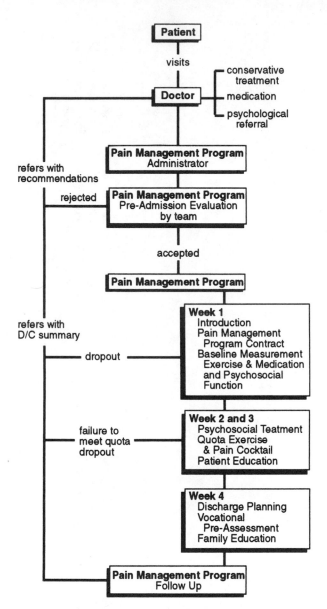

Fig. 8-3.   Structure of the Baylor College of Medicine Pain Management Program at the Methodist Hospital.

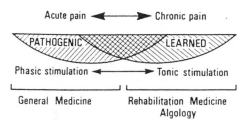

Fig. 8-4. **Nociceptive spectrum. (From Brena SF, Chapman SL. *Management of patients with chronic pain.* New York: SP Medical & Scientific Books, 1983, with permission.)**

Medication Management

Physicians have a long history of prescribing and chronic pain patients have a long history of using inappropriate medications, particularly narcotic medications. Studies show that patients are usually inadequately treated for acute pain syndromes and overtreated for chronic ones. In addition, some physicians mistakenly believe that giving medication on an as needed basis rather than on a scheduled dose basis results in less addiction. Physicians also tend to incorrectly label patients who respond to placebo as having a nonorganic type of pain. The philosophy of healthcare professionals regarding the use of opioid medication for treatment of chronic pain has gradually evolved over the years. At one time it was felt that patients with chronic noncancer pain should not be on opioid medication. However, with enlightened thinking and research, it is now felt that appropriate use of opioid medication can be a helpful strategy in some patients with chronic pain (Table 8.8). When the goal of pharmacologic management of a patient with chronic pain is to moderate or eliminate possible use of narcotics, tranquilizers, and hypnotic medications, it usually requires detoxification in an organized treatment program. No new narcotics, tranquilizers, or hypnotic drugs should be prescribed. Once the daily requirement for the patient is obtained over a few days, a "pain cocktail" approach is used on a time-contingent basis. The pain cocktail consists of methadone or a similar preparation of a dose equivalent to the currently used narcotic medication. It is mixed with a masking vehicle such as cherry syrup. The patient is fully informed in advanced that the drug will gradually be withdrawn but is not told the daily dose of the active ingredient. The cocktail is given at the dose and on the time schedule that the patient demonstrated in the daily requirement. Gradual reduction of the active ingredient with an equal increase in the masking vehicle is carried out over 3 to 6 weeks. Decrements are made slowly so as not to elicit withdrawal signs and symptoms. Eventually, the patient is receiving only the masking vehicle, and the cocktail is discontinued. The cocktail approach of gradual withdrawal can be used for tranquilizers and hypnotics as well as for narcotic medications (Table 8.9). Antidepressants, particularly the tricycle antidepressants, often offer a smoother treatment course for the patient with chronic pain. Correction of sleep disturbance and alleviation of depression may be accomplished with antidepressants

Table 8.8.   Narcotic Agonist Analgesics

Drug Equianalgesic Doses[a]	Intramuscular (mg)	Oral (mg)	Onset (minutes)	Peak (hours)	Duration (hours)	1/2 (hours)
Alfentanil	nd	na	immediate	nd	nd	1–2
Codeine	120	200	10–30	0.5–1	4–6	3
Fentanyl	0.1	na	7–8	nd	1–2	1.5–6
Hydrocodone	nd	nd	nd	nd	4–8	3.3–4.5
Hydromorphone	1.5	7.5	15–30	0.5–1	4–5	2–3
Levorphanol	2	4	30–90	0.5–1	6–8	12–16
Meperidine	75	300	10–45	0.5–1	2–4	3–4
Methadone	10	20	30–60	0.5–1	4–6	15–30
Morphine	10	60	15–60	0.5–1	3–7	1.5–2
Oxycodone (po)	na	30	15–30	1	4–6	nd
Oxymorphone	1	10	5–10	0.5–1	3–6	nd
Propoxyphene (po)	nd	130[b]/200	30–60	2–2.5	4–6	6–12
Sufentanil	0.02	na	1.3–3	nd	nd	2.5

nd, no data available; na, not applicable.
[a]Based on acute, short-term use. Chronic administration may alter pharmacokinetics and decrease the oral to parenteral dose ratio. The morphine oral to parenteral ratio decreases to 1.5–2.5:1 on chronic dosing.
After IV administration, peak effects may be more pronounced but duration is shorter. Duration of action may be longer with the oral route.
Rectal
Duration and half-life increase with repeated use due to cumulative effects.
Data based on intrathecal or epidural administration.
[*]HCl salt
Napsylate salt
Data based on IV administration.
From *Drug facts and comparisons*. St. Louis: Facts and Comparisons, Inc., 1993: 242a, with permission.

Table 8.9. Sample Pain Cocktail Regimen

Inpatient Days	Pain Cocktail Format
1–6 Baseline	Patient reports preadmission pattern of "one or two of the 50 mg tablets of Demerol two or three times a day, as needed, at home." Physician orders to nurse: "May have Demerol, prn pain, not to exceed three 50 mg tablets every 3 hours. Carefully record amount taken." Analysis of baseline data: Patient averaged 600 mg of Demerol per 24-hour period, averaging of 3- to 4-hour intervals between requests.
7–9 First cocktail	Prescription to pharmacists: Demerol, 1920 mg Bevisol, Plebex, or other liquid B complex, 12 ml; cherry syrup qs 240 ml Directions: Pain cocktail, 10 ml po q3h, day and night, not prn Nursing order: Pain cocktail, 10 ml po q3h, day and night, not prn Because contents of the pain cocktail are not on the label, a copy of the prescription must be kept in a separate pain cocktail book.
10–12	Decrease each daily total by 64 mg, 1/10 of original amount. A 3-day prescription is decreased by 64 × 3 or 192 mg. Prescription to pharmacists: Demerol, 1728 mg Bevisol, Plebex, or other liquid B complex, 12 ml; cherry syrup qs 240 ml Directions: Pain cocktail, 10 ml po q3h, day and night, not prn Nursing order: Pain cocktail, 10 ml po q3h, day and night, not prn
13–15	Prescription to pharmacists: Demerol, 1536 mg Bevisol, Plebex, or other liquid B complex, 12 ml; cherry syrup qs 240 ml Sig: Pain cocktail, 10 ml po q3h, day and night, not prn Nursing order: Pain cocktail, 10 ml po q3h, day and night, not prn
16–18	Prescription to pharmacists: Demerol, 1344 mg Bevisol, Plebex, or other liquid B complex, 12 ml; cherry syrup qs 240 ml Sig: Pain cocktail, 10 ml po q3h, day and night, not prn Nursing order: Pain cocktail, 10 ml po q3h, day and night, not prn

continued

Table 8.9.   *Continued*

Inpatient Days	Pain Cocktail Format

19–21	Prescription to pharmacists: Demerol, 1152 mg
	Bevisol, Plebex, or other liquid B complex,
	    12 ml; cherry syrup qs 240 ml
	Sig: Pain cocktail, 10 ml po q3h, day and
	    night, not prn
	Nursing order: Pain cocktail, 10 ml po q3h,
	    day and night, not prn

22–24	Prescription to pharmacists: Demerol 960 mg
	Bevisol, Plebex, or other liquid B complex,
	    12 ml; cherry syrup qs 240 ml
	Sig: Pain cocktail, 10 ml po q3h, day and
	    night, not prn
	Nursing order: Pain cocktail, 10 ml po q3h,
	    day and night, not prn

37–39	Prescription to pharmacists: Demerol 0 mg
	Bevisol, Plebex, or other liquid B complex,
	    12 ml; cherry syrup qs 240 ml
	Sig: Pain cocktail, 10 ml po q3h, day and
	    night, not prn
	Nursing order: Pain cocktail, 10 ml po q3h,
	    day and night, not prn (Maintain patient on
	    vehicle for 2 to 10 days, if all is going well,
	    inform patient and ask if continuation of ve-
	    hicle is desired.)

From Fordyce WE. *Behavioral methods for chronic pain and illness.*
St. Louis: CV Mosby, 1979, with permission.

in a single dose given at bedtime. Doxepin or amitriptyline (50 to 150 mg) can be used in doses smaller than those used to treat depression. Antidepressants, in addition, may act synergistically with some nonnarcotic analgesics and may enhance the effectiveness of physical modalities such as transcutaneous electrical nerve stimulation (TENS). Analgesia can be provided by nonsteroidal antiinflammatory drugs, acetaminophen, and occasionally muscle relaxants when used appropriately and should be used before narcotic medications are considered. The anticonvulsants carbamazepine, phenytoin, and valproic acid can also be effective in the treatment of neuropathic pain. Carbamazepine has been found to be useful in the treatment of trigeminal neuralgia, posttraumatic neuropathies, and phantom limb pain. Side effects that require routine monitoring with these medications include bone marrow suppression and hepatotoxicity.

Pain Modulation by Modalities

The complete eradication of chronic pain is rarely achieved and is not the goal of most interventions. The goal is the modification of pain to a more tolerable level. Pain modulation techniques often take advantage of the body's endogenous pain-modulating abilities first postulated and implied by the gate theory of pain of Melzack and Wall. Nonpharmacologic methods are usually adjunctive therapies and do not necessarily substitute for pharmacologic interventions. In the chronic pain population, optimal techniques are those that can be used by the patient in the home setting, are active rather than passive, and can be used for the shortest time possible or gradually weaned. Modalities should be used for the shortest time possible with gradual decreases in use as indicated. The physical modalities most used in treating chronic pain include heat, cold, biofeedback, and TENS. Modalities are used sparingly, and most have greater usefulness in acute and subacute pain conditions (Table 8.10). Occasionally they are used to treat acute pain superimposed on a chronic pain syndrome, particularly during the first week to help mobilize the chronic pain patient beginning the treatment program. Heat in the form of packs, pads, and whirlpool and cold in the form of ice packs are the most common modalities used to help treat pain. In the chronic pain patient, they may be employed before and after exercise, achieving their effects through their ability to modulate pain and promote muscle relaxation and sedation.

A trial of TENS is indicated in many neurogenic and musculoskeletal pain syndromes. Generally, it is found to be more effective in chronic pain patients without a history of significant surgical intervention and/or high narcotic use levels. The exact physiologic mechanism of TENS is not certain, but possibilities include the direct effects of stimulation of afferent nerves, modification of pain transmission at the level of the dorsal horn in the spinal cord, or the activation of supraspinal pain modulation centers mediated by endorphins. Before the rental or purchase of a TENS unit, a trial of therapy with appropriate positioning of electrodes and education in its use is indicated. Like most intervention techniques it has a significant placebo effect, and its effectiveness decreases significantly over time. Biofeedback can be used to provide instantaneous feedback to the patient with physiologic deficits such as muscle tension and skin temperature. Patients can then be taught to exert control over these and other functions mediated by both the somatic and autonomic nervous systems. In the patient with chronic pain it can be employed to facilitate relaxation, alleviate muscle tension and anxiety, demonstrate the role of the mind in modifying physical responses, and promote improved sleeping patterns. Although re-

Table 8.10.   Modalities Used in Chronic Pain

Nerve blocks
Trigger point injections
Spray and stretch techniques
Acupuncture
Hypnotherapy
Mobilization and manipulation
Surgical treatment

sults of treatment vary among individuals, the most successful responders seem to be patients with tension headaches, torticollis, musculoskeletal neck pain, and Raynaud's disease. Finally, patients must be educated in the management of the many controllable factors that can affect their pain level. These include, for example, the adverse effects of inactivity and deconditioning; poor body mechanics; the use of narcotics, sedatives, and tranquilizers; social withdrawal; inappropriate pacing of activities; and a host of others. It is particularly important to education patients regarding the nature of pain and the important differences in treatment between the approach to acute and chronic pain. Interventional procedures are an important component of the therapeutic armamentarium for chronic pain management. Some of these techniques play an especially important role when used as diagnostic procedures. Interventional procedures can be powerful tools when used and interpreted intelligently in the context of a multidisciplinary approach to chronic pain. They can also help prevent the development of chronic pain syndromes. The most commonly employed interventional techniques are listed in Table 8.11. Central and peripheral neuroaugmentation can be used in selected patients. Its mechanism of action is based on the notion that afferent input along low-threshold, large-diameter nerve fibers can exert a powerful inhibitory effect on nociceptive input conveyed along C fibers. This therapeutic modality may be indicated when other, more conservative measures have failed.

Exercise and Mobilization

One of the frequent components of the chronic pain syndrome is activity restriction resulting in deconditioning and the loss of strength and flexibility. There also may be significant abnormalities of static and dynamic posture and impaired biomechanics in sitting, standing, bending, and lifting. Exercises to strengthen and restore flexibility of specific muscle groups (e.g., Williams flexion exercises for the low back) and general conditioning exercises (e.g., cycling, walking, swimming) should be started at a low level and systematically increased to recondition the patient. As with the program of medication control, a behavior modification approach is used. The patient's level of activity and exercise is first determined over a few days. A goal is then set within the patient's ability and he or she is encouraged to achieve that level regardless of pain complaints. Every few days the goal is reset appropriately at a higher level (Fig. 8-5). Reinforcement is through daily positive feedback for accomplishing goals established. Patients are instructed in pacing themselves appropriately.

Psychosocial Intervention

Psychosocial issues relevant to the patient with chronic pain are identified through patient and family interviews, behavioral observation, and psychologic testing. Treatments used include group sessions, individual treatment, or behavioral interventions supported by the entire treatment team. Four problems requiring treatment are as follows:

1.   Pain behavior: chronic pain patients often are highly focused on their pain. Conversation may be dominated by references

Table 8.11. Commonly Used Interventional Treatments in Chronic Pain Syndrome

Treatments	Use/Comment
Nerve blocks	As diagnostic, prognostic, or therapeutic procedures
Diagnostic blocks	To ascertain source of pain, nerve pathway, or as tools for differential diagnosis
Prognostic blocks	Before neuroablative or neurolytic procedures to assess their possible effects
Therapeutic blocks	Can be performed with local anesthetics or with neurolytic agents
Trigger point injections	Treatment of myofascial pain
Facet or zygapophyseal blocks	Diagnostic or therapeutic
Epidural blocks	Useful especially when prolonged analgesia might be required for physical therapy, not for days but for weeks
Spinal blocks	Differential pain diagnosis
Neurolytic, epidural, and spinal techniques	Specific indications for the treatment of some intractable chronic pain syndromes
Sympathic nerve blocks	Effective therapeutic tools in dealing with sympathetically maintained pain
Chemoneurolysis Cryoneurolysis/ cryoanalgasia	Very effective in treatment of sympathetically maintained pain and cancer or noncancer chronic pain

to pain sensations, treatments, and pain-related physical limitations. Similarly, nonverbal behavior may be marked by grimaces, groans, limping, and so forth.

2. Depression: this is often present and may be reflected in mood, decreased libido, sleep disturbance, and social withdrawal. Grief about losses of physical abilities, social and family role, and previously enjoyed activities must be resolved. Antidepressants may be required in addition to psychologic therapies.

3. Stress: pain patients face multiple stressors, including pending litigation, uncertainty regarding the future of their economic and health status, and family or marital distress. Treatment may include training in stress management (e.g., relaxation techniques, problem solving) as well as marital, family, or vocational counseling.

4. Marital and family dysfunction: as time passes family members will alter their behavior in adapting to the chronic pain

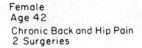

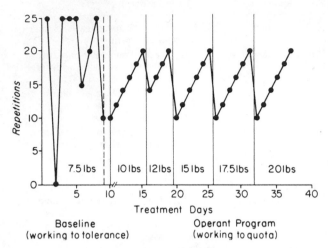

Fig. 8-5.   **Behavioral modification approach to exercise.** (From Fordyce WE. *Behavioral methods for chronic pain and illness.* St. Louis: Mosby, 1976:173, with permission.)

patient. Some of these adaptations may unwittingly contribute to the patient's pain behavior (e.g., giving attention to the patient's complaints, or taking over the patient's household duties when the pain is particularly bad). Enlistment of family cooperation in eliminating dysfunctional behavior patterns is essential in many cases.

Restoration of Functional Activity

Assessment of chronic pain patients' daily activities usually reveals multiple areas of deficits (Table 8.12). Remediation efforts involve the application of several key principles.

Activities to be worked on must be agreed on in advance. Patients will work best at activities that are important to them. Careful task analysis may reveal ways to simplify the activity, and principles of energy conservation and pacing should be observed. Physical activities require starting an exercise and activity program slowly and increasing the activity gradually (e.g., vacuuming initially may need to be done in 3-minute blocks). Activity diaries or other forms of monitoring progress can be used to help reinforce the activity program. Vocational counseling is an important component of the treatment program. Each patient should be evaluated to determine work history, educational background, vocational skills and abilities, and motivation to return to work. The vocational counselor can determine whether past work skills and current aptitudes can be transferred to alterna-

> ### Table 8.12. Typical Areas of Functional Activity Deficits in Chronic Pain Patients
>
> "Up time": excessive time spent in bed or reclining in chair or on sofa
> Upright sitting and standing tolerance
> Self-care: dressing, bathing, grooming
> Performance of household chores
> Performance of yard work
> Participation in avocational pursuits
> Task-oriented activities away from home: e.g., grocery shopping
> Activities away from home: social, family, community
> Vocational activities
> Driving

tive occupations if necessary. The vocational counselor can also work with the patient regarding legal rights and obligations for each state (e.g., worker's compensation) and help the patient set realistic vocational goals.

RESULTS

Several general and meta-analytic review articles have been published on the evaluation and treatment of chronic pain syndromes, as well as the efficacy of multidisciplinary pain treatment centers. Admittedly, there is no perfect study of multidisciplinary pain center treatment outcomes, but the data taken as an aggregate should not be summarily dismissed. Turk summarized the results of selected studies and reported the following facts about the efficacy of multidisciplinary pain centers:

1. Following treatment at a typical multidisciplinary pain center, the patient reported a reduction in pain ranging from 16% to 60%, which is comparable to the pain reduction reported following surgery. The pain reductions were reasonably maintained up to 5 years following treatment.
2. More than 65% of patients treated at multidisciplinary pain centers discontinued use of opioid medications and were still medication-free 1 year following discharge from the program. In contrast, patients not treated at such facilities reported an average reduction in medication of only 6% at 1 year following treatment.
3. On average, 65% of patients treated in multidisciplinary pain centers report increased activity at termination of treatment compared with 35% of patients not treated at these facilities.
4. The average return-to-work rate following treatment at multidisciplinary pain centers is 67% compared with 24% for patients not treated at those facilities. Approximately 43% more patients were working following treatment at multidisciplinary pain centers than before treatment.
5. Patients treated at multidisciplinary pain centers are three to six times less likely to be hospitalized later and have

significantly fewer surgeries for pain than those patients not treated at those facilities.

6. Studies that have investigated the closure rate of disability cases indicate that 64% to 89% of claims were settled by 3 months following discharge from multidisciplinary pain centers. This can be compared with 39% closure of claims following surgery.

7. Up to 86% of pending litigation cases have been reported as being resolved following treatment at a multidisciplinary pain center.

Outcome measurement for treatment of chronic pain can include use of medication, walking distance, strength, flexibility, setting tolerance, pain behaviors, vocational placement, and use of healthcare resources. The American Academy of Pain Medicine has developed an online computerized outcome program (digimed.com) to help demonstrate results of treatment by pain programs. When comparing one program with another, it is important to evaluate each program in terms of types of patients accepted, types of treatments offered, criteria for improvement, and follow-up time. Ideal pain rehabilitation candidates can achieve an 80% to 90% success rate. As the incidence of psychosocial problems and secondary gain issues increases, however, this rate drops to 40% to 50%. With major psychiatric or secondary gains, the success rate drops to 20% or less.

SUGGESTED READINGS

Arnoff GM. *Evaluation and treatment of chronic pain.* Baltimore: Williams & Wilkins, 1992.

Bloodworth D, Grabois M. Physical rehabilitation in chronic pain syndrome. In: Miller RD, ed. *Atlas of anesthesia,* vol VI, Pain management. Current Med, 1998;13.1–13.5.

Cutler RB, Fishbain DA, Rosomoff HL et al. Does nonsurgical pain center treatment of chronic pain return patients to work? *Spine* 1994;19:643–652.

Flor H, Fydrich T, Turk D. Efficacy of multidisciplinary pain treatment centers: a meta-analytic review. *Pain* 1992;49:221–230.

Grabois M, Garrison SJ, Hart KA et al, eds. *Physical medicine and rehabilitation: the complete approach.* Blackwell Science, 2000.

King J. Chronic pain. In: Grabois M, Garrison SJ, Hart KA et al, eds. *Physical medicine and rehabilitation: the complete approach.* Blackwell Science, 2000.

Melzack R. *Pain measurement and assessment.* New York: Raven Press, 1983.

Rueler J, Girard D, Nardone D. The chronic pain syndrome: misconceptions and management. *Ann Intern Med* 1980;93:588–596.

Sander SH, Rucker KS, Anderson KO et al. Clinical practice guidelines for chronic non-malignant pain syndrome patients. *J Back Musculoskel Rehab* 1995;5:15–120.

Tollison CD, Satterthwaite JR, Tollison JW. *Handbook of pain management.* Baltimore: Williams & Wilkins, 1994.

EMG

Jacqueline J. Wertsch and Gulapar Phongsamart

PRINCIPLES OF ELECTRODIAGNOSTIC MEDICINE

Electromyography (EMG) or electrodiagnostic medicine is the physiologic study of nerve and muscle. EMG evaluates the physiologic integrity of the peripheral nervous system and adds physiologic information to the history and physical examination. Electrodiagnostic medicine needs solid knowledge of musculoskeletal anatomy, nerve and muscle physiology, and kinesiology as well as technical knowledge of the instrumentation. We can use EMG as a tool to

- Help establish or narrow the differential diagnosis
- Help confirm the clinical diagnosis
- Provide additional physiologic details of severity, chronicity, and prognosis
- Follow the progression of disease
- Document improvement
- Perform research on physiology and kinesiology

Unlike radiologic studies that provide anatomic information, EMG provides physiologic information. Comparing the sensitivity of radiologic studies to the sensitivity of EMG is like comparing apples and oranges. Radiologic studies define the anatomy. EMG gives physiologic insight into the significance of the anatomic changes found. These diagnostic tests offer different points of view of the problem and are complementary. EMG may show physiologic changes even when no anatomic changes are seen. Signs and symptoms (pain, weakness, paresthesias) represent physiologic signals so the history and physical examination are critical in planning and interpreting the EMG examination.

Routine electrodiagnostic studies often consist of two main parts: nerve conduction studies (NCS) of the motor axons or sensory axons and needle EMG of skeletal muscles. Each part gives different information. It is not necessary to do both parts in all cases; what exact parts are done depends on the goals of the study. Clear goals based on the history and physical examination will lead to a clear, focused study plan. It is important to remember to gather information that might "prove you wrong" in addition to gathering information supportive of your clinical impression. For example, the history and physical examination may suggest carpal tunnel syndrome; however, it is still important to do some ulnar nerve studies to make sure that the abnormal median nerve studies do not simply represent a peripheral polyneuropathy.

BASICS OF INSTRUMENTATION

The core of an EMG machine is the differential amplifier that will show the difference between what is recorded at the E1 electrode (the so-called active) and what is recorded at the E2

Table 9.1.   Recording Parameters

	Low-Frequency Filter	High-Frequency Filter	Sweep Speed	Sensitivity
Sensory NCS	10 Hz	3 kHz	2 or 5 msec/div	10 or 20 μV/div
Motor NCS	3 Hz	10 kHz	2 or 5 msec/div	2 or 10 mV/div
Needle EMG	20 Hz	10 kHz	10 msec/div	50μV to 1mV/div
Single-fiber EMG	500–1,000 Hz	10–20 kHz	0.5–1 msec/div	200μV to 1mV/div

EMG, electromyogram; NCS, nerve conduction study.

electrode (the so-called indifferent). For EMG either a monopolar electrode (E1 is the needle, E2 is a disc on the skin) or a concentric (both E1 and E2 on the needle) electrode can be used. The most commonly used needle length is 37 mm, but 25-mm, 50-mm, and 75-mm needles are also available. The size or gauge of the needle must also be chosen; 28G or 26G are the most common. Numerous manuals exist offering details of electrode placement and stimulation sites for NCS. Table 9.1 gives typical recording parameters used during electrodiagnostic studies. Filter settings determine the frequency band of information that is allowed to pass or the "band pass." Both a high-frequency cutoff and a low-frequency cutoff must be chosen and can influence the information displayed on the screen in many ways (Table 9.2).

Table 9.2.   Effect of Changing Filters

	Onset Latency	Peak Latency	Amplitude	MUP Phases
Low-frequency Filter				
Increase	No effect	Decrease	Decrease	Increase
Decrease	No effect	Increase	Increase	Decrease
High-frequency Filter				
Increase	Decrease	Decrease	Increase	Increase
Decrease	Increase	Increase	Decrease	Decrease

MUP, motor unit potential.

NERVE CONDUCTION STUDIES (NCS)

NCS are based on the concept that once a nerve fiber reaches its threshold, there is propagation of an action potential along its length. NCS measure how long it takes for this impulse to travel a known distance. If the response is measured from another point along the nerve it is called a nerve action potential (NAP). This is most commonly done for sensory fibers and, therefore, called a sensory nerve action potential (SNAP). When motor nerve fibers are studied, the response is recorded from a muscle innervated by that nerve and called a compound muscle action potential (CMAP). Measurements that are routinely done include latency (either to onset or peak) and the amplitude of the response (baseline to peak or peak to peak). A conduction velocity can be calculated. Supramaximal stimulation is given to a nerve to make sure all axons are activated. Supramaximal stimulation is defined as 20% to 30% above the maximal intensity (the intensity at which the waveform stops growing in amplitude).

The optimal skin temperature for NCS should be at least 32°C for upper extremities and 30°C for lower extremities. As skin temperature drops, the CMAP amplitude increases and the CMAP latency and velocity prolong. Nerve conduction velocities in full-term infants are approximately one half of adult values. At age 5, nerve conduction velocities will be the same as normal adult then decline 1 to 2 m/second/decade.

NCS evaluate only part of the nerve fibers present in the peripheral nervous system. Nerve axons are divided into three major sizes: large myelinated A fibers (6 to 12 μm diameter), small myelinated B fibers (2 to 6 μm) and unmyelinated C fibers (0.2 to 2.0 μm). Routine NCS primarily evaluate the large myelinated fibers. Motor NCS evaluate A alpha fibers. Sensory NCS evaluate A alpha and A beta fibers. Therefore, NCS evaluate only a small component of the fibers in most nerves, which must be remembered during clinical interpretation of normal NCS.

Sensory NCS

A SNAP is the summated waveform recorded directly from the nerve. Onset latency reflects the interval between stimulation and the appearance of the SNAP (initial baseline deflection). In the past because of baseline noise, the peak latency was traditionally recorded. However, the peak latency does not measure the conduction time of the fastest conducting sensory axon. Therefore, it is recommended that both onset and peak latencies be recorded.

The amplitude of the SNAP is recorded from peak to peak. The amplitude of the SNAP reflects the cross-sectional density (not the number of axons) of the conducting sensory axons.

There are two ways to record SNAPs, orthodromically or antidromically. Orthodromic conduction is in the normally taken physiologic direction. Sensory information usually flows from the periphery to the spinal cord and central nervous system. An example of orthodromic sensory conduction would be stimulation of the sensory nerves on a finger and recording the SNAP over the median nerve at the wrist. Stimulation of the median nerve at the wrist and recording over the digital nerves on the fingers is in the opposite direction so is antidromic. The latency recording from orthodromic and antidromic studies at the same distance with the same E1-E2 interelectrode distance should be the same. The amplitude recording from an orthodromic study is about 25% to 35% smaller than that from the antidromic study.

The sensory neuron is in dorsal root ganglion. If the lesion is proximal to the sensory neuron (preganglionic lesion), the sensory neuron is not affected and its distal axon is still intact; therefore, sensory NCS will be normal even though clinical sensory may be abnormal. Examples of preganglionic lesions are radiculopathies, cauda equina lesions, and posterior column diseases. On the other hand, postganglionic lesions affect either sensory neuron or distal axon or both; therefore, sensory NCS will be abnormal. Examples of postganglionic lesions include plexopathy, CTS, ulnar neuropathy, peroneal neuropathy, and peripheral polyneuropathies.

Motor NCS

Most motor nerves are mixed nerves. For motor NCS the motor nerve action potential is recorded indirectly from muscle innervated by that nerve. The potential recorded from the muscle is the summation of action potentials recorded from many muscles and muscle fibers, called a CMAP or M wave. Traditionally, the CMAP onset latency reflects the arrival time at the muscle of the fastest conducting motor nerve fiber. This onset latency consists of latency of activation (0.1 msec), conduction time, and neuromuscular junction (NMJ) conduction (1.0 msec).

The CMAP amplitude is recorded from baseline to peak. The nerve conduction velocity (NCV) can be calculated by stimulating the nerve at two different points and then using the following formula:

NCV (m/sec) = distance ÷ latency difference (msec)

The CMAP onset latency and NCV provides information on the integrity of myelin sheath surrounding the nerve. Demyelinating disorders will result in prolonged latencies and slow conduction. The CMAP amplitude and morphology provides information on motor nerve axons. Axonal neuropathies will result in a decreased amplitude of the CMAP.

Late Responses

Late response is a broad term indicating a potential that has a longer latency than the M wave. The most commonly discussed late responses are the F wave, H wave, and the A wave (Table 9.3).

When a mixed nerve is stimulated in the arm or leg, the wave of depolarization spreads in both directions from the site of stim-

Table 9.3.   Late Responses

	H	F	A
Stimulation	Low	High	Low
Latency	Constant	Varies	Constant
Morphology	Constant	Varies	Constant
Size	Big	Small	Small

ulation. The wave of depolarization traveling to the motor neuron in the spinal cord will cause some (1% to 5%) of the motor neurons to backfire. The depolarization turns around and goes back down the axon, again resulting in a late response called the F wave because this was first recorded from foot muscles. Because only a small percentage of the motor neurons backfire each time, F waves are expected to have a small amplitude, varying morphology, and varying latency. Analysis of multiple sequential waves may be reported by minimum and maximal latencies, chronodispersion, and persistence. Large, persistent F waves have been noted in central nervous system disorders. F waves are useful to assess proximal conduction and may be the earliest finding in Guillain-Barré disease.

The H wave is widespread in infants until age 2 but can be recorded from only a few sites in adults. The H wave is comparable in latency and its presence is highly correlated with the Achilles reflex. It was initially described by Hoffman and named the H reflex by Magladery to honor Hoffman's work. The H wave comes in with low levels of stimulation and disappears with higher levels of stimulation. It has an amplitude and morphology similar to the M wave. The ratio of peak-to-peak maximum H to M (H/M) is a measure of motoneuron pool activation and excitability. H/M ratio for calf is normally less than 0.7. The H wave recorded from the soleus with tibial nerve stimulation has been described for evaluating S1 radiculopathies. Some authors have also described an H wave recorded from the flexor carpi radialis with median nerve stimulation. When two stimuli are given in a row, the amplitude of the second H wave will be smaller than the first. As the time between the stimuli is increased, there is a predictable change in the suppression of the second H amplitude that can be plotted as an H recovery curve. The H recovery curve and the H wave/CMAP amplitude (H/M ratio) have been used in physiologic studies of spasticity.

The A wave is seen when there is sprouting and axonal branching in a nerve axon. The A wave is also called an axon reflex. It will be small in amplitude and stable in morphology and latency. It can occur before or after the F wave. The A wave is created when a submaximal stimulus excites one branch of the axon but not the other and the antidromic impulse travels up to the branch point and turns around to travel distally along the second branch. With higher intensity stimulation the collateral branch will also be excited and the A wave will usually disappear because of collision. Proximal stimulation above the origin of the collateral sprout produces only an M response. Thus, a series of stimuli along the course of the nerve may localize the site of bifurcation. The A wave can be helpful in determining the site of focal nerve lesions.

Blink Reflex

The blink reflex is useful to evaluate cranial nerves V and VII and their connections in the pons and medulla. The blink reflex results from stimulation of the fifth cranial nerve and recording from muscles innervated by the seventh cranial nerve. It is easy to stimulate the supraorbital branch (ophthalmic division of the trigeminal nerve) above the medial eyebrow. Just like the clinical blink corneal reflex, this will elicit a bilateral blink (facial nerve motor efferent response). The facial nerve motor CMAP can be recorded

Table 9.4.   Blink Reflex

R1	R2	
−Ipsilateral	−Bilateral	
−11 msec	−Ipsilateral	31 msec
	−Contralateral	31 msec
−Pontine pathway	−Pons and medulla	
Bell's palsy		
−Abnormal R1 on affected side		
−Abnormal R2 on affected side regardless of stim side		
Trigeminal nerve problem		
−R1 abnormal on affected side		
−Both R2 ipsi & R2 contra abnormal when affected side stimulated		
Wallenberg syndrome		
−Affects lateral medulla		
−R1 normal		
−R2 abnormal		

Contra, contralateral; ipsi, ipsilateral; stim, stimulus.

from orbicularis oculi muscles. There is an ipsilateral early CMAP (R1 wave) and bilateral late CMAPs (R2 wave).

Repetitive Nerve Stimulation

Repetitive nerve stimulation is the technique of giving trains of supramaximal stimulations at a specific frequency (2 to 3 Hz) to a nerve while recording M waves from muscle innervated by that nerve. It is used primarily for evaluation of NMJ. Presynaptic and postsynaptic NMJ disorders will show different abnormal responses as noted in Table 9.5. Abnormal repetitive nerve stimulation is not a pathognomonic sign of NMJ disorders. Abnormal repetitive nerve stimulation can also be seen in many denervation disorders (e.g., amyotrophic lateral sclerosis), channelopathies, metabolic myopathies (e.g., McArdle's disease) and myotonic disorders.

NEEDLE EMG

A needle electrode inserted into a muscle can record the electrical activity generated by muscle fibers within that muscle. This electrode can detect changes in the electrical stability of the muscle membrane (such as those caused by neuropathic, myopathic, metabolic processes, or local trauma) and can also be used to examine the electrical properties of the muscle during voluntary contraction. The myotomal and peripheral nerve innervation pattern of abnormalities helps define the anatomic cause. Upper extremity and lower extremity myotomes and peripheral nerve supply are summarized in Tables 9.6 and 9.7.

The four major parts of the needle EMG examination are:

1. Insertional activity
2. Spontaneous potentials
3. Motor unit potential (MUP) morphology and stability
4. MUP recruitment

Table 9.5. Repetitive Nerve Stimulation

NMJ Disorders	Single Response	Repetitive 3Hz	Exercise	
			Immediate	After 2 Minutes
Normal	Normal CMAP	No change	No change	No change
MG	Normal CMAP	Decrement	Repaired decrement	Postactivation exhaustion
LEMS	Small CMAP	Decrement	Marked facilitation	Postactivation exhaustion
Botulism	Small CMAP	Decrement	Marked facilitation	Facilitation

CMAP, compound muscle action potential.

Table 9.6. Upper Extremity Muscles

Muscles	Roots	Nerves
Rhomboids	C5	Dorsal scapular
Supraspinatus	C5C6	Suprascapular
Infraspinatus	C5C6	Suprascapular
Deltoid	C5C6	Axillary
Biceps brachii	C5C6	Musculocutaneous
Brachioradialis	C5C6C7	Radial
Pronator teres	C6C7	Median
ECR	C6C7	Radial
FCR	C6C7C8	Median
Triceps (lateral head)	C6C7C8	Radial
Triceps (long head)	C7C8	Radial
FCU	C7C8	Ulnar
ECU	C7C8	PIN
EIP	C7C8	PIN
FPL	C8T1	Median
Intrinsic hand muscles	C8T1	Median/ulnar

Table 9.7. Lower Extremity Muscles

Muscles	Roots	Nerves
Iliopsoas	L2L3L4	Femoral
Adductor longus	L2L3L4	Obturator
Rectus femoris	L2L3L4	Femoral
VMO	L2L3L4	Femoral
Tibialis anterior	L4L5	Deep peroneal
Gluteus medius	L4L5S1	Superior gluteal
Semitendinosus/ membranosus	L4L5S1	Sciatic (tibial)
TFL	L5	Superior gluteal
Biceps femoris (long head)	L5S1	Sciatic (tibial)
Biceps femoris (short head)	L5S1	Sciatic (peroneal)
Tibialis posterior	L5S1	Tibial
Peroneus longus/brevis	L5S1	Superficial peroneal
EHL	L5S1	Deep peroneal
EDB	L5S1	Deep peroneal
Gluteus maximus	L5S1S2	Inferior gluteal
Gastrocnemius (lateral head)	L5S1S2	Tibial
Gastrocnemius (medial head)	L5S1S2	Tibial
FDIP	S1S2	Lateral plantar

The insertional activity and spontaneous activity gives information about the muscle cell membrane irritability. Analysis of the motor unit action potential morphology and stability will give information about primarily type I MUPs, which must be remembered when assessing for diseases that affect type II muscle fibers such as steroid myopathies. Motor unit recruitment is under central nervous system control but can reveal dropout of MUPs implying motor neuron cell and/or axon loss.

Insertional Activity

Inserting the needle electrode by very small increments into a resting muscle causes a burst of potentials referred to as insertional activity. In a normal muscle, the burst ceases the instant the insertion is stopped. If muscle fibers have abnormally increased membrane irritability, the potentials from these fibers may persist beyond the time during which the needle is being inserted and result in prolonged insertional activity. A common cause is a neuropathic condition, but many other types of disorders can also increase muscle membrane irritability including myopathic, inflammatory, local trauma, metabolic, and other conditions. Decreased insertional activity may be seen with loss of muscle fibers. Certainly, there can be loss of muscle fibers but the fibers remaining have increased muscle cell membrane irritability. There may be both decreased insertional activity and pockets of increased insertional activity.

Spontaneous Potentials

Normal muscle fibers at rest are electrically silent. With a pathologic condition, a muscle fiber might depolarize at rest with a resulting potential recorded by the needle and called a "spontaneous potential." Although numerous types of spontaneous potentials have been described, three types are most commonly encountered: fibs, positive waves, and fasciculation potentials. A fibrillation potential is the result of a spontaneous discharge of a single muscle fiber [spontaneous single fiber discharge (SSFD)]. Two forms are seen—spike potentials (sometimes referred to as fibs) and "positive waves." Grading of SSFDs is shown in Table 9.8. A fasciculation potential is the result of an involuntary spontaneous discharge of a single motor unit. This discharge can originate in the spinal cord or anywhere along the length of the motor axon. Fasciculation potentials look like MUPs but are differentiated by their firing patterns. Table 9.9 summarizes characteristics of spontaneous activities generated by different generators.

MUP Morphology and Stability

When an motor neuron in the brainstem or spinal cord is activated during voluntary or reflex muscle contraction, the wave of depolarization travels down its axon to excite, virtually simultaneously, all the muscle fibers supplied by that anterior horn cell. A needle electrode positioned in a muscle within that motor unit's territory will record the small potentials generated by muscle fibers that are within range of detection. However, because these muscle fibers discharge at approximately the same instant, they will be summated into a single larger waveform, the MUP. Every time the motor unit fires the MUP should look the same and,

Table 9.8.   Grading of SSFDs
(Positive Waves and Fibrillations)

Grade	Intensity
1 +	A few In 2 areas
2 +	Moderate number In 3 or more areas
3 +	Large number In all areas
4 +	Profuse, fill baseline Widespread, persistent In all areas

SSFDs, spontaneous single-fiber discharges.

Table 9.9. Spontaneous Potentials

Generator	Amplitude	Rate	Rhythm	Pathology
Arise from Single Muscle Cell				
End plate noise				
Miniature end plate potentials (MEPPs)	10–20 µVs	150–500 Hz	Irregular hissing	Normal
End plate spikes				
End plate potentials (EPPs)	100–300 µVs	50–100 Hz	Irregular sputtering	Normal
SSFDs				
Spike fibrillations (fibs)	15–1,000 µVs	0.5–10 Hz	Regular	Abnormal
Positive sharp wave (PSW)				
Myotonic discharge	20–200 µVs	20–80 Hz	Wax & wane in amplitude & rate	Abnormal
Arise from Motor Units				
Fasciculation potentials	Same as MUP	Variable	Irregular	Abnormal
Myokymic discharges	Same as MUP	Intraburst = 2–20 Hz Interburst = 1–5 Hz	Regular	Abnormal
Neuromyotoniac discharges	Same as MUP	150–300 Hz	Wane	Abnormal
Cramp	Same as MUP	Up to 150 Hz	Resembles interference pattern	Abnormal
Complex repetitive discharges (CRD)	Complex	50–100 Hz	Regular	Abnormal

MUP, motor unit potential; SSFDs, spontaneous single-fiber discharges.

therefore, be stable. Lack of MUP stability implies a pathologic condition. The amplitude and shape (or morphology) of a MUP is determined by the number and synchrony of the muscle fibers that are recorded. The MUP features that can be analyzed include amplitude, duration, complexity (phases, turns), and spectral content. If some muscle fibers are unable to discharge, the amplitude of the CMAP will be decreased and the smoothness of the waveform will be disrupted, resulting in a small, complex, or polyphasic MUP. Complex MUPs can be either myopathic or neuropathic and must be interpreted only with knowledge of all parts of the examination including MUP duration, recruitment, spontaneous activity, and the clinical examination. Small or large polyphasic MUPs of either short or long duration are seen in neuropathic disorders. These complex units may reflect either an evolving or healing process. If the small, complex polyphasic MUP has a short duration and is recruited out of proportion to the clinical muscle contraction, this may reflect a myopathic process. If a motor axon has reinnervated previously denervated muscle fibers belonging to another motor unit, initially the new branches are immature and slow so that the MUP may be increased in duration, small in amplitude, and polyphasic. With maturation, the MUP becomes shorter, larger, and less complex with old reinnervation giving large, even "giant" MUPs reflecting the fiber type grouping seen in neurogenic biopsies.

MUP analysis is playing an increasingly important part in the EMG examination and should be included in every study. The effect of needle type (monopolar or concentric) and filter settings chosen must be recognized in interpretation and use of reference values.

Motor Unit Recruitment

During voluntary muscle contraction, motor units are recruited in a very well-defined and unchanging order. The size principle of Henneman notes that the slow-firing, small, type I motor units are activated first, then subsequent motor units are recruited in order of increasing size. The initially recruited MUP starts firing at 5 to 7 Hz (onset frequency). The firing frequency of the initially recruited MUP will increase before the second MUP appears. The recruitment frequency, defined as the firing frequency of the first MUP when the second appears, is normally around 10 to 12 Hz (recruitment frequency). Thus, to increase the strength of a contraction, the motor units that are already activated will increase their firing rates before the next motor unit is recruited. This is referred to as temporal summation followed by spatial summation. Any process that prevents motor units from being activated, such as the loss of motor axons in a focal nerve lesion, disrupts this gradual progression from slower to faster firing frequencies, so that faster firing motor units are forced into service earlier than expected. Loss of these earlier MUPs, then, will result in increased onset and recruitment frequencies, which may be referred to as "dropout." For all muscle examined, onset frequency, recruitment frequency, and the recruitment ratio can be defined. The recruitment ratio should be about 5 and is calculated by the following equation:

Recruitment ratio = rate of fastest firing MUP ÷ number of MUPs
firing ≥ 5

CLINICAL APPLICATIONS

EMG/NCS studies are frequently ordered during workups of paresthesias, pain, or weakness. Common referrals include plexopathy, radiculopathy, focal entrapment neuropathies (CTS, ulnar, radial, peroneal, tarsal tunnel), motor neuron disease, peripheral polyneuropathy, or myopathy. There are numerous textbooks and manuals that detail the differential diagnosis, techniques, and reference values.

SUGGESTED READINGS

American Association of Electrodiagnostic Medicine. Mini monographs. Case reports and workshop handouts (available at www.aaem.net).

Brown WF, Bolton CF, ed. *Clinical electromyography.* Butterworth, 1993.

Buschbacher RM. *Manual of nerve conduction studies.* Demos Medical Publishing, 2000.

Campbell WC. *Essentials of electrodiagnostic medicine.* Williams & Wilkins, 1999.

DeLisa JA, Mackenzie K, Baran EM. *Manual of nerve conduction velocity and somatosensory evoked potentials,* 2nd ed. New York: Raven Press, 1987.

Dumitru D. *Electrodiagnostic medicine.* Hanley & Belfus, 1995.

Engel AG, Banker BQ. *Myology: basic and clinical.* McGraw-Hill, 1986.

Johnson EW, ed. *Practical electromyography,* 2nd ed. Baltimore: Williams & Wilkins, 1988.

Kimura J. *Electrodiagnosis in diseases of nerve and muscle: principles and practice.* FA Davis, 1989.

Lee HJ, DeLisa JA. *Surface anatomy for clinical needle electromyography.* Demos Medical Publishing, 2000.

Leis AA, Trapani VC. *Atlas of electromyography.* Oxford University Press, 2000.

Oh SJ. *Principles of clinical electromyography case studies.* Williams & Wilkins, 1998.

Preston DC, Shapiro BE. *Electromyography and neuromuscular disorders: clinical-electrophysiologic correlations.* Butterworth-Heinemann, 1998.

Spinner M. *Injuries to the major branches of peripheral nerves of the forearm.* Philadelphia: WB Saunders, 1978.

Sunderland S. *Nerve and nerve injuries.* Churchill Livingstone, 1978.

Geriatric Rehabilitation

Susan J. Garrison and Gerald Felsenthal

The goal of this chapter is to enable the resident at any level to formulate appropriate, individualized rehabilitative plans and goals for geriatric patients. After reading this chapter, the learner should be able to characterize various settings in which rehabilitative therapies may be delivered to a geriatric patient, including each setting's advantages and disadvantages; discuss motivation as applied to rehabilitative candidates; describe the concept of functional presentations of disease; and relate factors that influence the individualized rehabilitative plan for each of the following common geriatric rehabilitation diagnoses: hip fracture, osteoarthritis (OA), osteoporosis, stroke, and amputation.

DEFINITION

The population older than 65 years is generally considered to be the geriatric population. Medicare defines this as the age at which medical benefits are normally available. A special segment of the geriatric population older than the age of 85 is known as the old-old.

The difference in physiologic age compared with chronologic age may be amazing. A person may physically look and act much younger than his or her stated age. Of course, the opposite may be true. Also, from a psychologic perspective, people tend to become exaggerations of their adult selves as they age. Research has shown that people who live through their middle-age years without succumbing to major illness will live to be old. As one ages, however, chronic medical conditions accrue and may lead to functional impairment.

Candidates for any types of rehabilitative care should be physically well enough to participate in therapy sessions. If a patient cannot tolerate a rigorous program of 3 hours of therapy per day because of low endurance, the patient should be considered for admission to a skilled nursing facility (SNF; slower, not faster). Table 10.1 indicates settings for rehabilitative care.

Lack of motivation should never be used as a reason to exclude a person from therapies. The person is motivated to do something; however; it may simply be to stay in bed. Many older patients do not believe that they should exercise after a life of physical labor.

COMMON ISSUES

Functional decline is a common concept; as one ages, activities may be more difficult. This is particularly true for the elderly female, who may live up to a decade longer than her same-age spouse.

Besdine identified the concept of functional presentation of disease in the elderly. Whereas an adult may become acutely febrile in response to an acute infection, the elderly patient may become confused or begin falling rather than have a fever. Refer to Table 10.2.

Table 10.1.   Settings for Rehabilitative Therapies

Location	Advantages	Disadvantages
Acute care hospital	All patients eligible for therapies Therapy can be bedside or in department	Not a comprehensive rehabilitation team approach Lacks rehabilitation milieu No peer group Uses acute Medicare days
Acute inpatient rehabilitation, hospital-based or freestanding	Comprehensive team approach Therapeutic milieu Experienced nursing follow-through with activities Therapy can be bedside or in department	Not all patients are eligible for admission (must be able to participate in 3 hours of at least different therapies daily) Uses acute Medicare days Most expensive per day
Skilled Nursing Facility (SNF), hospital or nursing home based	Serves patients with both medical/surgical and/or PT, OT, or speech problems No requirement for 3 hours therapy per day Does not use acute Medicare hospital days Length of stay typically longer than acute rehabilitation Therapy can be bedside or in department	Sometimes less goal-oriented than acute rehabilitation Required by law to provide wheelchairs for use in the facility; patients cannot obtain their own until discharge Patients perceive a nursing home-like setting Nursing more likely to reinforce dependent patient behaviors Usual length of stay is 2–8 weeks
Long term acute care facility (LTAC), hospital-based or freestanding	Serves patients with both medical/surgical and/or PT, OT, or speech problems No requirement for 3 hours of therapy per day	Uses acute Medicare hospital days Usual length of stay is longer than SNF

continued

Table 10.1. *Continued*

Location	Advantages	Disadvantages
	Length of stay longer than SNF therapy can be bedside or in department	
Nursing home	Provides around-the-clock care Therapy available, but not required Therapy can be bedside or in department	Dependent role reinforced Patients become institutionalized Private pay or Medicaid
Home health care	Convenient Medicare and insurance allow Therapists can evaluate home setting for safety and support Eliminates transportation problems	Lacks equipment available in gym Only a certain number of visits allowed No peer group Family may interfere
Outpatient	Access to equipment and devices Covered by Medicare and most insurance Peer group More choices in locations, various therapists, and hours	Requires transportation

OT, occupational therapy; PT, physical therapy.
Adapted from Fox KM, Hawkes WG, Hebel JR, et al. Mobility after hip fracture predicts health outcomes. *J Am Geriatr Soc* 1998;46:169–173.

Cognitive performance in the geriatric population is another area of concern; most rehabilitation is based on the patient being able to learn compensatory skills for lost functional abilities. It is well known that standard rehabilitative techniques do not benefit severely demented patients. In fact, procedural memory, in which a person recalls and demonstrates physical abilities, may be of much more importance in geriatric rehabilitation than declarative memory, in which the person can recall therapists' names and list foods that were served at the last meal. Certainly, the effect of multiple medications, including those for pain, on cognitive performance should be considered in this population.

Table 10.2.   Functional Presentations of Disease

Stopping eating or drinking
Falling
Urinary incontinence
Dizziness
Acute confusion
New onset or worsening of dementia
Weight loss
Failure to thrive

Adapted from Besdine RW. The educational utility of comprehensive functional assessment in the elderly. *J Am Geriatr Soc* 1983;31:651–656.

Polypharmacy, the use of multiple medications, often results in compliance problems. Patients become confused over dose and scheduling and may forget to take their medications, causing potential adverse drug effects. The total number of medications should be from three to five. In addition, depending on financial status and insurance coverage, medications may represent a significant out of pocket expense. Refer to Table 10.3.

Appropriate nutrition is important because of the role it plays in maintaining good health and in allowing one to heal quickly from injuries as well as surgical procedures. The description "malnourished" can signify obesity as well as cachexia. Obesity creates problems with immobility and poor endurance because of the lack of conditioning. Those who are underweight are at risk for skin breakdown, low exercise tolerance, and peripheral edema because of low serum albumin levels. When referring to this population, the term *failure to thrive* describes a select group of patients who are near death.

Major muscle groups must be exercised to stay strong. This can be termed the disuse phenomenon, or "use it or lose it" concept. The geriatric patient must be encouraged to return to a routine home exercise program as soon as possible after it is interrupted by acute illness. Exercises should include strengthening, endurance, range of motion, and balance components. Each exercise program should be tailored for the individual.

Falls and subsequent injuries represent a threat to the functional abilities of this population. Typical reasons for falls include syncope, visual problems, peripheral vascular disease, poor balance, inappropriate footwear, and inappropriate use of gait devices. The use of sedative hypnotics in this age group has been shown to contribute directly to falls.

In today's world, virtually everyone works, including wives and daughters who once stayed at home and were available to care for elderly family members. Even if they live with younger relatives, elderly family members are sometimes left alone at home during the normal workday. Many adult women today find themselves providing care for elderly parents for a longer time than they spent caring for their children. Unfortunately, for some women

Table 10.3.   Steps to Writing Safer Medication Prescriptions for the Elderly

Action	Rationale
1. Start at two of the lowest recommended amounts and titrate up to the effect. Start low and go slow.	The response in the elderly is at a lower dosage than that required in the younger population.
2. Use a simple dosing regimen, with the fewest medications possible; encourage lifestyle modifications rather than drugs.	Noncompliance and the incidence of adverse drug reactions decreases with fewer doses of less medications.
3. Whenever adding a new medication or changing the dosing of a current one, make certain that the instructions are well understood.	Detailed information can assist in preventing problems.
4. Be aware of medication costs.	Patients are unlikely to be compliant with numerous expensive medications. They may continue to take a previously prescribed medication because it has already been purchased. Note: Medicare does not pay for medications.
5. Review patient medications, including over-the-counter drugs, periodically; eliminate those not being taken, attempt to keep the total number low. Dispose of them appropriately in your office.	This assists in preventing the possibility of drug-drug interactions, potentially reduces costs, and may prevent the accidental ingestion of medication. People are often hesitant to discard expensive medications, even when they are no longer using them. This also decreases the chances of sharing medications with another.
6. Create a written prescription record for the patient to keep in their possession.	Such a record is helpful to other physicians and pharmacists who may then review the list for possible drug problems. It is invaluable for the geriatric traveler and for ER visits.

continued

Table 10.3. *Continued*

Action	Rationale
7. Instruct home health nurses or aides to communicate directly with the physician about any medication problems.	The sooner a problem is recognized, the sooner action can be taken to correct the situation.

Adapted from Stein BE. Avoiding drug reactions: seven steps to writing safe prescriptions. *Geriatrics* 1994;49:28–36.

these care responsibilities exist simultaneously for many years. Refer to Table 10.4.

When providing care to a geriatric patient, be certain to talk directly to the patient whenever possible. Make certain that the individual's wants, needs, and goals are expressed to you. His or her input into the rehabilitation plan is essential for success. The presence of a third person in the room has been shown to diminish the amount of one-on-one interaction that the physician has with the patient.

Use of equipment can be troublesome; many elderly patients resist using gait devices or use inappropriate ones, such as "hand-me-down" canes and walkers. They may also request scooters or other types of electric mobility when standard wheelchairs are best. Remember that less is more. Too many adaptive devices may easily overwhelm people who are not "gadget tolerant." Interestingly, even though Medicare currently pays for ophthalmologic, dental, and auditory evaluations, it does not pay for corrective glasses, hearing aids, or dentures. Other areas of concern in this group include bracing, wheelchairs, gait devices, and environmental modifications such as the use of entrance ramps and grab bars in bathrooms.

TYPICAL GERIATRIC REHABILITATIVE DIAGNOSES, NEEDS, AND OUTCOMES

Hip Fracture

A hip fracture in this population is cause for concern; the mortality rate in the year following hip fracture ranges from 14% to 36%. An estimated 25% to 75% experience prolonged functional impairment following hip fracture. Four independent risk factors for nursing home residence 6 months after hip fracture include being single, incontinent, dependent in ambulation, and cognitively impaired. Poor balance following hip fracture is significantly associated with increased hospitalizations and mortality. The type of surgery, open reduction internal fixation as opposed to hemiarthroplasty or total joint replacement, is not a predictor of functional recovery following hip fracture. Refer to Chapter X.

Osteoarthritis (OA)

Tell your patients and their families that the medication you prescribe is for pain relief, not for the cure of OA. The drug of choice

Table 10.4. Housing Options for the Elderly

Site	Advantages	Disadvantages	Financial Implications
House or apartment	*most independent *private *personal belongings *familiar area *pets	*may not be accessible *lonely *upkeep *safety concerns	*mortgage or rent *utilities bills *paid care givers extra
with relatives	*comforts of home *probably familiar *access to kitchen *may have own room *companionship of siblings, children, or grandchildren *may have supervision	*not my home *may not be accessible *too much or too little activity *lack of privacy *implication of burden to family	*less expensive *paid care givers extra
personal care home	*allows some degree of independence *is a home setting *meals are prepared	*must live with strangers *must be able to take own medications *bathrooms shared	*one price for room and board *medication costs not included
assisted living	*allows some degree of independence	*must be able to ambulate to meals	*predominately private pay
nursing home	*typically long-term placement *structured setting *therapies available	*signals inability for self-care *institutional regimen	*private pay *Medicaid requires proof of indigence

for the treatment of OA is acetaminophen, up to 4,000 mg/24 hours. When this no longer provides relief, consider the use of nonsteroidal antiinflammatory drugs (NSAIDs). Various topical preparations, such as capsaicin and methyl salicylate may be helpful. Intraarticular joint injections of glucocorticoids should be limited to four. At that time, total joint replacement should be considered. Therapeutic modalities such as heat, cold, transcutaneous electrical nerve stimulation (TENS), and exercise may be helpful in pain management. Figure 10-1 details the management of OA in the geriatric patient.

Total Knee Replacement (TKR)

Indications for TKR in this population include varus angulation of greater than 10 degrees, ligamentous instability and any valgus deformity, or severe knee pain that is unrelieved by medications and back pain. The two postoperative TKR rehabilitation goals are to be able to ambulate household distances of 100 feet using a rolling walker, weight bearing as tolerated (WBAT) on the affected limb, and to achieve active range of motion (AROM) of the affected knee approaching full extension and 90 degrees of flexion, usually by postoperative days three to five.

Total Hip Replacement (THR)

THR is indicated in OA when nonsurgical strategies have failed to provide functional improvement and pain relief. Two thirds of THR patients are older 65 years at the time of surgery. Men who undergo THR are usually 65 to 74 years of age, whereas women are in the 75 to 84 year age range. Therefore, women typically have more advanced disease at the time of surgery. Postoperative THR rehabilitation involves teaching the patient independence in bed mobility and sit-to-stand and dressing while following hip precautions. These routinely include avoiding hip adduction, flexion, and internal rotation on the affected side following a posterior surgical approach. The patient also progressively ambulates to household distances WBAT on the affected limb using an assistive device such as a rolling walker. The geriatric patient is usually WBAT because the joint components are cemented into place. Other important aspects of rehabilitation include joint protection techniques, nutritional assessment, and instruction in a weight-reduction diet if the patient is significantly over ideal body weight. Resume any acetaminophen or NSAIDs that the patient was taking before surgery.

Osteoporosis

Osteoporosis is ubiquitous with aging. This discussion is limited to rehabilitation of the osteoporotic vertebral fracture. The onset is usually immediate after simple bending, twisting, or coughing. The rehabilitative problems include acute pain on movement with resultant immobility. This may progress to severe deconditioning and loss of functional ability.

Rehabilitation involves a gradual return to activities over time, as allowed by pain. These patients cannot tolerate trunk movement because of protective paravertebral muscular spasm. If the patient cannot participate in a rigorous inpatient rehabilitation program, he or she may be better served in a SNF, a long-term

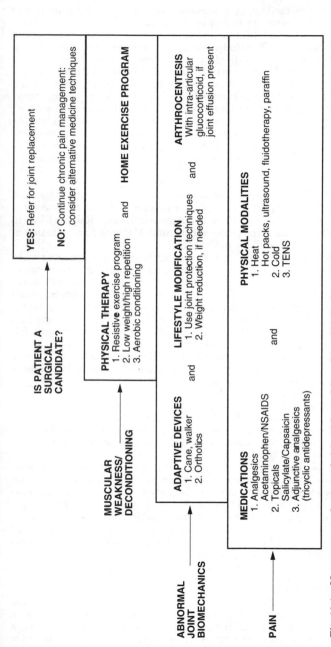

Fig. 10-1. Management of osteoarthritis. (Adapted from Ling SM, Bathon JM. Osteoarthritis in older adults. *J Am Geriatr Soc* 1998;46:222, with permission.)

acute care facility, or a nursing home temporarily if no one is available to care for him or her at home.

A typical rehabilitation program following an acute osteoporotic vertebral fracture includes bedrest in a position of comfort. Sitting should be limited to 10 minutes at a time for 7 to 10 days; time is added gradually as allowed by pain. Encourage as much ambulation as possible; for example, the patient should be up to the bathroom or bedside commode instead of using a bedpan. Treat localized paravertebral muscular spasm with local heat such as hot packs and ultrasound in addition to oral muscle relaxants (Flexeril), and TENS. Consider use of a thoracolumbar corset with rigid stays for support. Teach younger female family members that they may be at risk for the development of osteoporosis.

Stroke

Two thirds of the patients who sustain strokes are older than 65 years. The primary risk factor for stroke is age; the second is previous stroke. Age is not an outcome indicator. Rely on FIMs to predict the need and projected outcome of stroke rehabilitation in this population. Refer to Chapter 1.

Dynamic sitting balance, the ability to sit up unsupported without leaning back against something while using the upper limbs, is a good indication of the patient's ability to participate in an intensive stroke rehabilitation program. In stroke recovery, each patient follows an individual time line. Those who are slow remain slow, and those who regain abilities quickly do so quickly. Patients who do not recover dynamic sitting balance rapidly following stroke are not usually able to tolerate the intensive 3-hour therapy programs in acute care rehabilitation. Such patients may be better suited for a skilled nursing setting. Figure 10-2 details various locations for stroke rehabilitation therapies according to the individual patient's ability.

The goal of stroke rehabilitation is to teach compensatory skills to substitute for lost functional abilities, while natural muscular recovery occurs. The ability to learn is crucial in the stroke rehabilitation process. Identify cognitive strengths and weaknesses; then teach to the strengths.

Typically, unilateral hemispheric nonoperative stroke patients eventually regain some ability to ambulate, if they do not sustain a second stroke or die of some other cause first. Outpatient follow-up is important in this group; they may eventually be able to ambulate with additional inpatient rehabilitation several months following the acute stroke. They may also experience functional decline if they become medically ill; when stable, they may benefit from additional inpatient rehabilitative care to restore lost functional abilities. Refer to Chapter 19.

Amputation

In this population, amputation is usually a result of dysvascular problems, such as ischemia and diabetic or hypertensive neuropathy or a combination of the two. Whereas in the past a gangrenous leg often required transfemoral amputation in order for healing to occur, transtibial amputation is now the most common level as a result of revascularization techniques. Preservation

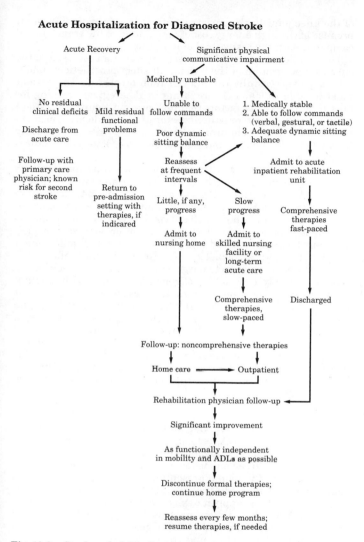

Fig. 10-2. Stroke rehabilitation decision tree.

of the knee joint in the geriatric patient is extremely important because of the high energy cost of ambulation of the transfemoral compared with the transtibial amputation.

The emotional effect of limb loss, the grieving process, and the cultural background of the patient all effect prosthetic rehabilitation. To successfully use a lower limb prosthesis, the patient must be able to learn. There is minimal caregiver training for prosthetic use. Other factors that may prevent a geriatric patient from participating in prosthetic restoration include previous neurologic deficits; poor endurance, longstanding, without possibility for much improvement; and significant hip or knee contractures of either leg.

The geriatric patient with an amputation must have enough upper limb strength to push up from a chair and must be able to bear weight on the remaining lower limb. Specific modifications in the prosthesis that provide more stability during ambulation include suspension methods, safety-type joints, and energy-storing feet. Some patients, particularly women who do not meet the qualifications for fabrication of a functional prosthesis, may benefit emotionally from a cosmetic lower limb. The limb allows the wearer to appear to have two legs while seated in a wheelchair.

Approximately 15% to 20% of geriatric patients with amputations will experience contralateral limb loss within 2 years. Four years after initial amputation, this number climbs to 40%. Despite limb revascularization techniques, this risk has not decreased over the past 20 to 30 years. It is, therefore, imperative to protect the remaining limb through meticulous foot care, use of an appropriate shoe, and maintenance of joint AROM and muscular strength. To decrease the risk of injury to the remaining limb before prosthetic restoration, limit hopping to room-to-room distances of less than 30 feet.

SUMMARY

The main rehabilitative diagnoses for the geriatric population include hip fracture, OA, osteoporosis, stroke, and amputation. These diagnoses may exist simultaneously. Individualize your rehabilitative plan to encompass comorbidities. Always consider the possibility of the functional presentation of disease. Consider the patient's desires first. Minimize equipment. Remember the use it or lose it concept and apply it to physical functioning, exercise, and cognition. When these issues are considered, clinical experiences in providing rehabilitative care to the geriatric population can be less complicated, more fun, and greatly rewarding.

SUGGESTED READINGS

Fried LP, Guralnik JM. Disability in older adults: evidence regarding significance, etiology, and risk. *J Am Geriatr Soc* 1997;45:92–100.

Garrison SJ. Geriatric stroke rehabilitation. In: Felsenthal G, Garrison SJ, Steinberg FU, eds. *Rehabilitation of the aging and elderly patient.* Baltimore: Williams & Wilkins, 1994:175–186.

Garrison SJ. Geriatric rehabilitation: caring for the aged. In: Grabois M, Garrison SJ, Hart KA et al, eds. *Physical medicine and rehabilitation: the complete approach.* Cambridge, MA: Blackwell Science, 2000:96:1788–1805.

Greene MG, Majerovitz SD, Adelman RD et al. The effects of the presence of a third person on the physician-older patient medical interview. *J Am Geriatr Soc* 1994;42:413–419.

Hanlon JT, Schmader KE, Koronkowski MJ et al. Adverse drug events in high risk older outpatients. *J Am Geriatr Soc* 1997;45:945–948.

Hesse KA, Campion EW. Motivating the geriatric patient for rehabilitation. *J Am Geriatr Soc* 1983;31:586–589.

Kane RA, Caplan AL, Urv-Wong EK et al. Everyday matters in the lives of nursing home residents: wish for and perception of choice and control. *J Am Geriatr Soc* 1997;45:1086–1093.

Ling SM, Bathon JM. Osteoarthritis in older adults. *J Am Geriatr Soc* 1998;46:216–225.

Norton R, Campbell AJ, Lee-Joe T et al. Circumstances of falls resulting in hip fractures among older people. *J Am Geriatr Soc* 1997;45:1108–1112.

Rantanen T, Era P, Heiikkinen E. Physical activity and the changes in maximal isometric strength in men and women from the age of 75 to 80 years. *J Am Geriatr Soc* 1997;45:1439–1445.

Sforzo GA, McManis BG, Black D et al. Resilience to exercise detraining in healthy older adults. *J Am Geriatr Soc* 1995;43:209–215.

Zorowitz RD, Adamovich BB. Assessment of communication. In: Grabois M, Garrison SJ, Hart KA et al, eds. *Physical medicine and rehabilitation: the complete approach.* Cambridge, MA: Blackwell Science, 2000.

Immobilization

Andy S. Chan and Carlos Vallbona

DEFINITION

Immobilization is defined as physical restriction or limitation of the body or its limbs. This may result from any of the following:

- Neuromusculoskeletal disorders and injuries, such as paralysis
- Orthopedic casts, body jackets, and splints
- Critical illness requiring bedrest
- Medical or caregiver neglect
- Prolonged stay in a reduced gravity position, such as sitting or recumbency
- Weightlessness in space, where movements are not restricted but occur without counteracting forces of gravity

Prolonged bedrest and inactivity reduce general metabolic activity. This results in decreased functional capacity of multiple body systems with clinical manifestations of immobilization syndrome. The metabolic consequences are independent of the cause for which immobilization might be prescribed. They are seen both in healthy volunteers and in patients with neuromusculoskeletal problems. The outcome, however, depends on the degree and duration of immobilization. After space flights, astronauts demonstrate a decrease in muscle strength, with individual variations. In a patient who has a neurologic or musculoskeletal deficit, the effects of immobilization result in further reduction of functional capacity. This causes severe disability. It takes longer to restore these patients to their maximal functional potential. In general, it will take at least as long to recover as it took to become deconditioned despite participation in a maximal strengthening program. In many cases, it will take twice as long or longer to recover to the previous baseline. Recovery of strength occurs much more slowly than loss of strength.

Awareness of the deleterious effects of prolonged bedrest allows for judicious planning of physical activities, exercise, and rest, thereby preventing immobilization syndrome. The clinical manifestations of immobilization are summarized in Table 11.1. Some are self-explanatory. Others are described later because they influence patient management. Rehabilitation measures to counteract or prevent disability resulting from immobilization are described at the end of each section.

DELETERIOUS EFFECTS OF PROLONGED IMMOBILIZATION

Musculoskeletal System

Strength

The scientific literature suggests that, with total immobility, strength gradually decreases by 0.7% to 1.5 % per day to a maximum of a 25% to 40% decrease in overall strength. The decrease

Table 11.1. The Immobilization Syndrome: Clinical Manifestations

Central nervous system
Altered sensation
Decreased motor activity
Autonomic lability
Emotional and behavioral disturbances
Intellectual deficit

Muscular system
Decreased muscle strength
Decreased endurance
Muscle atrophy
Poor coordination

Skeletal system
Osteoporosis
Atrophy of articular cartilage
Decrease in tendon/ligament strength
Fibrosis and ankylosis of joints

Cardiovascular system
Increased heart rate (adrenergic state)
Decreased cardiac reserve
Orthostatic hypotension
Phlebothrombosis

Respiratory system
Decreased vital capacity (restrictive impairment)
Decreased maximal voluntary ventilation (restrictive impairment)
Regional changes in ventilation/perfusion
Impairment of coughing mechanism

Digestive system
Anorexia
Constipation
GERD

Endocrine and renal effects
Increased diuresis and extracellular fluid shifts
Decreased sensitivity to insulin
Increased natriuresis
Hypercalciuria
Electrolyte imbalances
Renal lithiasis

Integumentary system
Atrophy of the skin
Pressure ulcers

GERD, gastroesophageal reflux disease.

appears to be greatest after the first week. Furthermore, different muscle groups show a variable decrease in strength. The antigravity muscles and larger muscles, particularly those in the lower limbs, lose strength disproportionally. Interestingly, in as little as 24 hours of immobilization, muscle fiber atrophy has been demonstrated in animal studies. Disuse atrophy has also been reported to start in as little as 4 hours of immobilization.

Muscle atrophy is dependent on the degree and the cause of inactivity and disuse. In the case of lower motor neuron dysfunction with chronic irreversible flaccid paralysis, muscle bulk is reduced by 90% to 95%. In upper motor neuron disease with resulting spasticity, muscle bulk decreases by only 30% to 35% because the increased tone actually prevents complete atrophy. The atrophy involves both Type I and II fibers, but Type I fibers are predominantly involved in immobilization atrophy. If recovery does not occur, muscle fibers are replaced by connective tissue. This process of collagen reorganization may begin after as little as 1 week of immobilization and will predispose to contracture formation. Positioning also plays an important role. Muscles, which are immobilized in a shortened position, will also be predisposed to a more rapid decline.

Endurance

The decrease in strength and concomitant effects of immobilization on the cardiovascular system results in decreased endurance.

Joints

Immobilization also affects the joints. The hyaline cartilage in joints receives its nutrition through the influx and efflux of synovial fluid caused by joint loading and unloading. During immobilization, this process stops. The hyaline cartilage is then dependent on simple diffusion to obtain nutrients. Unfortunately, the needs of the cartilage exceed the capacity of simple diffusion. Although qualitative data is not available at this time regarding the extent of articular changes in humans, studies in immobilized animals indicate a decrease in overall thickness of articular cartilage of 9% after 11 weeks.

Contracture is a loss of range of motion (ROM) in a joint. It may result from several causes, such as tightness of connective tissue, muscle, and joint capsule, as well as a joint disorder. However, in an immobilized person, mechanical factors are most important. If a muscle is chronically maintained in a shortened position, the muscle fibers and connective tissue adapt to the shortened length, causing contracture on the relaxed side of the joint. A muscle held in shortened position for only 5 to 7 days will demonstrate shortening of the muscle belly because of contraction of collagen fibers and decrease in muscle fiber sarcomeres. If this position continues for 3 weeks or more, the loose connective tissue in muscles and around joints will gradually change into dense connective tissue, causing contracture.

Contributing factors, such as edema, hemorrhage, spasticity, paralysis, pain, muscle imbalance, soft tissue injury, and advanced age, compound and enhance formation of contractures. Muscle imbalance is the most important contributing factor. In the immobile patient, lower limb contractures are most common, usually involving the hips, knees, and ankles (two-joint muscles). In the upper limbs, the wrists, shoulders, and elbows are at risk. Similar pathophysiologic changes may occur in the joints of the spine, especially in the cervical and lumbar regions. Development of contractures is one of the most severe, yet in most cases preventable, disabilities that result from immobilization. Contractures have a major influence on the functional outcome of rehabilitation. Be aware. Anticipate and take measures to prevent contractures. Prevention is preferable to treatment, and is much more cost effective.

Osteoporosis

The stimulus of weight bearing, gravity, and muscle activity on bone mass maintains the balance between bone formation and resorption. Several enzymatic factors also play a part. Prolonged bedrest leads to bone atrophy that involves both organic and inorganic bone components. Increased urinary excretion of calcium and hydroxyproline as well as increased excretion of calcium in stool result in a decrease in total bone mass, especially from the weight-bearing bones. In contrast to senile osteoporosis that develops from the marrow outward, immobilization osteoporosis is more marked in the subperiosteal region. In addition, disuse osteoporosis is most apparent in cancellous bone at the metaphysis and epiphysis and later extends to the entire diaphysis.

Up to a 1% loss of vertebral mineral content may occur per week of immobilization. After 12 weeks of bedrest, bone density is reduced by 40% to 45% and by 50% by the 30th week. Osteoporosis may lead to compression fractures of vertebral bodies and weight-bearing long bones with minor trauma, as well as predisposing the patient to wrist and hip fractures. Incidentally, osteoporosis may not be evident initially on plain x-ray films and may require more specialized techniques such as DEXA for quantification and diagnosis.

Neurologic System

Although immobilization does not directly affect the neurologic system, disorders of coordination, balance, and affect may occur. In a patient who has a central nervous system (CNS) lesion causing incoordination, the effects of immobilization can make it appear worse. Focal compression neuropathies are another common complication. These are most often secondary to positioning, such as foot drop from peroneal nerve compression.

Cardiovascular System

Effects of immobility include increased sympathetic tone (adrenergic state), increased heart rate, decreased cardiac efficiency, postural hypotension, and phlebothrombosis. Heart rate increases one beat per minute per 2 days of bedrest in healthy volunteers. Blood volume decreases by 7%. Maximum oxygen uptake (VO_2 max) decreases 27% after 20 days of bedrest. Although initially the hematocrit is noted to rise because of the loss of plasma volume, after 2 to 4 weeks an anemia will develop. The combined effect of these factors is a reduction in cardiac efficiency and intolerance to upright posture, resulting in dizziness or faintness on attempting to stand. Most of these effects can be noted to occur during the first

4 to 7 days of bedrest. Note, however, that cardiac output, total peripheral resistance, maximum heart rate, and resting systolic and mean blood pressure are not affected. There is also no change in oxygen uptake at rest.

Phlebothrombosis, also known as deep venous thrombosis (DVT), is a known risk. Lymphatic and venous stasis occurs in the lower limbs resulting from a lack of calf muscle pumping action. Other contributing factors usually associated with immobility include paralysis, postsurgical state, congestive heart failure, obesity, advanced age, hypercoagulable state, and dehydration. All increase the risk of phlebothrombosis, and pulmonary embolus as a hypercoagulable state may result from these pathophysiologic changes.

Respiratory System

Bedrest causes mechanical restrictive impairment as a result of decreased overall strength and a reduction of intercostal, diaphragmatic, and abdominal muscle excursion in supine breathing. The costovertebral and costochondral joints and the abdominal muscles may become fixed in an expiratory position, further reducing maximal inspiration. This results in a decrease in vital and functional respiratory capacities causing regional differences in ventilation/perfusion ratio, poorly ventilated as well as overly perfused areas, and arteriovenous shunts. If increased metabolic demand occurs, hypoxia results. Mucociliary function is also impaired. Mucus secretions accumulate in the dependent respiratory bronchioli, leading to atelectasis and hypostatic pneumonia.

Digestive System

Anorexia, gastroesophageal reflux disease (GERD), and constipation are the result of decreased metabolic demand, endocrine changes, and decreased gastric and intestinal motility.

Metabolic Effects

Marked hypercalcemia may occur several weeks after immobilization with a peak at 2 to 4 weeks. This is most often seen in young adult men after trauma. It is associated with hypercalcemic metabolic alkalosis and may lead to renal failure and ectopic calcification. It manifests clinically as headache, nausea, vomiting, anorexia, abdominal pain, lethargy, constipation, and weakness. Other circulating chemicals affected by immobilization include nitrogen, phosphorus, sulfur, sodium, potassium, magnesium, zinc, and chloride.

Renal System

Renal function demonstrates a decrease in the glomerular filtration rate, the ability to concentrate urine, and increased excretion of phosphorous.

Skin

Skin atrophy results from inadequate nutrition. Pressure ulcers, a dreaded complication of immobility, are better prevented than treated. They occur over bony prominences such as the sacrum, ischium, trochanter, and heel. They result from prolonged pressure causing ischemic necrosis of soft tissue overlying the bony prominences. A Stage I pressure ulcer may begin in as little as 2 hours. Edema, malnutrition, anemia, hypoalbuminemia, and paralysis are contributing factors.

MANAGEMENT OF COMPLICATIONS

The best management of immobility is prevention. When this is not possible, the following management of potential complications is indicated.

Musculoskeletal System

Physical therapy should begin at bedside and progress to the therapy department emphasizing progressive mobilization. Isometric, isotonic, and aerobic exercises may be used singly or in combination. It is noted that overly strenuous exercise of atrophic muscle may result in muscle damage. Passive range of motion (PROM) and subsequently active assistive range of motion (AAROM) and active range of motion (AROM) of all major joints is necessary, at least once to twice daily. Stretching of the muscles delays atrophy. Indeed, even immobilization of a muscle in a stretched position appears to decrease the amount of resulting atrophy. Modalities, such as heat, may be used before ROM for maximum benefit. Botulism toxin, motor point blocks, or nerve blocks may also be used to correct muscle strength imbalances. These interventions will allow for greater ROM than previously possible provided that a fixed contracture has not already formed. In more severe cases of contracture, serial casting and ultimately surgical intervention may be necessary.

Positioning of the patient in bed is extremely important. In the supine position, the trunk should align with the hips, knees, and ankles in a neutral position with the toes pointing toward the ceiling. The shoulders should be in 30 degrees of flexion and 45 degrees of abduction, the wrists in 20 to 30 degrees extension, and the hands in the functional position. This can easily be achieved with the use of pillows, trochanter rolls, or resting splints. Refer to Fig. 11-1. A prone position or side-lying position may also be used. Position changes every 2 hours may be necessary in quadriplegic patients with insensate skin and in comatose patients. (Refer to Chapter 15.)

Osteoporosis can only be prevented by weight bearing. Use a standing frame or tilt table with patients who are unable to stand unsupported. Begin a general endurance program, including strengthening and coordination exercises. Encourage functional activities if the patient is able to cooperate. Refer to Chapter 12.

Neurologic System

Teach independence in transfers and wheelchair propulsion to patients who are not ambulatory. Make a referral to occupational therapy for activities of daily living (ADLs), application of splints, and upper limb care. Avoid sensory deprivation. Encourage the patient to interact with staff, other patients, and family members. Order recreational therapy for psychosocial integration, resocialization, and adjustment to independent functioning.

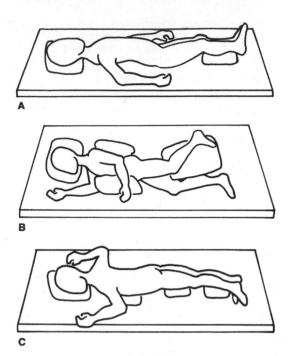

Fig. 11-1.   Appropriate bed positioning. A: Supine: elevate the calves to remove pressure from the heels. B: Side-lying: decrease trochanteric pressure by positioning the legs as shown. C: Prone: provide pressure release for the iliac crests and knees by using the illustrated arrangement of pillows or foam. (From Donovan WH et al. Pressure ulcers. In: DeLisa JA, et al., eds. *Rehabilitation medicine,* 2nd ed. Philadelphia: JB Lippincott, 1993:726, with permission.)

Cardiovascular System

Early mobilization is encouraged. However, if this is not a possibility, sit the patient in a chair. In addition, isometric exercises have been shown to be effective. Supine exercises have not been found to be effective. In severe cases of orthostasis, tilt-table conditioning should begin as soon as the patient is stable, beginning at a 30-degree tilt for 1 minute. Gradually increase the tilt 10 degrees every 3 to 5 days or earlier as tolerated, until the patient is able to tolerate a 70-degree tilt for 30 minutes. Then progress to standing and, finally, ambulation. Refer to Chapter 7.

Prevention is first line treatment for phlebothrombosis. Use knee or thigh-high elastic stockings or elastic wraps in all bedridden patients. Consider the use of external intermittent compression of the lower limbs. Low molecular weight heparin, low-dose heparin, or oral anticoagulation may be indicated in patients at high risk for venous thrombosis.

Respiratory System

Chest physical therapy with deep breathing exercises, incentive spirometer, assisted coughing, and/or chest percussion may be indicated, depending on the patient's needs. See Chapter 16.

Digestive System

Prescribe a stool softener and/or dietary fiber supplement to prevent constipation. Review the medication list. Try to eliminate or change drugs that may adversely affect motility such as narcotics, anticholinergics, and so forth. Ask the patient. Keep track of bowel movements as part of the daily routine.

Metabolic Effects

Isometric and isotonic exercise have been shown to increase peripheral sensitivity to insulin, particularly in the noninsulin-dependent diabetic patient. Monitor electrolytes and correct as necessary.

Renal System

If difficulties with voiding arise, manage the bladder with an external catheter or intermittent catheterization, depending on the patient's needs.

Skin

Accurate assessment of bed mobility is critical, especially in insensate patients. Interventions may include specialty mattresses, manually turning the patient, prefabricated ankle-foot orthoses, and other pressure relieving devices/splints, as well as careful attention to areas prone to breakdown. Adequate nutrition and proper hydration are essential. Prealbumin level is a marker of current nutritional status. Bear in mind that even a grossly obese patient may be malnourished.

CONCLUSION

Immobilization affects multiple systems. The effects of immobilization may occur within a few hours of onset. Prevention of complications is key; recovery may require a prolonged period of time. Even partial immobilization can have bad effects. Proper positioning and early mobilization including ROM, sitting, isometric, isotonic, and aerobic exercises are useful in preventing complications. All interventions are not necessary in all patients. In addition, other management may be indicated in specific patients. Interventions should be individualized. For example, in spastic patients, a more aggressive ROM exercise three to four times per day may be necessary, along with management of spasticity. Bed positioning changes may not be feasible in some patients; special beds may be necessary. Refer to Chapter 15.

In some cases, bedrest is necessary for a short period, such as after acute myocardial infarction, cardiac dysrhythmia, or septic shock. Evaluate your patient from a rehabilitation standpoint, but obtain agreement from the referring physician before initiating an aggressive mobilization program. Problems related to immobility can, and should, be prevented.

SUGGESTED READINGS

Buschbacher R, Porter D. Deconditioning, conditioning, and the benefits of exercise. In: Braddom R, Buschbacher R, Dumitru D et al, eds. *Physical medicine and rehabilitation,* 2nd ed. Philadelphia: WB Saunders, 2000:702–726.

Cardenas DD, Stolov WC, Hardy R. Muscle fibers numbers in immobilization atrophy. *Arch Phys Med Rehabil* 1977;58:423–426.

Dietrick JE, Whedon GD, Shorr E. The effects of immobilization upon various metabolic and physiologic functions of normal man. *Am J Med* 1948;4:3–36.

Fournier A, Goldberg M, Green B et al. A medical evaluation of the effects of computer-assisted muscle stimulation in paraplegic patients. *Orthopedics* 1989;7:1129–1139.

Haler EM, Bell KR. Contracture and other deleterious effects of immobility. In: DeLisa JA, ed. *Rehabilitation medicine: principles and practice.* Philadelphia: JB Lippincott, 1988:448–462.

Kasper CE, Talbot LA, Gaines JM. Skeletal muscle damage and recovery. *AACN Clin Issues* 2002;13:237–247.

Kottke FJ. The effects of limitation of activity upon the human body. *JAMA* 1966;196:117–122.

Muller EA. Influence of training and inactivity on muscle strength. *Arch Phys Med Rehabil* 1970;51:449–462.

Nicogossian AE. Overall physiologic response to space flight. In: Nicogossian AE, ed. *Space physiology and medicine,* 2nd ed. London: Lea & Febiger, 1989:139–153.

Sliwa J. Acute weakness syndromes in the critically ill patient. *Arch Phys Med Rehabil* 2002;81:S45–S52.

Spencer WA, Vallbona C, Carter RE. Physiologic concepts of immobilization. *Arch Phys Med Rehabil* 1965;46:89–100.

Steinberg FU. The immobilized patient. In: *Functional Pathology and Management.* New York: Plenum, 1980.

Tardin C, Tabary JC, et al. Adaptation of connective tissue length to immobilization in lengthened and shortened positions in cat soleus muscle. *J Physiology (Pare's)* 1982;78:214–220.

Vallbona C. Bodily responses to immobilization. In: Kottke FJ, Stillwell GK, Lehmann JF, eds. *Krusen's handbook of physical medicine and rehabilitation,* 3rd ed. Philadelphia: WB Saunders, 1982.

Vallbona C. Immobilization syndrome. In: Halstead LS, Grabois M, Howland CA, eds. *Medical rehabilitation.* New York: Raven Press, 1985:290.

Vanwanseele B, Lucchinetti E, Stussi E. The effects of immobilization on the characteristics of articular cartilage: current concepts and future directions. In: *2002 OsteoArthritis Research Society International.* Elsevier Science Ltd.

Limb Fractures

Fae H. Garden

DEFINITION

A fracture is a structural break in a bone, an epiphyseal plate, or a cartilaginous joint surface. Although damage to bone is often immediately obvious, damage to the surrounding soft tissues may escape early clinical detection. Damaged soft tissue associated with a fracture is of great clinical significance and may ultimately affect clinical outcome. This chapter focuses on adult limb fractures, their aftercare, and rehabilitation.

TERMINOLOGY

Refer to Fig. 12-1.

Transverse fracture: the long axis of bone and fracture plane are perpendicular. Usually caused by a direct blow or pure angular force being applied to the bone. The bone segments in transverse fractures often remain aligned.

Spiral (or Oblique) fracture: produced by a twisting force to the long axis of bone that causes fracture along shear lines. The long axis of bone and fracture plane form an angle. These fractures are difficult to align and may become unstable.

Comminuted fracture: more than two fracture fragments present. There is splintering of the bone ends. Usually caused by direct trauma.

Greenstick fracture: an incomplete fracture produced by angulatory forces. The opposite cortex is intact. Occurs in children.

Buckling (torus) fracture: a fracture in which one cortex is compacted while the opposite cortex is intact. Occurs in children.

Compression fracture: decreased length or width of bone segments caused by impaction of trabecular bone.

Avulsion fracture: fracture produced by traction forces on bone through the enthesis. A sudden, strong contraction tears away a portion of bone.

Stress fracture: small cracks in bone that develop as a result of repeated fatigue. Discontinuity of bone can usually be avoided by stopping the repeated stress.

Pathologic fracture: interruption of bone at an area that has been weakened by a pathologic process, such as tumor or infiltrative process.

Closed (simple) fracture: fracture surface is not in contact with the skin or mucous membranes.

Open (compound) fracture: fracture surface communicates with skin or mucous membranes.

ANATOMY

The load-bearing capacity of bone can reach up to 10 to 20 times body weight. This is made possible by the elastic properties of bone that allow it to bend slightly when load is applied.

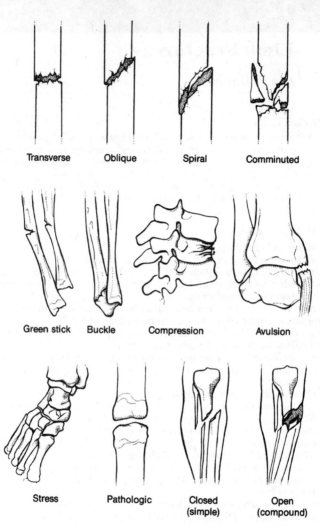

Fig. 12-1.   Types of limb fractures.

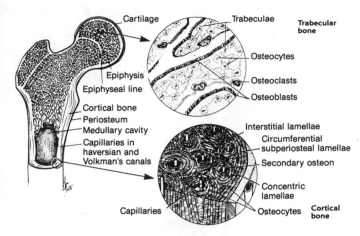

Fig. 12-2.   Composition of bone.

Bone is composed of a compact cortical layer that forms the outer shell and a spongy, interior trabecular meshwork. Although both cortical and trabecular components contribute to overall bone strength, cortical bone is able to resist compression or shearing forces better than tension forces.

The ratio of cortical to trabecular components in the adult skeleton is about 4:1. Vertebrae are mostly composed of trabecular bone, whereas long bones such as the radius and ulnar are approximately 90% cortical. See Fig. 12-2.

The periosteum becomes weaker and less osteogenic with age. Periosteal tearing at the time of a fracture may interfere with surgical reduction procedures. Decreased periosteal osteogenesis in adults results in slower fracture healing and may contribute to delayed union and nonunion.

EPIDEMIOLOGY

In the United States, fractures represent nearly 10% of all reported injuries. A 1976 National Health Survey estimated that for every 10 persons in the United States, fractures account for more than 6 days of restricted activity each year. In addition to huge economic costs, fractures can result in permanent disability and premature death.

Limb fractures occur most often in young men and older women. In the United States, the most common fracture among white women up until age 75 are Colles' fractures (fracture of the distal radius with posterior displacement of the fracture fragment). After age 75, hip fractures become more frequent. Nearly half of all hip fractures occur in persons older than 80 years. More than 75% of all hip fractures occur in women. The cause and pathophysiology of hip fractures resulting from osteoporosis is discussed Chapter 12.

Patients with Colles' fractures rarely require hospitalization or rehabilitation services. Hip fractures, especially in the geriatric population, are associated with high rates of morbidity and

Table 12.1.   Causes of Limb Fractures

Falls
Crush injuries
Motor vehicle accidents
Bicycle accidents
Auto/bicycle/pedestrian accidents
Sports injuries
Fights
Repetitive stress or fatigue
Spontaneous/idiopathic

mortality. The ability of a person to regain ambulation after his or her fracture has been associated with survival.

CAUSE AND PATHOPHYSIOLOGY

Bone is strongest when subjected to symmetrical compression forces. Excessive bending or torsional loads leads to tension failure and fracture. The most common direct cause of limb fractures is a fall. These falls usually occur at home and frequently involve heights of less than 6 feet. See Table 12.1.

Bone pathology, especially as a result of osteoporosis, may predispose an individual to sustaining a limb fracture. See Table 12.2.

Table 12.2.   Factors Contributing to Limb Fractures

General
Osteoporosis
Osteogenesis imperfecta
Osteitis deformans (Paget's disease)
Metabolic
Vitamin C deficiency (scurvy)
Vitamin D deficiency (rickets)
Hyperparathyroidism
Osteomalacia
Inflammatory
Osteomyelitis
Rheumatoid arthritis
Ischemic
Avascular necrosis
Neoplastic
Primary tumors of bone
Metastatic carcinoma
Neuromuscular
Spinal cord injuries
Anterior horn cell disease
Myopathies

Table 12.3. Factors Affecting Fracture Healing
Patient age
Amount of fracture displacement
Type of fracture
Location of fracture
Blood supply to fracture
Coexisting medical conditions

ASSESSMENT OF FRACTURE HEALING

There is a great deal of variation in fracture healing time from one individual to the next. The location of the fracture also affects the time needed for bone union. See Table 12.3.

Motion at the fracture site can delay bone union. Fractured bones are typically immobilized one joint above and one joint below the fracture site.

In an uncomplicated fracture, microscopic evidence of healing can usually be seen at the fracture site within 15 hours of injury. Radiographic evidence of callus formation is apparent at about 4 weeks following injury. Callus is made up of a mixture of cartilage and woven (fibrous) bone. Callus formation and its progressive replacement by stronger, remodeled osteomal bone may continue for several years. The state of fracture healing is determined by clinical examination and radiographic assessment. Even when the patient and the examiner fail to detect movement or pain at the fracture site, the fracture line will still be visible on x-ray film. Although immobilization may no longer be required, the bone should not be exposed to excessive stress. Clinical and radiographic assessment should continue on a periodic basis until the fracture line is no longer visible and callus formation has occurred. Age effects fracture healing time. Fractures in older persons tend to heal more slowly than those of a similar type and site in children.

REHABILITATION EVALUATION

The physiatrist must communicate effectively with the patient as well as with the referring surgeon. Elicit a detailed history, including prefracture functional status and support systems. Review radiographs and pertinent laboratory values before commencing therapies.

Inspect the affected limb carefully. Document presence or absence of edema, trophic changes, muscular atrophy, pressure ulcers, and/or clinical evidence of deep venous thrombosis (DVT). Palpate peripheral pulses above and below the fracture site. Perform a careful neurologic examination to rule out sensory or motor deficits as a result of peripheral nerve injuries. Note any pain elicited by palpation, movement, or weight bearing of the affected limb. A manual muscle test to determine strength will not be accurate in the early phase of postfracture rehabilitation

because of pain and swelling and may even result in fractur
displacement. Document initial passive and active range o.
motion in joints proximal and distal to the fracture site, as well
as the patient's ability to contract muscles voluntarily in the
affected limb.

TREATMENT

Descriptions of splinting and fracture reduction techniques
may be found in most orthopedic surgery textbooks.

The major goal of rehabilitation management in fracture aftercare is restoration of the patient's normal activity level. See
Table 12.4. Patients with lower limb fractures, particularly fractures of the femoral head and neck and traumatic musculoskeletal injuries are those most commonly referred for rehabilitation
services. Rapid mobilization lessens the deleterious effects of immobility on the cardiopulmonary and musculoskeletal systems.
After the initial immobilization period, consider using a fracture

**Table 12.4. General Rehabilitation
Measures for Limb Fractures**

Goal	Measures
Reduce pain	Oral, nonnarcotic analgesics Modalities: heat, massage, TENS, fluidother- apy (heat should not be applied until hemo- stasis is assured)
Reduce edema	Active, assisted exercises Elevation of distal and proximal aspects of the limb Hydrocollator packs Whirlpool bath Gentle massage Compression garments
Restore range of motion and strength	Active, assisted exercises Neuromuscular reeducation Resistive exercises (when appropriate) Modalities: heat followed by stretching of con- nective tissue Resistive exercises (when appropriate) Modalities: heat followed by stretching of con- nective tissue
Return to independence in self-care and ADLs	Adaptive equipment prescription; raised toi- let seat, reacher, chair cushion, bathtub bench, long-handled bath sponge, hand- held shower nozzle Ambulatory aids: walker, cane, crutches

TENS, transcutaneous electrical nerve stimulation.
Susan J. Garrison (Ed.): Handbook of Physical Medicine and Rehabilitation
Basics. Philadelphia: J.B. Lippincott Company, 1995.

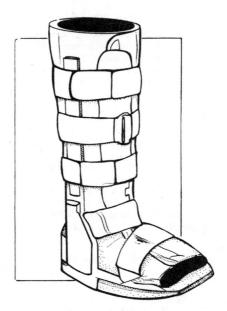

Fig. 12-3.   Orthotic cast.

orthosis to facilitate ambulation and to allow progressive weight bearing. Fracture orthosis are most commonly prescribed for fractures of the tibia and distal femur. See Fig. 12-3. The decision to resume normal activity levels should be made jointly by the physiatrist, orthopedic surgeon, therapist, and patient. Weight-bearing status and length of immobilization varies according to the type of fracture, its location, and treatment. The following general guidelines pertain to hip fractures. Surgeons often differ in their choice of postoperative rehabilitation protocols. It is good clinical practice to determine the local standard of care of the referring orthopedist before commencing rehabilitation management.

Femoral neck fractures, either subcapital, intercapsular, or transcervical, are frequently associated with mild groin pain that may refer to the knee. Endoprosthetic replacement is often necessary because of the risk of avascular necrosis.

A patient with an intertrochanteric fracture may experience more severe pain and present with apparent shortening and external rotation of the affected extremity. Surgical intervention [open reduction and internal fixation (ORIF)] using pins and plates or a compression screw is often necessary.

Preoperative Care Guidelines

Examine unaffected joints, opposite leg, and upper limbs.
Exercise to strengthen hip abductors (if appropriate).
Discuss postoperative therapy and goals with patient.

Postoperative Care Guidelines (Day 2 to 3)

Determine whether cemented or noncemented prosthesis was used.

Examine for postoperative complications: sciatic or peroneal nerve paresis, hematoma, or DVT. Make note of the type of DVT prophylaxis used (Coumadin, Lovenox, Fragmin, etc.).

Patients with total hip arthroplasty should avoid hip adduction, internal rotation, and flexion past 90 degrees in the affected limb. An abduction pillow helps maintain proper position while in bed and sitting. A knee immobilizer brace may also be used to restrict unwanted movements.

Weight bearing as tolerated (WBAT) in parallel bars may begin in patients with cemented hip prosthesis. Initially, many patients are unable to fully weight bear because of pain and reduced proprioceptive feedback.

Patients with noncemented prosthesis should be restricted to touch-down or non-weight-bearing for the first 6 weeks. The same applies to fractures treated by ORIF.

Active assisted exercises may begin in the normal anatomic plans of motion.

Postoperative Care Guidelines (Day 4)

Progress to three-point gait with standard walker crutches (cemented prosthesis) and advance to WBAT.

Non-weight-bearing or touch-down weight-bearing with standard walker or crutches if noncemented prosthesis or ORIF.

Isometric exercises for the quadriceps should be taught before discharge.

Outpatient Care Guidelines (6 to 12 Weeks Postoperatively)

Obtain radiographic evaluation of the surgical site.

Advance to a cane if cemented prosthesis was used.

Advance to partial weight bearing with standard walker or crutches if noncemented prosthesis was used.

Begin low-weight, isotonic exercises to strengthen thigh and hip muscles.

During the program of fracture rehabilitation, therapeutic modalities are often applied externally to reduce pain and facilitate movement. Superficial heat modalities in the form of hot packs, cold packs, vapo-coolant spray, paraffin baths, and fluidotherapy can help relieve pain and muscle tension. Improved range of motion is also a treatment goal.

Deep heat in the form of ultrasound may be helpful to relieve contractures of muscle or joint. The use of ultrasound is contraindicated directly over the fracture site or over a metal implant.

COMPLICATIONS

Nonunion at fracture site—little or no callus formation is seen at the fracture site.

Delayed union—fracture segments are mobile 3 to 4 months after the initial injury.

Failure of a fracture to unite after 4 months may be due to factors such as age, overall health, and motion at the fracture site. Electrical stimulation to enhance osteogenesis and bone grafting are accepted treatment techniques.

eripheral Nerve Injuries

Minor stretch injuries and swelling can result in neuropraxia. Nerve conduction studies are abnormal. Recovery typically occurs within 10 weeks after the injury if pressures are removed. More severe stretch injuries and direct nerve trauma may result in axonal degeneration. Surgical repair of lacerated peripheral nerves may be necessary.

Osteomyelitis

An active infection of the bone, osteomyelitis, can be caused by contaminants introduced at the time of trauma or from hematogenous spread.

Avascular Necrosis

In avascular necrosis, bone dies because of a lack of blood supply.

Fat Embolus

A fractured long bone can release globules of fat. These travel into the pulmonary system and cause obstruction. Fat embolism typically occurs during the first 4 hours to 4 days posttrauma.

Compartment Syndromes

Unrelieved swelling in the tight osteofascial compartments of the limb leads to ischemia of the enclosed muscles and nerves. Peripheral pulses in the affected limb should be monitored closely. The signs and symptoms of compartment syndrome can be summarized by "the four Ps"—pain, pulselessness, puffiness, and pallor. A patient who experiences severe pain with passive stretch and loss of muscle strength should be suspected of having developed compartment syndrome. Persistent use of analgesics for pain control can mask these symptoms and delay necessary surgical decompression. Careful, repeat physical examination should be performed in patients complaining of persistent pain or sensory/motor loss. Displaced supracondylar fractures of the humerus can be complicated by a compartment syndrome and lead to development of Volkmann's contracture, in which the muscles of the flexor forearm are shortened and the fingers contracted. Forearm pronation and elbow flexion contractures are also frequently present.

Skin Complications

Immobilization without appropriate pressure relief and incorrect application of a fracture cast can result in development of a pressure ulcer. Both of these complications are iatrogenic and preventable.

Reflex Sympathetic Dystrophy (RSD)

RSD is a syndrome of pain, hyperesthesia, vasomotor disturbance, and dystrophic changes in the skin and bone of an affected extremity. RSD that occurs after soft tissue trauma with predominant findings of bony atrophy is referred to as Sudeck's atrophy of bone. The diagnosis of RSD is primarily clinical and the disorder typically progresses in stages. Paravertebral sympathetic ganglior block is a widely used treatment. Pain management includir selective use of opioids and gabapentin (Neurontin) plays an important role in RSD treatment. Reports of successful treatment of symptoms using physical therapy, transcutaneous electrical nerve stimulation (TENS), corticosteroids, and phenoxybenzamine have appeared in the literature.

SUGGESTED READINGS

Cummings SR, Kelsey JL, Nevitt MC et al. Epidemiology of osteoporosis and osteoporotic fractures. *Epidemiol Rev* 1985;7:178.

Demopoulous JT. Rehabilitation in fractures of the limbs. In: *Current therapy in physiatry.* Philadelphia: WB Saunders, 1984.

Garraway WM, Stauffer RN, Kurland LT et al. Limb fractures in a defined population. Part I. Frequency and distribution. *Mayo Clin Proc* 1979;54:701.

Garraway WM, Stauffer RN, Kurland LT et al. Limb fractures in a defined population. Part II. Orthopedic treatment and utilization of health care. *Mayo Clin Proc* 1979;54:708.

Gradisar IA. Fracture stabilization and healing. In: Gould JA, Davies GJ, eds. *Orthopedic and sports physical therapy,* 2nd ed. St. Louis: Mosby, 1990.

Hoaglund FT, Duthie RB. Fracture and joint injuries. In: Schwartz SI, ed. *Principles of surgery,* 6th ed. New York: McGraw-Hill, 1994.

Knapp M. Aftercare of fractures. In: Kottke FJ, Stillwell GK, Lehmann JF, eds. *Krusen's handbook of physical medicine and rehabilitation.* Philadelphia: WB Saunders, 1982.

Miller CW. Survival and ambulation following hip fracture. *J Bone Joint Surg* 1978;60A:930.

Opitz JL. Total joint arthroplasty: principles and guidelines for postoperative physiatric management. *Mayo Clin Proc:* 1979;54: 602–612.

Salter RB. *Textbook of disorders and injuries of the musculoskeletal system,* 2nd ed. Baltimore: Williams & Wilkins, 1983.

Schwartzman RJ, McLellan MD. Reflex sympathic dystrophy, a review. *Arch Neurol* 1987;44:555.

Waugh T. Arthroplasty rehabilitation. In: Goodgold J, ed. *Rehabilitation medicine.* St. Louis: Mosby, 1988.

Wild D, Nayak U, Isaacs B. Description, classification and prevention of falls in old people at home. *Rheumatol Rehabil* 1981;20:153.

Zuckerman JD, Newport ML. Rehabilitation of fractures in adults. In: Goodgold J, ed. *Rehabilitation medicine.* St. Louis: Mosby, 1988.

Neuromuscular Diseases

Maureen R. Nelson

Neuromuscular diseases encompass a variety of disorders with abnormalities from the anterior horn cell, nerve, neuromuscular junction, and muscle. Therefore, this chapter covers a spectrum of diseases from spinal muscular atrophy and amyotrophic lateral sclerosis (ALS) to botulism and myasthenia gravis (MG), and to myopathies, including Duchenne muscular dystrophy (DMD) and dermatomyositis (DM).

MYOPATHIES

The myopathies are a group of muscle diseases whose common primary symptom is proximal limb muscle weakness. There are a variety of myopathies including the dystrophies, congenital myopathies, metabolic myopathies, endocrine myopathies, and inflammatory myopathies. The one that is best studied and has the most specific information is DMD; therefore, this is our prototype and starting point.

Duchenne Muscular Dystrophy (DMD)

DMD is an X-linked recessive myopathy leading to an abnormality of the protein dystrophin. Dystrophin is a part of the cytoskeleton, and because of its abnormality there is membrane instability. The incidence of DMD is 1 per 3,500 live male births with a prevalence approximately 3 per 100,000 live males. Approximately one third of the cases of DMD are secondary to spontaneous mutation. The location of this mutation is on the XP21 locus, the short arm of the X chromosome. DMD is rare in females but can be seen in a girl with Turner syndrome or an X autosomal translocation or break at the XP21 locus. Female carriers also can have elevation of muscle enzymes and mild muscle weakness.

The history in DMD is classically that of a 3- to 5-year-old boy with clumsiness; frequent falls; and poor, and perhaps delayed, walking. Physical examination shows calf pseudohypertrophy in 80% of the boys, with fatty and fibrotic replacement of the muscle. Gower's maneuver is frequently seen because of hip weakness. The gait is frequently wide-based with toe walking. Reflexes are absent or decreased. Twenty-five percent of boys have nonprogressive decrease and IQ below 75. Cardiac abnormalities may be seen with abnormality of the posterior basal area and left ventricular wall.

Laboratory evaluation shows an elevated creatine kinase (CK) level up to 300 to 400 times normal. Because of atrophy of the muscle fibers, this level decreases as the child ages. Seventy percent of the female carriers have a mild elevation of CK. Other muscle enzymes may also be elevated. Electrocardiogram (ECG) shows an abnormality in two thirds of the boys, most commonly with a tall right precordial R wave. Electrodiagnostic evaluation shows a normal sensory nerve conduction studies and motor nerve conduction studies with decreased amplitude of the compound muscle action potential (CMAP) that worsens as the disease progresses. The electromyogram (EMG) early on may show increased insertional activity, fibrillations, and positive sharp waves along with complex repetitive discharges (CRDs) and short-duration low-amplitude polyphasic (myopathic) motor units with satellite potentials. There may be early recruitment. Muscle biopsy shows fibrosis, necrosis, and phagocytosis. The microscopic immunochemistry shows absent dystrophin in the sarcolemma of skeletal muscle fiber. DNA screening shows specific genetic lesions that are family specific.

The DMD gene is a large locus with over 2 1/2 million base pairs on the human X chromosome. Its large size is believed to lead to its high mutation rate. The size of the genetic lesion does not lead to severity of the disease, but the severity of the disease depends on whether the mutation leads to the ability to produce any dystrophin.

Other problems in DMD involve weakness of skeletal muscle and respiratory muscle, contractures of limbs, restrictive lung disease, and scoliosis. Later there may be upper gastrointestinal (GI) tract dysfunction and gastric hypomotility.

Treatment

There is no cure for DMD; therefore, treatment addresses each of the known systems' problems. Vigorous exercise programs, with range of motion to minimize contractures, are a key early intervention. Bracing is also used to assist with prevention and minimization of contractures by use of nighttime splints and with increased positioning and function by daytime bracing. Surgical release of contractures is also undertaken in an attempt to prolong function. Scoliosis is present in approximately 75% of patients, and bracing is not effective in improving positioning or delaying worsening of the curve. Surgery for scoliosis must be undertaken with consideration for both the degree of spinal curvature and the respiratory function. Common recommendations are for spinal stabilization before the percentage of normal forced vital capacity (FVC) is less than 35% to 30% and commonly when the curve is no worse than 35 degrees. If the respiratory function is worse, there are severe difficulties with removal from ventilatory assistance. Mobilization postoperatively is generally initiated on the second day because of the risk of weakness after any period of immobilization in boys with DMD.

Medications are being studied to find maximal benefit with minimal side effects. Currently it is know that independent ambulation can be prolonged in boys who use prednisone, but side effects of cushingoid facies, increased appetite, weight gain, hyperactivity, cataracts, gastritis, behavioral changes, acne, and bone loss limit the use. Deflazacort, a derivative of prednisone, is used in some children as well with less benefit and less side effects than with prednisone. Steroids do not prevent the eventual weakness of DMD. Cyclosporine may also result in some delay in the weakness, and it is generally clear within 2 weeks if this drug will be effective in the child.

Monitored resistive exercise programs can show short-term increase in strength and a delay in progressive weakness in boys with DMD. Boys with greater strength initially have more potenal for improvement. A key precaution is to prevent a decrease in muscle function secondary to overwork weakness.

Bracing can be used extensively in boys with DMD. AFOs and ischial weight-bearing KAFOs are frequently used for maximizing gait. The KAFOs may be used with locked knees. Night bracing is done as well for maximized positioning and stretching program. For ambulation, a combination of surgical tendon release with bracing and therapy is commonly used. Bracing for upper extremities also can be critical in maintaining function because the proximal weakness. Fine motor ability is generally relatively preserved with proximal strength loss. Wrist extensor strength is generally found to be decreased by the age of 8 years. There is also frequent ulnar deviation contractures of the wrist, and this combination decreases activity of daily living (ADL) function. Bracing can be used to minimize the deformity and to improve function. Proximal weakness can be treated by use of a balanced forearm orthosis (BFO), which gives the ability to move the arm proximally while using the functional hand. Minimal elbow flexion contracture of 15 degrees or less can be a benefit in ADL performance.

Ventilation is one of the key areas of treatment in boys with DMD. In boys with no ventilatory assistance, the median age of death is approximately 20 years of age, mostly from chronic respiratory disease. With assisted ventilation, survival has been noted to increase by approximately 6 years. Ventilatory options are many. Vital capacity (VC) is maximal at approximately 10 years of age, and this level can help predict the progression of restrictive disease. Patients with maximum VC below 1,200 mL die on average at age 15.3 years without ventilatory assistance, but those with a plateau more than 1,700 mL live to approximately age 21 without assistance. Those with a peak FVC of more than 2,500 mL have slower progression of respiratory disease with a decrease of 4% of FVC per year compared with 10% for those with a peak FVC less than 1,700 mL. Even with ventilatory assistance, patients with DMD have a progressive decrease in VC.

Respiratory assistance is typically initiated when the VC is decreased to approximately 10% to 20% of the predicted normal or when the boy has symptoms of nocturnal hypoventilation and hypercapnia. These symptoms include irritability, morning headaches, sleepiness, nausea, and decrease in daytime energy. Because the respiratory drive is decreased during sleep there is an increased risk at this time. If PCO_2 levels are increased during the day, there is likely dramatically increased PCO_2 at night. Treatment is generally initiated with noninvasive negative or positive pressure ventilation at night.

With the use of negative pressure ventilation, the ventilator performs part of the work of breathing and rests the respiratory muscles during sleep. It is hoped that sufficient rest is obtained so that the muscles may then work effectively during the day. Negative pressure ventilators give an intermittent flow of negative pressure into the tank that results in negative interpleural pressure and generates airflow, which ventilates the lungs. An iron lung is an example of a negative pressure ventilator. Noninvasive intermittent positive pressure ventilation may be done with a nasal or mouth access, generally with a mouth seal or nasal seal. A pneumo belt is also noninvasive positive pressure ventilation. These devices also are generally initiated at nighttime. Invasive positive pressure ventilation is with a tracheostomy and positive pressure ventilator. Potential problems with tracheostomy include increased risk of infection, fistula, or stenosis. This also makes suctioning, pulmonary toilet and speech more difficult. This also limits activities and living situations that may be available because a tracheostomy is considered an open wound.

The purpose of the assisted ventilation treatment for these boys with restrictive lung disease is to assist with the mechanical work of ventilation not to give oxygen.

Pulmonary care for boys with DMD also includes influenza vaccine beginning at age 6 months, pneumococcus vaccine beginning at 2 years, and excellent chest physical therapy during any respiratory infection.

Another critical area of treatment in boys with DMD is psychosocial management. This is an extremely difficult disease for the boy and his family, and the boy and family require support and assistance. There can be predictable variations in grief and stress during the disease process, many of which are predictable and related to such things as the onset of wheelchair use and ventilatory assistance. Early on boys tend to have a fear of falling and later they tend to have a fear of dying. Counseling should be available to the boys and the families throughout. A proper educational environment and support in the school system is also critical with proper placement in classes that provide stimulation and are neither too easy nor too difficult.

Complications of DMD include osteoporosis secondary to disuse and, secondarily, pathologic fractures. Fractures are treated traditionally but immobilization of the body must be avoided because of the high risk of additional weakness. Obesity may also become a complication during the transition of walking to wheelchair mobility because of the increased energy efficiency of movement in a wheelchair. In addition, food may become a substitute for other pleasures that are more difficult to attain. Later on in the course of the disease, weight loss may be a dramatic problem because of hypercatabolic protein metabolism, most commonly in 17 to 21 year olds.

Patients with DMD and other myopathies have been reported to have malignant hyperthermia during general anesthesia. There is tachycardia, cardiac arrhythmia, unstable blood pressure, cyanosis, fever, rigidity secondary to severe muscle contractures, and convulsion. There may be resultant metabolic acidosis with myoglobinuria and then renal failure. The mortality rate is 60%. These problems can be induced by the use of halothane and succinylcholine. Treatment is to discontinue the anesthetic agents and administer 100% oxygen, cool the patient, and give bicarbonate for metabolic acidosis and dantrolene for muscle relaxation. The classic hyperthermia defect is not present; it is likely that the defect is due to the abnormality of the muscle cell membranes.

Prognosis

The clinical course of DMD is progression in all areas except for cognitive deficit. There is progression of weakness of the muscles, progression of scoliosis, progression of restrictive lung disease, and progression of contractures. There is a decrease in the functional capacity. Those boys who are weaker die from respiratory failure and pneumonia, and those who are stronger die from cardiac failure. Respiratory assistance can prolong survival. A study looking at quality of life showed that patients with DMD were just about as satisfied with their life as a group of healthcare professionals who were surveyed at the same time. A vast array of ventilatory options are currently available to help make quality of life better than previously possible. There is a good deal of research going on for boys with DMD including trials with myoblast implantation and gene transfer. Even if the myoblast transfers were successful in skeletal muscle, cardiac muscle treatment would still be a problem. Any treatment that replaces dystrophin must also replace the large complex of glycoproteins called dystrophin-associated proteins (DAPs), which are another major structural component of the cytoskeleton. The DAPs are missing in all muscle fibers in boys with DMD. Therefore, these also must be accounted for in any type of treatment.

Other Dystrophies

There are several other types of muscular dystrophies. Becker's muscular dystrophy (BMD) has a mutation of the same gene that causes DMD but is a more slowly progressive and milder X-linked disorder. There is generally an onset of weakness in boys between 10 to 15 years of age. They may also have cardiac disease and generally have milder findings throughout than boys with DMD. They have an abnormal quantity and quality of dystrophin on muscle biopsy but have at least 5% of normal amounts. The survival is to middle adulthood and can vary from the 20s to 60 years of age. The treatment is with range of motion exercises, bracing, structured weight training program, and surgical release of contractures.

Facioscapulohumeral dystrophy (FSH) is an autosomal dominant myopathy with a spectrum of severities within the same family because of complete penetrance but variable expressivity. There is a normal lifespan. There is weakness generally in the shoulder girdle and anterior portion of the leg. Onset can be in infancy, in which case the course is more severe or in the teens or later. Most commonly facial weakness is first noted. The molecular defect is at chromosome 4q35 markers. There are no ECG abnormalities. The CK maybe elevated two to four times normal and an EMG may show changes as in DMD and BMD. Biopsy shows an increased variability in size of fibers and small fibers called tiny fibers. Treatment is with orthoses, supervised strengthening, and, occasionally, scapular stabilizing after a careful preoperative evaluation. There may be a problem with dry eye secondary to facial weakness, and artificial tears may be helpful; if very serious, plastic surgery may be required.

Limb-girdle dystrophy (LGD) is a group of disorders with weakness at the hips and shoulders and with various inheritance patterns. Cardiopulmonary difficulties may be present and intellect is normal. CK is only mildly increased up to 10 times normal. Clinical course may vary, but ventilatory assistance and a modified strength training program may be beneficial.

Myotonic dystrophy (MD) is an autosomal dominant disease with progressive muscle weakness that is generally worse distally.

There is a classic atrophy of the face, jaw, anterior neck, and distal limb muscles. Myotonia is characteristically found. Myotonia is a delayed relaxation of muscle contraction, which is often interpreted by patients as muscle stiffness. This may be worsened by cold. There is onset of weakness in young adulthood with symmetrical slowly progressive weakness. A long face and nasal voice are often noted. The presenting complaint may be weakness of the hands or feet or stiffness and cramps of the muscles. On examination, myotonia of the muscle can be found with percussion, but this is more difficult to find as the disease progresses. Cataracts are present in 90% of the patients. Also common are abnormalities of the smooth muscle, including the uterus, esophagus, and the bowel musculature leading to constipation. Cardiac abnormalities include cardiomyopathies and conduction defects with pacemaker useful in approximately one half of the patients. Thus, any exercise must be carefully monitored. Males have degeneration of testicular tubular cells with low sperm formation and low testosterone, with females having frequent amenorrhea; infertility occurs in both genders. Mental retardation is frequent. Infants born to mothers with MD generally have a more severe form called congenital MD. These children have mental retardation and respiratory difficulties and motor delay. They have hypotonia and facial paralysis with the upper lip described as having an inverted V or tented appearance. The EMG classically shows myotonic discharges, which have a waxing and waning of amplitude and frequency similar to a motorcycle or a dive-bomber. CK is increased and muscle biopsy shows internal nuclei and atrophy of type 1 fibers. Genetic abnormalities on chromosome 19 with an unstable repeat at 19q13.3. Some families show "anticipation" in which each generation has a clinically worse manifestation than the previous generation. Treatment includes orthoses, medications if myotonia is severe, and cardiac medications or pacing.

Emery Dreifuss muscular dystrophy (EDMD) is another X-linked recessive dystrophy that has a classic triad of early contracture, particularly of the elbows; cardiac conduction defects; and slowly progressive weakness and atrophy in a humeral peroneal distribution. The severity of the cardiac disease is much worse than the myopathy. CK is normal to moderately increased. The genetic abnormality is on Xq28.33, and the abnormal gene product is a nuclear protein called emerin. Treatment is generally with a pacemaker for cardiac disease, as well as bracing and stretching exercises.

Other Myopathies

Other types of myopathies include congenital myopathies, which are a group of slowly progressive or nonprogressive myopathies that present as hypotonia or weakness during infancy and generally show improvement later; metabolic myopathies primarily involving glycogen storage and the utilization; endocrine myopathies including hyperthyroidism, hypothyroidism, thyroid disease, and corticosteroid myopathies, which improve with improvement of the endocrine status; infectious myopathies, which include myopathies from trichinella and human immunodeficiency virus (HIV); toxic myopathies, which include acute and chronic alcoholic myopathy; and inflammatory myopathies including polymyositis (PM), DM, d sarcoidosis. PM and DM are generally discussed together, though they appear to have different causes. These are acquired myopathies with acute or subacute course with pain and muscle aches commonly present. DM is more common in childhood and middle age with a bimodal distribution but can occur at any age. It is frequently associated with collagen vascular disease, and, in adults, it is associated with cancer. DM has a classic rash that frequently is present before any other signs are noted and that is seen during and after muscle weakness. There is a classic rash over the eyelids and cheeks and periorbital edema. There also may be an erythematous rash over any exposed part of the body, especially extensor surfaces of the joints. There may be calcinosis, particularly in children with DM in whom it has been reported in 50% to 75%. This consists of calcium deposits beneath the skin that sometimes extrude through the skin. These generally resolve spontaneously but can be a chronic problem. Commonly early in the course of the disease there are nonspecific complaints of weight loss, anorexia, malaise, and fever.

Raynaud's phenomenon is seen in 20% of patients. Dysphagia may be seen, and other collagen vascular diseases may be present. There is proximal weakness of the hips, shoulders, and anterior neck muscles. Reflexes are generally normal, and there may be mild muscle atrophy. There may be minimal muscle palpation tenderness. CK is elevated in 90% of patients, with myoglobin and erythrocyte sedimentation rate increased as well. Ninety percent of patients show abnormal EMG with CRDs; fibrillations; positive sharp waves; and small, brief polyphasic potentials. Muscles with moderate weakness and the paraspinal muscles classically exhibit abnormalities on EMG. There is no correlation of the severity of EMG findings and the severity of this disease. There is correlation of the amount of spontaneous activity and the course of the disease, so this may be helpful in following sequentially for a response to treatment. Magnetic resonance imaging (MRI) shows a swelling of the muscles particularly in the thigh. Muscle biopsy shows necrosis, phagocytosis, inflammatory cells, and degeneration.

The clinical course is variable: there may be complete recovery after one episode, there may be a remitting and relapsing course, or there may be a chronic course. This last form commonly has pulmonary function compromise, and mortality is 15% to 30% in chronic PM and DM.

The severity of weakness at the beginning of the disease, the CK level, and the biopsy results do not correlate with outcome. Treatment of DM and PM is with steroids, most commonly prednisone, as early in the course of disease as possible. Other immunosuppressants may be used including methotrexate, cyclophosphamide, azathioprine, and chlorambucil. Cyclosporin also may be used. Cataracts have been described in approximately 30% of patients using steroids for more than 12 months. Treatment also includes range of motion and stretching programs to prevent contractures while the muscles are extremely weak. Monitored resistive exercise program can help regain strength.

NEUROMUSCULAR JUNCTION DISORDERS

Neuromuscular junction abnormalities are manifest in botulism and in MG. **Botulism** is an acquired abnormality caused by

the botulinum toxin that is released by the anaerobic bacter.
Clostridium botulinum. Babies may ingest the bacteria and fo.
the toxin in their intestinal tract, whereas older individuals mus
ingest the toxin. There is a presynaptic abnormality with toxin
binding irreversibly to the presynaptic membrane, inhibiting
acetylcholine release. Physical findings are of a descending paralysis with frequent involvement of the cranial nerves. Upper limbs
and lower limbs become weaker over time, and there is hyporeflexia or areflexia. Ventilatory assistance may be required. In infants there is frequently a history of constipation, occasionally
honey ingestion, poor suck in feeding, and lethargy. In infants
this is most common between 1 and 6 months of age. Diagnosis is
confirmed by isolation of the *C. botulinum* organism from stool
samples.

Repetitive nerve stimulation shows an incremental response at
50-Hz stimulation and usually at 20 Hz as well. There may be a
decremental response at 2 to 3 Hz repetitive nerve stimulation.
EMG may show short-duration, low-amplitude, polyphasic potentials and infrequently shows positive waves and fibrillations.

Botulinum types A, B, and E are most commonly responsible for
adult poisoning, generally after ingestion of raw or inadequately
cooked or canned vegetables, meat, or fish. An infected wound may
also provide the toxin. The toxin is heat sensitive, and botulism is
more common at high altitudes. In adults clinical symptoms may
begin 1 or 2 days after contamination of food or 1 or 2 weeks after
wound contamination. Initial findings may be diarrhea, nausea,
and vomiting; weakness may first manifest with decreased extraocular movements and ptosis and with pupils fixed and dilated.
Dysarthria and dysphagia may also be seen. There may be constipation and urinary retention. Cardiac and respiratory failure may
be present. Diagnosis in adults may be confirmed by culture of suspected food. Electrodiagnostic findings include CMAP with small
amplitude, with decrement at least 10% with slow-rate (2 to 3 Hz)
repetitive stimulation. There is some facilitation of muscle response with fast-rate (20 Hz) repetitive stimulation. There may be
significant true incremental response at high-rate repetitive stimulation or with 10 seconds of maximal voluntary contraction. These
findings are variable depending on the severity of the disease. The
electrophysiologic findings correlate with the severity and progression of the disease. The affected muscles most commonly show
abnormalities. On single-fiber EMG testing, jitter is increased, and
blocking is present with slightly decreased fiber density.

Myasthenia Gravis (MG)

MG is a postsynaptic neuromuscular junction disorder that results from inadequate numbers of acetylcholine receptors, widened
synaptic space, and simplified postsynaptic membranes. There is a
bimodal distribution of incidence with women in their 20s, men in
their 30s and both in their 70s. In younger presentation there is a
female to male ratio of 7:3, but in the older age group the ratio is
1:1. Clinically MG manifests as fluctuating weakness with abnormal fatigability that improves with rest. There is generally weakness confined to specific muscle groups, most commonly ocular,
bulbar, and proximal limb muscle groups. If severe, the progression
of weakness may become generalized. Diplopia at the end of the

y is a common first complaint. Speech may also fatigue, which may be relieved with rest. Visual complaints are the most common presenting problems, particularly diplopia and ptosis, and one third present with dysphagia. Neck and proximal limb weakness is a first complaint in approximately one fourth of patients.

Physical examination shows normal sensation and reflexes. Motor examination should include an attempt to fatigue the patient, particularly by having the patient repeatedly open and close the eyes (if ptosis) and by repeated forceful jaw closure, and resisted mouth opening, resisted eye closure, and resisted neck flexion and extension. Observation of strength and endurance in doing repetitive movements may be useful. The administration of small amounts of edrophonium (Tensilon) results in clinical improvement in a number of disorders other than MG; therefore, edrophonium administration indicates only a potential neuromuscular junction transmission failure and not specifically MG. Electrodiagnostic examination shows normal sensory nerve conduction studies and motor nerve conduction study with normal or decreased CMAP amplitude. There are varied results depending on the severity and distribution of the disease. Various muscles may show various responses. There may be decrements on low-rate repetitive stimulation (2 to 3 Hz) with greatest difference between the first and second response. Postexercise, the decrement may decrease and the CMAP may immediately increase with subsequent further decrement at several minutes following exercise and repair to the initial finding approximately 5 to 6 minutes postexercise. If the patient is unable to exercise, high-frequency stimulation at 20 to 50 Hz may also show immediate increased amplitude and decreased decrement. There may be variable patterns found, however, depending on the specific patient and specific muscles tested. A decrement greater than 10% in adults, however, does indicate faulty neuromuscular transmission. The EMG study may be normal or may show positive sharp waves and fibrillations in less than 15% of the patients, most likely those with more severe disease. In MG, single-fiber electromyography is classically reported with findings of increased jitter and blocking present with slightly increased fiber density.

There are also a heterogenous group of congenital myasthenic syndromes, which are genetic or transient abnormalities. The transient form is secondary to transfer of maternal ACh receptor antibodies and will resolve. There are four genetic myasthenic syndromes: (a) familial, secondary to defects in ACh synthesis and mobilization; (b) decreased number of ACh receptors or end-plate ACHR deficiency; (c) defect in ACh breakdown by acetylcholinesterase (end-plate ACHE deficiency); and (d) prolonged open time of the ACh receptor channel (slow channel syndrome). These show various responses to repetitive stimulation and edrophonium test and repetitive response to single maximum stimulus. Decrements of at least 10% at 2-Hz stimulation is seen in all types; however, this may only be present in muscles that are weak clinically. Stimulated single-fiber EMG may be performed in this group by having a stimulating monopolar electrode at the motor point to obtain muscle twitch. Stimulated single-fiber EMG has variability in one end plate as opposed to two end-plate variability in traditional single-fiber EMG and shows a smaller jitter.

ANTERIOR HORN CELL DISEASE

The anterior horn cell disease classically described in adults i amyotrophic lateral sclerosis (ALS) or Lou Gehrig's disease. The most commonly described anterior horn cell disease in childhood is spinal muscular atrophy (SMA). A variation presenting in infancy is known as SMA type I, Werdnig Hoffman disease; a type presenting in older children is called SMA type II, Kugelberg Welander disease.

SMA is the most common peripheral neuromuscular cause for a floppy baby. Infants with SMA type I are described as having a floppy body and a lively facial expression, with frog-leg position of the leg and jug-handle position of the arms. Tongue fasciculations and paradoxical breathing are frequently noted. The infant may present with respiratory and feeding problems and shows a failure to progress with gross motor development; these infants are never able to sit independently. Nerve conduction studies normally show decreased motor amplitude and possibly decreased velocity with normal sensory studies. The EMG findings are fibrillations; positive sharp waves; decreased numbers of the motor unit potentials with increased firing frequency; and large-amplitude, prolonged-duration motor units with polyphasicity. These have been described as 5- to 15-Hz spontaneous rhythmic motor unit activity in resting muscles. At least three limbs should be electrodiagnostically studied.

Laboratory studies in SMA show an elevated CK. The gene abnormality in SMA is the survival motor neuron gene (SMN), which appears to be abnormal in all types of SMA and most severely abnormal in type I.

Babies with SMA type I have hyporeflexia and atrophy. There is a risk of aspiration secondary to weakness; feeding and respiratory status require careful monitoring and frequent assistance. Infants with SMA have an abnormality in chromosome 5q13.

Prognosis for SMA type I is poor with frequent prenatal onset or onset at less than 3 months of age; lifespan without ventilatory support is 2 years or less. There are other SMA types with later onset and milder course; those less severely affected live to adulthood.

Treatment for infants with SMA type I is range of motion and proper positioning including use of supported seating and possible bracing for avoiding contractures. Gastrostomy tube may be used for a feeding program to maximize safety. Bowel program may be required. Education and counseling for families is critical.

ALS is an anterior horn cell disease in adults. There is focal asymmetrical weakness initially noted over weeks and months, with bulbar complaints most common initially. The distinguishing factor in ALS is that upper neuron signs, including spasticity, accompany weakness. This is believed to be due to a multifactorial process including genetic predisposition with environmental triggers. A familial form accounts for approximately 5% of those with ALS; incidence is approximately 2 per 100,000 and prevalence is 5 per 100,000. There is a male to female prevalence of 2:1, with mean survival of 2 1/2 years after diagnosis and an average age of diagnosis of 62 years. Those with onset before 40 years have a longer lifespan (approximately 8 years).

The common complaints are cranial nerve weakness, which generally spares extraocular movements, along with hand and wrist weakness, neck extensor weakness, and a decrease in the ability to dorsiflex or evert the feet. Foot drop may be a presenting complaint in the minority of patients, but most eventually develop this difficulty. Dysphagia is a problem in most patients, particularly those with severe bulbar involvement. A feeding evaluation and guidance is critical with common use of pureed food or soft solid food and, at times, gastrostomy tube feedings. Management of secretions may also eventually be a problem. There may also be dysarthria with progressive difficulty with speech leading to the possible use of augmentative communication systems. Speech therapy may improve the production of speech and may prolong the time before augmentative communicative devices are needed. Muscle contractures also may be problematic and use of range of motion program and splinting may be beneficial. Oral antispasticity medication may be more difficult to manage because of the combination of weakness and spasticity with potential side effects causing significant deficits. The use of botulinum toxin is not recommended although phenol injections may be used.

Cognition is generally maintained in ALS. Because of the rapidly progressive and fatal course, there may be emotional difficulties in adjusting to the physical loss and dying. Counseling should be available for the patient and family.

SUMMARY

Neuromuscular diseases are an extremely varied group of problems with causes including anterior horn cell disease, neuromuscular junction disorders, and muscular disease. There is also a spectrum of ages involved. Diagnosis and management of these diseases provides a challenge in maintaining function, maximizing safety, and preventing complications through the course of the disease process, which are an excellent opportunity for the physical medicine & rehabilitation team to assist the patients and families.

SUGGESTED READINGS

Braddom RL, ed. *Physical medicine and rehabilitation,* 2nd ed. Philadelphia: WB Saunders, 2000.

Brook MH. *A clinician's view of neuromuscular diseases.* Baltimore: Williams & Wilkins, 1986.

Dubowitz V. *A color atlas of muscle disorders in childhood.* London: Wolfe Medical Publications, 1989.

Dumitru D, ed. *Electrodiagnostic medicine,* 2nd ed. St. Louis: Hanley & Belfus, 2001.

Grabois M, Garrison SJ, Hart KA et al, eds. *Physical medicine and rehabilitation: the complete approach.* Malden, MA: Blackwell Science, 2000.

Jones HR, Bolton CF, Harper CM, ed. *Pediatric clinical electromyography.* Philadelphia: Lippincott-Raven, 1996.

Osteoporosis

Susan J. Garrison

DEFINITION

Osteoporosis is loss of skeletal bone that may result from a variety of factors.

Any person who is immobilized over a prolonged period will experience some degree of osteoporosis. Refer to Chapter 10. Advanced age is a factor in osteoporosis. Remarks here mainly address postmenopausal osteoporosis, but overall concepts may be applied to most situations.

ANATOMY

Trabecular bone is more affected than cortical bone. Spinal vertebrae are usually affected first. Typically, these are the lower thoracic and upper lumbar (T6 to L1). If lesions are higher than this, neoplasm must be considered. Thoracic vertebrae sustain wedge-shaped fractures, whereas crush fractures are common in lumbar vertebrae. See Fig. 14-1.

Thoracic wedge fractures create the typical "Dowager's hump" of kyphoscoliosis. The arms and legs lose their normal proportion to the axial skeleton and appear to be longer. Loss of height resulting from vertebral collapse may be as much as 5 to 8 in. This phenomenon may progress until the lower rib cage rests on the anterior iliac crests. See Fig. 14-1.

EPIDEMIOLOGY

In the United States, osteoporosis affects one in four women older than 60 years, and virtually all white women by the age of 90. At that age, a white woman has at least a 30% chance per year of hip fracture. Estimated costs are $4 to $10 billion per year for patients with symptomatic fractures. In many instances, death results from complications related to hip fracture; the mortality rate of those affected in the first year postfracture are 12% to 20% higher than for matched populations without fracture.

Some of the risk factors for postmenopausal osteoporosis are listed in Table 14.1. Premenopausal peak bone mass may be related more directly to premenopausal estrogen exposure and genetic predisposition than to environmental factors.

ETIOLOGY/PATHOPHYSIOLOGY

Normally, the process of bone mineralization remodels 10% to 30% of the skeleton yearly. See Table 14.2.

Reduced bone mineralization is ubiquitous with age. Until early adulthood, more bone is built than absorbed. By the fourth decade, both men and women experience a gradual loss of bone. However, after menopause, women are six times more affected than men. Women lose 0.5% to 1% of their peak bone mass yearly for approximately 20 years after menopause. The rate of bone loss slows after the age of 65 years.

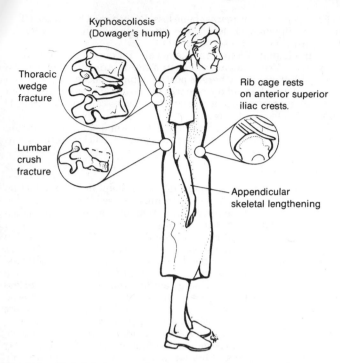

Fig. 14-1. Skeletal changes of postmenopausal osteoporosis.

Table 14.1. Some of the Risk Factors for Osteoporosis

Fair-skinned, white female
Positive family history
Thin, small-framed
Surgical removal of ovaries/early menopause
Endocrine disorders
Older than age 50
Smoking
Alcohol abuse
High-protein diet
Sedentary lifestyle

Table 14.2. Bone Mineralization Process

1. Osteoclasts absorb bone
2. Osteoblasts produce collagen matrix
3. Calcium and phosphorus crystals laid down in matrix

Estrogen protects against bone loss. Parathyroid hormone (PTH) and 1,25 dihydroxycholecalciferol are other contributing factors to bone formation and resorption.

An inadequate dietary intake of calcium may contribute to osteoporosis. Premenopausal calcium needs are considered to be 800 to 1000 mg/day, whereas postmenopausal needs are 1,200 to 1,500 mg/day. Secondary hyperparathyroidism may result from reduced absorption or increased excretion of calcium. Vitamin D deficiency also is a factor.

PTH levels increase when dietary calcium is deficient, calcium absorption is defective, or estrogen is absent. PTH maintains constant calcium plasma levels by depleting skeletal stores.

ASSESSMENT

Routine radiographic evaluation is not helpful in the detection of osteoporosis, because bone loss must exceed 30% before it becomes apparent. Bone mass measurement may be accomplished through the use of photon absorptiometry, which measures low-energy gamma rays of radionuclide through bone. Single-photon absorptiometry is used to evaluate the wrist or heel (cortical bone). Dual-photon absorptiometry (DPA) is used for spinal vertebra assessment. Ultrasound of the patella has been shown to measure a property of bone fragility that is distinct from bone mass; it is less expensive than DPA but is not widely used. Computed tomography (CT) scanning using a phantom device for comparison is more appropriate but has drawbacks of expense, radiation exposure, and availability. There is as yet no standard for bone mass measurement, and little to be gained by obtaining routine lateral x-ray films of the thoracic and lumbar spine. Dual x-ray or photon absorptiometry are common methods of evaluation.

Diagnosis is usually made on symptoms of gradual or sudden onset backache and/or change in bodily habitus. It may take up to 4 weeks for an acute compression fracture to become apparent on routine x-ray film. It is important that a timely diagnosis be made, so that bone trauma and resultant pain can be minimized, family members at risk can be followed, and other causes of bone loss such as osteomalacia can be eliminated. See Table 14.3.

EVALUATION

On physical examination, note general bodily habitus, kyphoscoliosis, and any other scoliosis. Usually there is not tenderness

Table 14.3.   Other Causes of Bone Loss
Osteomalacia
Hyperparathyroidism
Hyperthyroidism
Immobilization
Multiple myeloma
Metastatic carcinoma
Chronic anemia

ectly over the vertebral spinous process. Cervical or lumbo-
cral paravertebral muscles may be in chronic spasm. Observe
,ait for shuffling or poor balance. A patient who has sustained a
recent vertebral fracture may be unable to sit or stand for a prolonged period because of pain. This pain may be radicular in a
thoracic pattern related to the level of the fractured vertebrae.

TREATMENT

Treatment encompasses two aspects: medications for those
known to be at risk and rehabilitative management of the patient
who has general back pain or who has experienced an acute spinal
vertebral fracture.

Drug Therapy

The two main objectives are to decrease the rate of bone loss
and increase the rate of new bone formation.

Estrogen replacement, given as cyclic therapy (0.635 mg of con-
jugated estrogens for 21 days, followed by 7 days of progestin) is
recommended in the perimenopausal period. However, the protective effect may last only 2 to 3 years. There is little evidence
that it is helpful in osteoporotic women older than age 65. The
risk of endometrial cancer must be considered; however, progestins
may have a protective effect against breast cancer.

Calcitonin reduces bone turnover by inhibiting osteoclasts.
Salmon calcitonin, given as 50 to 100 units intramuscularly daily,
or human calcitonin, 0.5 mg intramuscularly every other day, is
commonly used. An intranasal calcitonin spray may also be used
in some cases. Calcitonin is used for therapy of diagnosed osteoporosis; its use in prevention is under investigation.

Use of supplemental calcium is controversial. Typical diets do
not provide the 1,500 mg/day postmenopausal requirement. Caution must be used in patients who are known to form kidney
stones. There may be poor intestinal absorption of sufficiently
provided dietary calcium in the aged patient.

Vitamin D should be supplemented only if the patient is deficient. Do not use combination calcium/vitamin D tablets; the
ratio may lead to vitamin D toxicity. The recommended dosage
of vitamin D is 400 to 800 units per day. Some sources advocate 5
to 10 minutes of sunshine three times per week, rather than supplementation. Use of calcitrol, the biologically active vitamin D
metabolite, is controversial, and requires further research.

Fluoride therapy is used to stimulate new bone formation.
Given as sodium fluoride, 40 to 100 mg/day, the larger doses result in fragile bone formation, which is more likely to fracture.
Side effects include gastrointestinal (GI) disturbances, inflamed
joints, recurrent vomiting, and anemia. Do not use this as a routine treatment. Sodium fluoride is not approved by the Food
and Drug Administration (FDA) for treatment of osteoporosis
at this time.

Etidronate (Didronel) administered orally on an intermittent,
cyclic basis has been shown in some studies to increase bone mineral content and decrease the rate of new vertebral fractures. Coherence therapy, known as activate, depress, free, repeat (ADFR)
involves use of oral phosphate as an activator of bone remodeling,
followed by etidronate, and finally a drug-free period of several

weeks. The cycle is then repeated. This method is still unde. going study.

In hypertensive women at risk, another consideration is the use of thiazide diuretics that lead to tubular reabsorption of calcium. Adequate clinical studies have not yet established the role of these medications.

Use of anabolic steroids for osteoporosis requires further study and should be avoided, because of androgenic effects and problems associated with liver function and plasma lipoproteins.

Alendronate sodium (Fosamax), an antiresorptive, normalizes the rate of bone turnover and increases bone mass, especially in the lumbar spine. Patient compliance with administration is critical because of the risk of esophageal irritation. Use of risedronate (Actonel), 5 mg per day, in women with postmenopausal osteoporosis has been shown to decrease fracture incidence.

Rehabilitative Treatment

Chronic back pain may result from compression fractures or kyphotic/scoliotic changes. Posture can be addressed by several means. A posture training support (PTS) by CAMP may be used to improve posture in an effort to prevent or lessen osteoporotic skeletal problems. See Fig. 14-2. For more involved cases, a back support device can be used, such as a semirigid dorsolumbar support with shoulder straps or a custom-made jacket. Proper back exercises emphasize extension and omit flexion maneuvers. See Figs. 14-3 and 14-4. Chronic pain management techniques may be helpful. See Chapter 8.

Acute back pain secondary to osteoporotic vertebral fracture follows a typical course, shown in Table 14.4. General preventive measures are shown in Table 14.5.

Severe kyphotic posture causes fatigue easily because of ligamentous stretch and reduced vital capacity. A back support device should be worn. Stooping should be discouraged. Chest expansion may be improved by deep breathing exercises, pectoral stretching, and thoracic spine extension.

OUTCOMES

The typical postmenopausal osteoporotic woman is at great risk for fracture-related complications. However, these can be minimized with patient education and appropriate drug therapy where indicated. Women at risk should be followed perimenopausally to assess the need for estrogen replacement. Encourage young women to routinely perform weight-bearing exercises and obtain sufficient daily amounts of dietary calcium.

FOLLOW-UP

The patient with postmenopausal osteoporosis requires intermittent follow-up for management of sporadic acute injuries, prescription of therapies, and instruction in appropriate exercises. Routine plain x-ray films are not indicated. Ongoing patient education and psychologic support is necessary.

ACKNOWLEDGMENT

With grateful acknowledgment to Mehrsheed Sinaki, MD, MS for her revisions to this chapter.

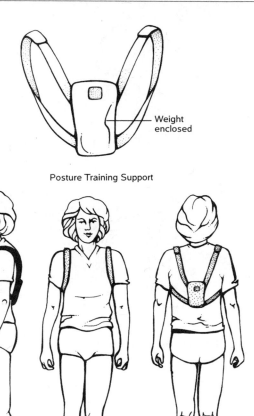

Posture Training Support

Fig. 14-2. Posture training support by CAMP.

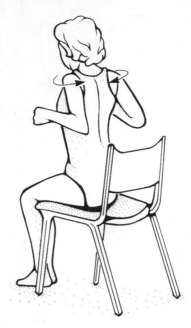

Fig. 14-3.   Seated position: back extension exercise.

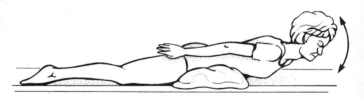

Fig. 14-4.   Prone position: back extension exercise.

Table 14.4.   Acute Back Pain

Bed rest (position of comfort) 7–14 days
Hospitalization not usually required
Analgesics, including oral narcotics for severe pain or non-
    steroidal antiinflammatory drugs for mild to moderate pain
Modalities: heat, massage, TENS
Back support
Cane in opposite hand if pain unilateral

TENS, transcutaneous electrical nerve stimulation.

Table 14.5. Osteoporosis: General Preventive Measures

Avoid heavy lifting and bending
Proper shoes: rubber heels or cushion soles; avoid high heels
Use cane for stability
Weight-bearing exercise throughout life (walking, bicycling)
Appropriate drug therapy
Proper nutrition

SUGGESTED READINGS

Ambrus JL, Hoffman M, Ambrus CM, et al. Prevention and treatment of osteoporosis. One of the most frequent disorders in American women: a review. *J Med* 1992;23:369–388.

Armamento-Villareal R, Villareal DT, Avioli LV, et al. Estrogen status and heredity are major determinants of premenopausal bone mass. *J Clin Invest* 1992;90:2464–2471.

Avioli LV. Significance of osteoporosis: a growing international health care problem. *Calcif Tissue Int* 1991;49:S5–7.

Avioli LV. Osteoporosis syndromes: patient selection for calcitonin therapy. *Geriatrics* 1992;47:58–67.

Brixen K, Nielsen HK, Charles P, et al. Effects of a short course of oral phosphate treatment on serum parathyroid hormone (1-84) and biochemical markers of bone turnover: a dose-response study. *Calcif Tissue Int* 1992;51:276–281.

Felson DT, Sloutskis D, Anderson JJ, et al. Thiazide diuretics and the risk of hip fracture. *JAMA* 1991;265:370–373.

Heaney RP, Avioli LV, Chesnut CH, et al. Osteoporotic bone fragility. *JAMA* 1989;261:2986–2990.

Melton LJ, Chrischilles EA, Cooper C, et al. Perspective: how many women have osteoporosis? *J Bone Miner Res* 1992;7:1005–1010.

National Institutes of Health Consensus Development Panel: Osteoporosis. *JAMA* 1984;262:799–802.

Pacifici R, McMurtry C, Vered I, et al. Coherence therapy does not prevent axial bone loss in osteoporotic women: a preliminary comparative study. *J Clin Endocrinol Metab* 1988;66:747–753.

Simmons JW, Norwood SM. Calcitonin and osteoporosis. New mechanisms of pathophysiology. *Orthop Rev* 1987;16:718–725.

Sinaki M. Prevention and treatment of osteoporosis. In: Braddom R, ed. *Physical medicine and rehabilitation.* Philadelphia: WB Saunders, 2000:894–912.

Sinaki M, Nicholas JJ. Metabolic bone diseases and aging. In: Felsenthal G, Garrison SJ, Steinberg FU, eds. *Rehabilitation of the aging and elderly patient.* Baltimore: Williams & Wilkins, 1994: 107–122.

Sinaki M, Wahner HW, Offord KP et al. Efficacy of nonloading exercises in prevention of vertebral bone loss in postmenopausal women: a controlled trial. *Mayo Clin Proc* 1989;64:762.

Storm T, Thamsborg G, Steiniche T et al. Effect of intermittent cyclical etidronate therapy on bone mass and fracture rate in women with postmenopausal osteoporosis. *N Engl J Med* 1990;322:1265.

Pediatric Rehabilitation Medicine

Margaret A. Turk

Rehabilitation management of children with physical and cognitive impairments is a challenge that requires integration of the identification of functional capabilities, the selection of the best intervention strategies, an understanding of growth and development, and an appreciation of the continuum of care. Some of the more frequently encountered disabling conditions of childhood treated by physiatrists are cerebral palsy (CP) and other brain injury, spina bifida (SB) and other spinal cord dysfunction/injury, developmental delays, muscular dystrophy, congenital brachial plexus palsy, and hypotonia. This chapter provides general information regarding the diagnosis and management of children with disabilities, with specific information about the two most common reasons for referral to a pediatric physiatrist, CP and SB.

General rehabilitation and evaluation principles are the cornerstone of management. However, keep in mind the following aspects of pediatric rehabilitation medicine that are unique to treating children:

- Do not treat children as though they are little adults. Awareness of normal development and understanding age-appropriate emotional needs are essential for therapeutic interactions with children with disabilities and their families.
- Use knowledge of normal growth patterns, functional developmental milestones, and possible deviations for diagnosis and for development of a comprehensive treatment plan to facilitate achieving the maximal functional status of each child.
- Monitor general health and functional status for both improvement and decline of skills. This also includes recognition of common complications, associated conditions, or secondary conditions. Prevention strategies may be helpful.

  - Childhood disabilities or illnesses can affect growth. There may be generalized growth retardation because of failure to thrive, oral motor dysfunction, endocrine abnormalities, or anticipated short stature (e.g., Down syndrome, CP).
  - Chronic constipation and gastroesophageal (GE) reflux are common in children with multiple disabilities and chronic conditions.
  - Asymmetric motor control and function may produce significant leg and arm length discrepancies. With awareness of growth trends and radiographic bone age determination, changes in orthoses, wheelchairs, and devices can be planned, as can timing for treatment of leg length discrepancies or scoliosis.
  - Significant loss of skills should not be anticipated in childhood onset disabilities, unless the diagnosis is one of the pro-

gressive disorders. Any unanticipated loss of skill at any age
must be evaluated.

–Secondary osteoporosis (immobility osteoporosis) is only now
being recognized as a common secondary condition for children with motor impairments. At present, there are no studies that suggest specific interventions (including supported
standing); however, adequate dietary calcium and vitamin D
should be maintained.

–Strengthening exercises are important to maintain and improve function. Children with spasticity or weakness can participate in these exercises, although appropriate modifications
may be needed and precautions taken. Adaptive sports and
recreation should be considered. Promoting a routine activity
program early in life may increase the chances of continuing
that activity into adulthood.

–Psychosocial development should also be monitored. Issues
of sexuality and sexual functioning must be addressed in
adolescents with disabilities.

- Use age-appropriate assessment and measurement tools to
  evaluate functional status or outcomes of interventions.
- Remember that rehabilitation of children, in contrast to that
  of adults, is often focused on *new* learning of appropriate
  motor and social skills appropriate for their age or developmental level, through use of adaptive strategies and functional
  capabilities.
- Educate parents and care providers not only about the disabling condition of their child but also about what constitutes
  a therapeutic environment.
- Recognize that there is three-way communication (child,
  parent/care provider, physician) in the typical patient-physician
  relationship for a child with a disability. During adolescence
  the relationship may begin to become more traditional, and by
  young adulthood the clinician must request permission to
  share information with parents and care providers.
- Acknowledge that interventions and attitudes promoted during childhood will have effects on adult functioning and self-
  assessment of capabilities, in a positive and negative manner.
- Use federal and state laws to ensure appropriate medical,
  rehabilitation, and education services for children with disabilities.
- Treat adults with childhood-onset disabilities first and fore-
  most as adults.

GENERAL PEDIATRIC REHABILITATION
MEDICINE COMPONENTS

Diagnosis and Assessment

Children with motor abnormalities, developmental delays, and
disabilities are referred to the physiatrist for diagnosis as well as
for development of a rehabilitation plan. A complete history must
include prenatal, natal, and perinatal information; developmental
skill attainment; a family history; details of the illness or injury
causing the disability; premorbid functional level when appropriate; and general observations or concerns of the family (Table 15.1).
Information regarding the attainment of developmental milestones
is a useful tool in determining a diagnosis. Achieving head control

Table 15.1. Information Often Reported by Careprovider Indicating Possible Motor Disorder in Infants and Toddlers

Report of Careprovider	Development History
Irritable	1. Nonsequential development
No cuddling—stiff	"Head control" using extension
or arches back	<2 mo
Startles or is jittery	Rolls with extensor posturing
Favors one side	<3 mo old
Floppy; held in vertical,	Head and chest up on forearms
"slips" through hands	in prone prior to head control
Problems with feeding	Walking with support before
Early head control	crawling
Keeps hands fisted	2. Developmental delay
"Scissors" when held vertical	
"W" sits	
Stands or walks on toes	

is a common milestone evaluated in infants; delay in attaining head control can be a marker for pathology of either the peripheral nervous system or central nervous system (CNS). In older infants and toddlers, motor skill attainment can provide insight into motor control and weakness; attainment of hand dominance, coordination, transitions, and walking skills offer insights into causes of delays.

A physical examination requires observation of function as well as a hands-on examination. Observations can be made while taking the history, which allows the infant or child (and parent) to become comfortable. The examination is both passive (e.g., tendon and primitive reflexes, tone assessment, and passive range of motion) and active (e.g., strength, movement patterns and motor control, posture, functional capabilities, and gait). Knowledge of normal growth and development patterns, possible deviations, and presentation of typical pediatric diagnoses is helpful. The examination is organized by the history, observations made, and the differential diagnosis developed.

In the infant, use of developmental reflexes is a practical method of evaluating function. Asymmetry of primitive reflexes can denote focal weakness, as in a brachial plexus injury. Generalized hypotonia can be documented with absence of or limitation in typical reflexes (Moro reflex) or delay in onset of expected reflexes (body righting reflex). Persistence of reflexes denotes delay in maturation of central motor control and emergence of postural reflexes (Table 15.2).

Demonstration of reported skill attainment allows observation of quality of movements and provides information regarding focal and generalized problems. The presence of a Gower sign denotes proximal weakness. Using extension of lower limbs to achieve standing indicates hypertonia. "W" sitting shows the need to maintain a wider base of support for limited trunk control from hypotonic or

Table 15.2. Primitive and Postural Reflexes

Reflex	Onset	Persistence
Primitive reflexes		
• Moro	Birth	Fades 4–6 mo
• Asymmetric tonic neck (ATNR)	Birth	Fades 6–7 mo
• Symmetric tonic neck (STNR)	Birth	Fades 6–7 mo
• Palmar grasp	Birth	Fades 5 mo
• Plantar grasp	Birth	Fades 12–14 mo
• Automatic walking	Birth	Fades 3–4 mo
Postural reflexes		
• Head righting prone	2 mo	Persists with volition
• Head righting supine	3–4 mo	Persists with volition
• Body righting	4–6 mo	Persists with volition
• Protective extension responses	Sit: forward 5–7 mo	Persists with volition
	Sit: lateral 6–8 mo	
	Sit: backward 7–8 mo	
	Stand: 12–14 mo	
• Equilibrium reactions	Sitting 6–8 mo	Persists with volition
	Standing 12–14 mo	

hypertonic conditions. Coordination assessment is by observation of gross and fine motor skills in children younger than 2 to 3 years; at age 3 and older, the performance of complex tasks can be more qualitatively examined. The physical examination provides a basis for a differential diagnosis and directs a rehabilitation program.

Laboratory and radiologic testing can be employed. Electrodiagnostic studies (EDX) may also be indicated for diagnosis and prognosis. EDX can be particularly helpful in the management of neuropathies and other lower motor neuron pathologies, as in congenital brachial plexus injuries, congenital band entrapments, or arthrogryposis congenita multiplex.

There are a variety of standardized assessment tools used to identify delays in development. The Denver Developmental Screening Test may identify deviations in development, and, because it is a screen, further detailed and specific diagnostic testing is indicated. Other commonly used assessment tools include the Bayley II (developmental delay for 0 to 42 months of age), the Peabody Motor Scales (motor delay for 0 to 83 months), the Vineland Adaptive Behavior Scales (developmental delay and mental retardation for 0 to 19 years), and the Hawaii Early Learning Profile (developmental delay for 3 to 6 years). There are instruments developed for assessment and follow up of children with disabilities. The Gross Motor Function Measure (GMFM) was developed specifically to measure change over time in children with CP, ages 5 months to 16 years of age. The Pediatric Evaluation of Disability Inventory (PEDI) identifies functional limitations and disabilities in age-appropriate independence skills for children ages 6 months to 7.5 years. The WeeFIM (Pediatric Functional Independence Measure) measures burden of care in ages 6 months to 12 years and can track outcomes across health, development, and community settings.

Comprehensive evaluations of the child with a disability are multidisciplinary. In addition to the physiatric history and examination, functional assessment using standard tools is done, general therapist assessments are completed, vision and hearing may be evaluated, and intellectual level or learning capability is assessed. This comprehensive approach is needed to establish a treatment plan. The plan must be goal directed.

Medical management may also require a team approach, particularly for children with associated conditions, pathologies, and impairments. Contact with the primary care provider allows an encompassing management of health and rehabilitation.

Therapy Settings

Therapy services may be provided in a typical hospital or clinic setting, particularly when only one discipline is involved. However, more commonly, therapy services involve many disciplines and require a team involvement, often in more educational or home settings. Infants and children receive services in a variety of settings that support other age-appropriate needs. Therapy can be provided in a typical outpatient setting, and when single services are prescribed, they are often provided in that setting. However, more commonly, and in particular when multiple services are required, home or school settings are available.

Early intervention (EI) is a family-centered system of programs, mandated by the federal government, for children 0 to 3 years old with developmental delay. The program provides parent education for managing the child at home, support for coping and improved infant-caregiver interaction, and treatment to promote developmental skills. The EI team is composed of education and medical professionals; developmental assessments are completed and tied to goals determined by the professionals and the family. Therapists provide hands-on treatment and instruct the family or caregivers in positioning and handling techniques to promote developmental progress. The programs are effective in supporting families and minimizing complications. It is not scientifically supported that the programs prevent disability or produce brain reorganization in the presence of CNS injury.

Preschool programs can support therapy and training programs, and children with disabilities are often encouraged to participate in segregated (preschools developed for children with disabilities) or inclusive (preschool programs not directed to children with disabilities but that encourage consult or direct therapy within their setting) programs. Therapy goals are directed to mobility, age-appropriate self-care (including feeding, drooling, and toileting), play, and family involvement.

School programs are mandated by federal law to provide education programs with needed support personnel, resources, and facilities to children with handicapping conditions and within the least restrictive environment. Local school systems' responses to this mandate and their options for support differ from region to region and may not be consistent even within a single state. However, there is a committee on special education (CSE) within each system, and routine meetings are held among school staff, families, and advocates or consultants to determine goals and services. Therapy goals for school-aged children with disabilities who are in mainstream inclusive programs are geared to function and participation in school activities. Children with more severe disabilities are provided services to encourage basic developmental function. Cognitive and learning impairments resulting from brain injuries may be supported with typical programs for learning disabilities and may also involve occupational and speech and language therapies. In the adolescent and teenage years, the focus of the program may change from an academic approach to a transitioning approach, which encourages life skills or vocational opportunities. Any change to the program requires review and a vote at the CSE; the parent or guardian is an active participant of the committee. Services are provided until age 21.

Rehabilitation Services

Treatment programs should be goal directed. There may be multiple therapies involved or focused to one discipline, depending on the impairments and treatment goals. The pediatric physiatrist should have a global view of the rehabilitation plan (Fig. 15-1) to ensure that all elements support functional progress. Basic health and general rehabilitation goals must precede special-

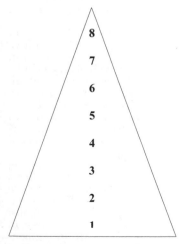

8. **Skill Acquisition/Motor Control** CI, FES, sEMG, facilitation
7. **Endurance**-practice, home program, repetition in contexts, sports
6. **Balance**-aquatic therapy, NMES, assisted weight bearing
5. **Strength**-TES, NMES, resistance exercises, aquatic therapy, sports
4. **Flexibility**-positioning, stretching, massage, aquatic therapy, tone management
3. **Maintain Biomechanics**- orthotics casting, BTX, surgery, TES, NMES
2. **Diet** – Nutritional assessment, G-tube, weight management
1. **Rest and Regeneration** – Goal setting, tone management, interval therapy

Fig. 15-1. Pyramid of rehabilitation care. Adapted from Logan L. Facts and myths about therapeutic interventions in cerebral palsy: integrated goal development. *Phys Med Rehab Clin N Am* 2002;13:979–989.

ized motor control skill goals. The child and family should be a part of goal determination and prioritization.

There are **systems of therapy** that have been developed for children in certain diagnostic groups, particularly children with CP or other neurologic conditions (Table 15.3). These systems have been developed empirically using theoretic constructs to explain clinical observation, but there is little evidence to support any one method in particular. The most commonly employed system is the Bobath or neurodevelopmental treatment (NDT) approach, in which the goals are to promote typical developmental progress, maintain biomechanical alignment, and facilitate automatic movement reactions. Although NDT was initially developed for use in children and adults with CP or hemiplegia, its use has expanded to other neurologic conditions. NDT promotes positioning and movement to decrease hypertonicity, while assisting development of fundamental movement patterns. Movements are controlled proximally while stressing rotation and balance in antigravity posture. Techniques are also employed for oral motor control in feeding and articulation. Most therapeutic programs involve a combination of therapy systems with other techniques and functional approaches.

Traditional exercises such as strengthening, stretching, endurance, coordination, and balance are modified for developmental levels. For the younger child, play, adaptive toys, and games can provide strengthening, coordination, and balance activities. Strengthening exercises are appropriate for all disabilities, although limitations, types of exercises, and expected outcomes must be defined. Flexibility exercises are also a part of the program, and parents are often instructed in these exercises early in a therapy program (Fig. 15-2). Use of modalities may be helpful for flexibility, particularly for children with joint diseases. Documentation of strength, range of motion, endurance, balance, and coordination allows assessment of the therapy program and need for possible changes.

Functional training programs use motor learning theories and strategies and focus activities on clear goals. The cognitive level and learning styles of each child must be taken into account. Motor activities may be broken down into individual components; instruction, modeling, and repetition of the components and full task may allow a more coordinated and automatic motor performance. Feedback can be provided verbally and visually. Therefore, purposeful routine age-appropriate activities coupled with clear instructions and explanations of expectations are the cornerstone of this approach. This strategy is used for a variety of motor tasks such as self-care, transfers, and walking.

Modalities can be used with children. Heat and ice can be useful for stretching activities and for pain management. Biofeedback or surface electromyography (sEMG) may be used to improve motor control in a variety of conditions such as CP, Guillain-Barré, brachial plexus injuries, and spinal cord dysfunctions. Neuromuscular electrical stimulation (NMES) can be used in children as young as 18 months of age to assist with strengthening and motor control; a trigger switch can be particularly effective in gait training. Reciprocal stimulation of agonists and antagonists can be helpful in spasticity, but the effect may not be long lasting. Threshold electrical stimulation (TES), a low-

**Table 15.3. Common Systems of
Therapy in Pediatric Rehabilitation**

Treatment Approach	Candidates for Treatment	Features of Treatment
Phelps method	Children with neurologic conditions	Combined treatments for polio with movement patterns, tone reduction; extensive bracing and use of adaptive equipment; emphasis on self-help skills
Deaver method	Children with disabilities	Bracing to limit all but 2 motions of a limb; voluntary motion to perform ADLs; use of assistive devices
Rood	Any age with neurologic conditions	Linking sensory and motor systems; stimulation with brushing, ice to activate, facilitate, or inhibit; goal for movement and posture to be automatic
Neuro-developmental treatment (NDT)	Any age with CP or other neurologic conditions	Goals to promote typical development progress, maintain biomechanical alignment, facilitate automatic movement reactions; kinesthetic feedback by handling; family involvement with carryover into ADLs and home activities
Sensory integration (SI)	Preschool and school-aged children with learning disabilities or autism	Techniques focus on providing appropriate and varied types of sensory experiences (e.g., tactile, proprioceptive, kinesthetic, visual, auditory) to facilitate controlled motor output
Conductive education (CE)	Preschool/school-aged children with CP or other neurologic conditions	Integration of education and therapy approaches using verbal, sequence, and rhythm reinforcement to facilitate motor responses

continued

Table 15.3. *Continued*

Treatment Approach	Candidates for Treatment	Features of Treatment
Constraint-induced therapy (CI)	Any age, neurologically based asymmetric function, able to tolerate constraint of the more functional limb	Restraining the more functional upper limb promotes function and use of the less functional limb
Locomotor training	>2 years old with walking impairment	Partial body support with mobile or stationary body harness to facilitate walking
Doman-Delacato method	Any age with CP or other neurologic condition	Theory is that passive primitive patterned movements applied regularly through day improves motor development; involves periods of rebreathing CO_2, fluid restrictions, and assisted breathing to ↑ cerebral O_2; remains controversial
Vojta method	Any age with CP	Activating reflex movement and locomotion allows development of normal sequential mobility and posture; subcortical brain holds these patterns

ADLs, activities of daily living; CP, cerebral palsy.

intensity nighttime stimulation, has been used to promote motor function, particularly of trunk and proximal musculature in children with CP.

Children with disabilities should be encouraged to engage in a **routine exercise** program, particularly as they approach adolescence. The routine activities in which some children with disabilities engage (e.g., walking or propelling their wheelchairs) cannot be equated to routine exercise programs in which their nondisabled peers engage. Children with disabilities maintain their level of performance but do not challenge their cardiovascular or musculoskeletal systems to improve their level of performance or prepare for unexpected challenges with routine activities. Specific interventions must be instituted to provide these challenges. Exercise

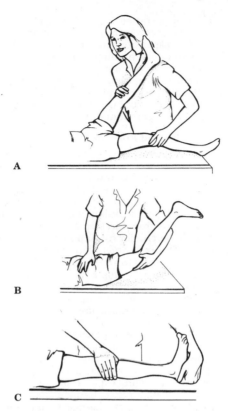

Fig. 15-2. **Passive stretching of the lower limb. A: Hamstrings (stabilize opposite limb) B: Iliotibial band (stabilize pelvis) C: Heel cord (keep knee extended). (Adapted from Vignos PJ. Rehabilitation in progressive muscular dystrophy. In Lichr S, ed. _Rehabilitation and medicine._ New Haven, CT: Elizabeth Lichr, 1958, with permission.)**

programs can be as varied for children with disabilities as they are for those without disabilities. Routine strengthening or conditioning can be home, school, or health club based. Recreational and sports activities should be promoted; many regions have adapted sports and recreation programs, and individual adaptations can be made as well. A few examples are swimming or aquatic therapy to allow flexibility, strengthening, and functional programs and rollerblading to increase proximal strength. Exercise programs should be designed to maintain or increase the endurance required to accomplish daily activities through the growth period.

Parental involvement in the rehabilitation program is key. Parents provide the day-to-day carryover of therapy programs. Beginning in the EI programs, parents are instructed in a variety of handling techniques, functional strategies, and exercises. They also provide the transportation to medical, therapy, and recreational programs outside of routine school activities. Parents have the expected parent responsibilities of providing structure and routine for their families, maintaining appropriate living arrangements, and providing all other support activities. Consequently it is important to recognize that labor-intensive therapy activities may not receive the high priority placed by the therapeutic team. Goals should be decided on and prioritized by the rehabilitation team, which includes the parent and child.

Equipment for Health and Function

Many pieces of equipment are available and/or requested for the care and rehabilitation of a child with a disability. Many children requiring high **medical technology** are now supported in a home environment. Pulmonary and nutritional support equipment can be safely and competently used and serviced within homes. This requires family training, home nursing, prevention strategies, maintenance procedures, and back-up plans.

Equipment may be helpful for **hygiene and day-to-day care.** There are a variety of bathing and toileting devices available, appropriate for specific age and functional needs. Transfer aids are helpful for the adolescent or young adult who can provide minimal to no assistance. Hospital beds may not be required; however, use of railings or other bed adjustments can prevent falls. Mattresses to better distribute pressure may be indicated for children who are unable to change their own bed position or are at risk for pressure sores. Modifications to highchairs may be required to provide trunk support or to inhibit tone and allow dining with the family. Car seats provide safety in transportation.

Positioning devices may provide age-appropriate supported positions to allow environmental exploration and promote general development. Corner seats, Preston feeder seats, or Rifton chairs may be prescribed depending on the needs and function of the child. Supported standing devices (e.g., prone standers, supine standers, standing tables and frames) are often used in therapy programs, with goals of improving head or trunk support, improving upper limb function, or the like. They do allow a different position for function and possibly provide a prolonged stretch of tight muscles to manage contractures but have no proven influence on bone density or growth, cardiopulmonary function, urinary function, or gastrointestinal function. Children who require significant support because of contractures with hypertonia or hypotonia may require more specialized positioning devices.

Children with delayed motor development may benefit from some type of **wheeled mobility.** Goals for use of the device should be defined: enhance function, provide support, allow exploration of the environment, limit deformity, and provide safe transportation. The prescribing physician must understand the features and problems of the device, the function and prognosis of the patient, the community and family issues, and the funding restrictions; decisions require discussion with patient, family, therapists, and other care providers. Prolonged use of strollers should be avoided, but, if they must be used, modifications should provide a good base of support and needed head and trunk support. Child-sized wheelchairs are available from a number of manufacturers, and prescription depends on function and growth expectation. The goals of seating inserts are to provide support and enhance function rather than to correct deformities. When choosing a dependent mobility base, the needs of the child and primary care provider must be considered. Children with good trunk and upper limb strength and control can achieve high performance in wheelchairs similar to adults. Therefore, the frame (e.g., lightweight vs. standard) and the child's position in a manual wheelchair (e.g., best access to the hand rims) should be considered. Power mobility should be considered for young children to allow independence and promote self-initiated behaviors. Children as young as 24 months can learn to safely propel power wheelchairs. Wheelchair safety includes frame/base maintenance, adjustments for growth, good judgment for modifications, and car/bus security.

Orthoses are commonly considered for children with disabilities. There are a variety of types of ankle foot orthoses (AFOs) that can be prescribed. Besides the traditional solid ankle AFOs, there are dynamic AFOs (DAFOs), spiral AFOs, articulating AFOs (that can be fitted with posterior or anterior stops), and floor reaction AFOs, and others. Supramalleolar foot orthoses (SMOs) have trimlines that provide medial-lateral stability, but allow ankle dorsiflexion and plantar flexion. Footplates providing tone reduction or support may be incorporated into the braces or may be used as foot orthoses (FOs) or shoe inserts. KAFOs (knee-ankle-foot orthoses) or HKAFOs (hip-knee-ankle-foot orthoses) are prescribed for children with weakness that requires knee and/or hip control; the parapodium was developed for children with SB and provides trunk through lower limb support. A sitting, walking, and standing hip (SWASH) orthosis has been used successfully to support the pelvis in sitting or to maintain hip abduction in walking or standing; use of AFOs with the SWASH is usually not recommended. Thoracolumbosacral orthoses (TLSOs) may provide trunk support, but their ability to limit progression of neuromuscular scoliotic curves has been questioned. Limiting trunk flexibility with a TLSO potentially reduces some independent functional skills (e.g., adjusting footrests, operating the brakes, propelling the wheelchair). For children with torticollis and/or plagiocephaly, there is information to support use of a molding helmet before age 12 months or closure of the calvarial sutures and a tubular orthosis for torticollis (TOT) for active neck positioning once head control has been achieved; both require appropriate measurement and fitting.

There are a variety of **walking aids.** Walkers are commonly used for children with motor impairments first beginning to walk. The traditional anterior walker requiring pushing may be used; however, a posterior walker promotes trunk extension that is an important consideration for children with CP in particular. Walkers can be adjusted and modified with forearm supports, seats, wheels with and without locks, and brakes. Canes and crutches should be considered for use at age and function appropriate times.

Splints are often fabricated for upper limb and hand positioning; however, they usually provide only passive support and in and of themselves usually do not limit progression of deformities. Aside from burn management in children, splinting has not been evaluated well. Thumb-in-palm deformities seen in congenital hydrocephalus or spastic CP may respond to soft splints, neoprene sleeves, or kineseotape that allow hand function and prehension with sensory feedback. Goals for splinting should be defined and revisited to ensure usefulness.

Assistive devices include high- and low-technology devices. Augmentative and alternative communication (AAC) devices are varied and features to consider are physical interface, communication output, and language features. The level of cognition, language development, and prognosis for skill acquisition must be taken into account in prescription. Adaptive interfaces have been developed to allow environmental control to maximize independence. High-technology devices obviously can be costly. High complexity of the device may limit its usefulness by the child or family. Users of AAC must be able to incorporate the device use in all levels of communication, which is difficult and often not successful.

Prostheses and their components should be prescribed with knowledge of available components and their features, of developmental skill attainment for timing of prescription, of the child's family and support, and of the fabrication and fitting issues. Many factors influence long-term use of a prosthesis. In general, the higher the limb deficiency, the less likely the child will find the prosthesis useful.

There is a variety of equipment available, and often multiple options may be useful in a single setting. The prescribing physician should use other professionals and consumers or their family members for information about possible alternatives. Decisions regarding equipment cannot be made in a void.

Psychosocial Issues

Psychosocial development in children with disabilities is influenced by a variety of factors. Individual characteristics such as cognition, coping strategies, personality, and self-esteem can affect or be affected by family relationships, peer relationships, societal attitudes, community resources, and education resources. Medical factors also influence psychosocial adjustment; the length and number of hospitalizations within the first 6 years of life have been shown to negatively correlate with self-esteem at age 12 years in children with SB. Issues of continence, independence in mobility, and ability to communicate and be understood may be barriers to socialization. Family support is pivotal to psychosocial adjustment, and the role of the family must change during transitions to adulthood.

Adolescents begin to ask questions about sexuality, and sex education should be available to them as it is to their nondisabled peers. Often adolescents and young adults with disabilities have limited opportunity for socialization and sexual activity. Adults with childhood onset disabilities often report fewer dating experiences or sexual encounters. They also report less use of contraception and protection with sex. Gynecologic examinations should proceed at an age-appropriate time, and positioning, technique, and accessibility must be taken into account.

Adult Issues

Adults with childhood-onset disabilities often report pain, fatigue, and change in function as their most important medical issues related to function. Although there may be a modest change in function with age for people with "nonprogressive" conditions, there should never be significant change in performance. Significant change necessitates medical evaluation.

Pain is the most common medical complaint, and cause of the pain must be determined. Musculoskeletal causes may relate to biomechanics and ergonomics, weakness, and overuse as it does in the general population. Radiculopathies and peripheral nerve entrapments must also be considered. Appropriate evaluation, diagnostic testing, and treatment should be afforded adults with childhood-onset disabilities just as it is for their nondisabled peers. There may need to be modifications to approaches because of positioning issues, hypertonia, and contractures. Manual medicine techniques, trigger point injections, epidural injections, and cognitive coping strategies all have been used successfully for pain management in appropriately selected adults with childhood-onset disabilities having pain complaints.

Osteoporosis (secondary or immobility) is likely common in adults with motor impairments. It obviously becomes a more important issue in the face of fracture management. Fractures are more commonly seen in limbs, often proximal long bones in those who do not walk. Prevention strategies such as adequate calcium and vitamin D intake, adjustment of transfer techniques, and modification to activities should be routine. DEXA scans can be done, but interpretation is not well defined because comparison is made to nondisabled norms at present. Significant osteoporosis has been treated with accepted interventions such as bisphosphonates.

Health promotion, especially exercise, should be offered to adults with disabilities. Exercise programs at home or in the community may prevent the typical complaints of pain and fatigue. Often aquatic programs allow more active exercise and movement. Exercise or recreational equipment can be modified.

CEREBRAL PALSY

Definition

CP is not a specific disease but refers to a group of nonprogressive disorders affecting motor function, movement, and posture. CP is the result of a developmental abnormality or a one-time nonprogressive injury to the immature brain (onset from conception to age 5 or 6 years). It is a lifelong motor dysfunction, although functional limitations can change over a lifetime because of growth and development. The incidence of CP is approximately 1 to 2 per 1,000 live births (about 3,500 new cases per year) and it is distributed equally between the sexes, among the races, and across national boundaries. CP is among the more common causes for motor disabilities in children and also in adults with congenital onset disabilities.

The manifestation of CP varies greatly, ranging from extremely mild motor control problems to almost total lack of voluntary motor control involving limbs, trunk, and head. The types of CP are described by the neurologic or physiologic pattern of muscle tone and topography of body dysfunction (Table 15.4), and relate to the location and extent of the nonprogressive lesion. Hyperto-

Table 15.4.	Classification of Cerebral Palsy
Physiologic	Hypertonia: Spasticity
	Dystonia
	Rigidity
	Ataxia
	Hypotonia
Topographic	Hemiparesis
	(Monoplegia—likely missed hemi)
	Diparesis
	Quadriparesis
	(Triparesis—most functional limb
	involved)
	(Double hemiparesis—upper limbs
	much more involved than lower limbs)

nia is the common abnormal muscle tone or physiologic pattern seen in CP and is defined by abnormal increased resistance to imposed movement about a joint. It is described as spasticity, dystonia, rigidity, or a combination of these. It is now more commonly believed that spasticity is often not isolated and that there is an associated dystonic feature or "posturing." Diplegia is the most common topographic presentation. Typical topographic presentations and anticipated outcomes for function are described in Table 15.5.

There are conditions commonly associated with CP (Table 15.6), which often influence classification by severity. A simple traditional system of severity uses mild (no limitations to typical activities), moderate [limitations in activities of daily living (ADLs) and possible use of assistive devices], and severe (moderate to severe limitations). The Gross Motor Functional Classification System (GMFCS) can be used to describe the functional capabilities of children from infancy to 12 years, over five levels (level I least involved) based on age-appropriate self-initiated movement with emphasis on trunk control through sitting and walking.

Risk Factors and Etiology

The causes of CP encompass all the causes of brain injury during the prenatal, perinatal, and postnatal periods. There is overwhelming evidence now that 70% to 80% of CP is prenatal in origin and often multifactorial. Prematurity is the most common risk factor for CP, with periventricular leukomalacia the pathology seen on diagnostic studies (Tables 15.7 and 15.8). The cause of CP is often unexplained in a large proportion of patients.

Diagnosis and Assessment

The diagnosis of CP is based on the history, clinical examination, and diagnostic studies when indicated. Taking a careful history of pregnancy, labor, delivery, and the immediate neonatal period provide information on risk factors for CP. A developmental history in a toddler or child gives insights on quality of motor

Table 15.5. CP Presentations and Anticipated Outcomes

Classification	Anticipated Outcome
Hemiparesis—same side upper and lower limb involvement	Walk by age 3 years Independent in ADLs High risk of seizures Less common cognitive problems Common shortened involved limbs Common contractures involved limbs
Diparesis—lower limbs involvement greater than upper limbs; may be asymmetric	Walking depends on motor development (trunk control, protective responses) and absence of primitive reflexes Walking expected if sitting by age 2 years or crawling by age 2.5 years Typical crouched gait Usually independent in ADLs Possible learning disabilities Seizures less common Hip pathology common; monitor for scoliosis Common equinovalgus ankle May choose wheelchair mobility
Quadriparesis—all four limbs involved; often hyptonic trunk with spastic limbs	Usually requires a wheelchair for mobility Usually dependent for many ADLs, or requires set-up to perform Seizures more common Cognitive and learning problems common Often dysarthria or feeding problems Common hip dislocation and scoliosis

ADLs, activities of daily living; CP, cerebral palsy.

control and age achievement of milestones. The clinical examination is tailored to the age of the child and includes an active (e.g., assessment of movement patterns, asymmetry of function, motor control, posture, functional capabilities, and gait) and passive [e.g., range of motion (ROM) to demonstrate limited range, contractures, or asymmetries; tone assessment with Ashworth or Tardieu; deep tendon reflexes (DTRs); and presence of primitive reflexes] evaluation. Often the infant with CP may be hypotonic, with spasticity developing by age 6 to 9 months, and athetosis or dystonia after a year of age. In general, a diagnosis of CP is suggested by failure to accomplish motor milestones at the expected time, persistence of primitive reflexes beyond the time at which they are expected to disappear, poor motor control or paucity of movement in affected limbs, and abnormal muscle tone in affected limbs. Often repeated examinations are required to make

Table 15.6. Conditions Associated with Cerebral Palsy (CP)

Mental retardation	Incidence ~ 50% (all levels); most common in quadriparesis
Seizures	Incidence ~ 50%; frequent in hemiparesis, common in quadriparesis
Poor nutrition	Associated with more severe presentations, quadriparesis with poor oral motor function, reflux
Gastrointestinal: reflux, constipation	Common in more severe presentations, especially quadriparesis
Visual impairment	Strabismus common Hemianopsia—consider in hemiparesis Visual perception—noted with learning
Hearing impairment	Higher risk when associated with infectious or hyperbilirubinemia etiology; associated with medications
Sensory impairment	Cortically mediated—more common in hemiparesis or quadriparesis; can be neglect or hypersensitivity
Pulmonary conditions	Associated with: prematurity (bronchopulmonary dysplasia); aspiration with significant oral motor dysfunction
Dental problems	Malocclusions associated with deformities; gingival hyperplasia associated with medications; enamel dysgenesis; caries seen with poor tolerance mouth care, feeding issues, drooling

the diagnosis, and by 8 months the presence of three or more abnormal signs in neurologic status, motor function, primitive reflexes, and posture is highly predictive of CP.

Laboratory tests and imaging can help categorize the type of CP, identify the cause, and sometimes predict the clinical course. The infant can be tested for metabolic, genetic, infectious, and endocrine etiologies. Ultrasound of the brain is most useful in the newborn period and commonly used in premature infants. A computed tomography (CT) scan of the brain may be helpful in diagnosing congenital malformations, hydrocephalus, and intracranial hemorrhages; a magnetic resonance imaging (MRI) allows better visualization of leukomalacia and other white matter changes; however, it is of limited use in premature infants. An electroencephalogram (EEG) is helpful if seizures are suspected. Evoked potentials (visual evoked potentials, brainstem evoked potentials) may assist in identifying and managing sensory deficits.

A comprehensive evaluation of the patient with CP is multidisciplinary, including health assessments, functional skills (motor and cognitive), sensory assessments, and family needs and support evaluations. General standardized scales as previously noted

Table 15.7. Risk Factors Associated with Cerebral Palsy (CP)

Time	Risk Factor
Pregnancy	Maternal medical problems/bleeding Multiple fetuses Poor maternal nutrition Infection Teratogens Genetic factors
Delivery	Fetal distress Multiple births Abnormal presentation
Neonatal	Prematurity Low birth weight Hypoxia Ischemia Intraventricular hemorrhage (IVH) Periventricular leukomalacia (PVL) Infection Chromosomal abnormalities

may be helpful, and instruments specific to CP can follow development and change with interventions, such as the GMFM. The GMFCS is used to describe and follow functional capabilities.

Medical Management

Associated conditions (Table 15.6) or their management can influence general health, ability to participate in rehabilitation strategies, prescription of equipment, and functional status. Nutritional status must be addressed routinely; children with significant impairments from CP commonly are undernourished and require tube feedings and fundoplications to maintain adequate nutrition and growth. There are some preventive strategies that can be initiated to influence other secondary conditions and health-related problems, particularly in the older child or young adult. Medications should be considered for the management of

Table 15.8. Pathologies for Cerebral Palsy (CP)

Prematurity—Periventricular leukomalacia
                    Periventricular hemorrhagic infarct
Malformations
Hypoxic ischemic encephalopathy
Stroke
Infection
Bilirubinemia (rare)
Unknown

seizures, drooling, and tone control (see later). More recently botulinum toxin injection (BTX) into the secretory glands has been studied to manage drooling.

There can be other medical comorbidities unrelated to the CP that can affect health and function.

Rehabilitation Management

Therapy Systems and Approaches

Therapy and rehabilitation programs for children with CP are often instituted early in life with EI. Programs will change with goal achievement and progress over time. A variety of methods and techniques (Table 15.3) can be employed, which are modified depending on the age and goals of the child. Selected components of many methods are often combined to develop an individualized goals directed rehabilitation program. In particular, NDT often comprises the base of therapy interventions for children with CP. Techniques can be applied to gross and fine motor tasks, as well as to oral motor functions.

More recent conceptualization of the motor impairment of CP includes tone abnormalities, insufficient force generation (weakness), abnormal extensibility, poor selective control and regulation of motor activity, and limited ability to learn unique movements. Consequently, more traditional therapy modalities are also included in the individualized therapy program. Strengthening activities such as progressive resistive, isometric, and isokinetic training programs can be employed to address the underlying weakness. Balance and coordination training should progress with repeated task practice. Functional training in needed daily activities (e.g., toileting, transfers, dressing) involves repetition and use of compensatory strategies. Kineseotaping has been used in conjunction with postural and functional activities and is tolerated better than traditional athletic taping. Constraint-induced therapy in children with hemiparetic CP has been studied, as has locomotor training with partial body weight support in children with diplegic and quadriparetic CP, both with success.

Electrical stimulation has gained some recent acceptance as a modality to consider for modifying hypertonia and enhancing motor function and control. NMES and sEMG can be used as it is in adult populations, to modulate spasticity, assist with strengthening, and initiate or trigger muscle groups for active use during function. It can be particularly effective in conjunction with tone-reduction techniques. TES continues to be more controversial but has been proven effective as an adjunct to posterior rhizotomy in decreasing tone and improving motor function.

Feeding problems can be assessed clinically, through a modified barium swallow study and with fiberoptic endoscopic evaluation of swallow (FEES). Clinical assessments can be effective, although silent aspiration should be considered with the history of recurrent pneumonias. Positioning, changes in textures and consistencies, use of adaptive feeding products, and method of presentation all can improve oral feeding. Oral motor control problems affecting feeding are usually noted within the first 3 to 6 months of life, and modifications of oral feeding should progress with improved motor control.

Communication problems may be related to decreased motor control problems (articulation, phonation, or breath control issues; see Table 15.9) or may be language based (cognitive or learning problems). Hearing also influences speech production, and hearing screens should be completed on children with delayed speech production. Speech and language therapies can assist with identification of limitations, direct work on motor or cognitive activities, or use of assistive devices.

Tone Management

Abnormal tone is the hallmark of CP. Hypertonia is the most common presentation, although a small percentage of children may be hypotonic or present initially with hypotonia. Hypertonia can be further described as spastic, dystonic, or rigid (Table 15.10). Management options are noted in Table 15.11. Often multiple techniques are used serially or as adjuncts to each other. Tone management should begin early and should change with improved motor control and improved function. Routine measures should be used to monitor progress and change. Range of motion

Table 15.9. Speech and Voice Disorders in Cerebral Palsy (CP)

Area of Control	Manifestation	Speech Production
Respiratory control	Rapid breathing	Infancy—lack of vocalization
	Shallow inspiration	Limited number of syllables per utterance
	Reduced exhalation	Poor initiation voice Unable to sustain vocalization
	Poor control respiratory muscles	Breaks in speech Unable to modulate loudness
Oral motor control	Limited control of lip closure, tongue placement, soft palate movement, jaw movement	Reduced articulation targets
	Poor control vocal folds	Breathy voice, hypernasality, or changes in pitch, loudness, quality during speech
	Increased body tension during phonation	Slow speech rate, "spastic dysarthria," facial grimacing with speech

Adapted from Molnar G, Alexander MA, eds. In: *Pediatric rehabilitation*, 3rd edition. Baltimore: Williams & Wilkins, 1999.

Table 15.10. Hypertonia

Spasticity	Dystonia	Rigidity
Increasing resistance with increasing velocity of stretch	Resistance at low velocity	Resistance at low velocity
	No change of resistance with direction	No change with speed or angle
Varies with direction of joint movement	Co-contraction with rapid reversal of direction immediate	Co-contraction with rapid reversal immediate
	Attains an involuntary posture	No involuntary posturing
Resistance rises rapidly above speed or joint angle threshold	Worsened with voluntary movement	
	Varies with arousal or emotion	

Adapted from Sanger TD, et al. Classification and definition of disorders causing hypertonia in childhood. *Pediatrics* 2003;111:89–97.

and the Ashworth and Tardieu scales offer passive measures; the GMFM, physiologic measures, motion analysis, and achievement of skills or goals provide active assessments.

Although tone can be modified, a change in functional activity cannot be expected, particularly without adjustment to existing programs or initiation of postintervention activities. Strengthening of agonist muscles requires the ability to activate those muscle groups. NMES can sometimes assist with strengthening programs, both through sensory feedback and activation. Use of casting, dynamic splints, or kinesotape may also be helpful. Selective dorsal rhizotomy (SDR) is the only management option that has identified the need for aggressive physical therapy (PT) following the procedure through research, although theoretically PT programs should be modified and possibly increased following any intervention. Braces likely requires changes.

Tone management must be considered in the treatment of pain complaints secondary to hypertonia. Painful dislocating hips often respond to oral medications or BTX, along with more standard pain management strategies. BTX to paraspinal muscles have also proven helpful in back pain management and positioning.

Mobility Aids: Orthotics and Wheelchairs

Orthotics should be prescribed with particular goals in mind. These may include providing optimal joint alignment, allowing selective motion, protecting weak muscles, preventing contractures, controlling abnormal tone and the associated deviations, enhancing function, and protecting postoperative results. AFOs are commonly prescribed for children with CP. A child with hypertonic diplegic CP with a typical crouched gait likely will not change to a foot flat gait with these AFOs. The braces can assist with tone modification and developmental progression and may

Table 15.11. Hypertonia Management in Cerebral Palsy (CP)

Intervention	Candidate	Side Effects	Postcare
Positioning or splinting	Generalized ↑ tone for positioning, focal for splints; any age	Not long-lasting	Monitor pressure areas, progression of contractures; may not enhance function
Oral medications	Generalized ↑ tone; any age usually ≥2 yr	Lethargy, ↑ drooling or change in feeding	Strengthening; adjustment to seating or switch use; adjustment therapy program
Intrathecal baclofen (ITB)	Generalized ↑ tone with reasonable trunk control; ~ age 4 yr or ≥ 40#; catheter tip placement dependent on upper limb involvement	Infection; spinal leaks; malfunction; reimplant ~ q 6 yrs; tied to medical center for refills	Therapy to achieve goals; change to seating, positioning, orthoses; strengthening
OT/PT/ST	Generalized or focal ↑ tone; goal dependent; any age	None	Focused on goals
Serial casting	Focal ↑ tone; usually used with other interventions (e.g., post-botulinum toxin injection) but can be done alone; any age	Pressure areas	Appropriate orthotic prescription to maintain correction and improved function; adjustment other devices; modify therapy program

continued

Table 15.11. *Continued*

Intervention	Candidate	Side Effects	Postcare
Botulinum toxin injections (BTX)	Focal ↑ tone; any age, typically beginning 12–18 mo	None; resistance possible if <3 mo between injections	Strengthening; NMES or surface EMG; orthoses, splints, casting; functional program; position change
Phenol injection	Focal ↑ tone; any age	Nerve block— dysesthesia with mixed nerves Motor point block— pain at site	Strengthening; NMES or surface EMG; orthoses, splints, casting; functional program; position change
Orthoses	Focal ↑ tone; any age	Pressure areas; changes for growth	Match choice of brace to goal
Selective dorsal rhizotomy (SDR)	Lower limb ↑ tone with good trunk control and strength, usually ages 4–7 yr	Infection; spinal leaks; urinary changes; long-term scoliosis development	Extensive PT/OT required; TES/NMES
Orthopedic surgery	Focal ↑ tone with deformity, contracture, or dislocation; any age usually > 4 yr	Infection; nonunion of bony surgeries; overcorrection; repeat may be needed if performed in younger age group	PT; position changes

EMG, electromyography; NMES, neuromuscular electrical stimulation; OT, occupational therapy; PT, physical therapy; TES, threshold electrical stimulation.

be more useful following tone management interventions. In particular, hypertonia responds well to footplates fabricated within the brace as is commonly seen with DAFOs and SMOs. When ankle deformity is present (e.g., ankle valgus secondary to a tight gastrocsoleus mechanism), serial casting before casting for the brace fabrication may allow a better fitting and more functional brace. Bracing principles used for lower motor neuron conditions likely will not be effective for children with CP.

HKAFOs or KAFOs are not usually prescribed for children with CP. Twister cables were designed many years ago to assist with hip abduction and foot eversion. However, they have fallen out of favor because their passive design does not provide long-lasting change in walking. A SWASH orthotic provides pelvis and hip support for sitting or walking, although long-lasting response to bracing alone is unknown. Use of posterior or reverse walkers promotes trunk extension, much needed for children with CP.

Mobility devices should be considered early. An appropriate prescription requires knowledge and understanding of the patient's function, growth potential, family concerns, and device features. Independence in mobility is associated with increased self-esteem; therefore, power mobility for children with CP may be considered at a young age. Inserts require routine adjustment.

Orthopedic Surgery Considerations

Surgical intervention was once central to the overall rehabilitation management of children with CP. Use of BTX and ITB has changed decision making regarding management of dynamic and static deformities and performance changes with age. Surgery continues to hold a place of importance, but interventions must be timed appropriately and goals must be clearly defined. Often, surgery is considered after tone management or positioning strategies have been used successfully for some time but can no longer maintain alignment or function. Therefore, in some centers, children receive surgery at older ages than had been seen previously.

Management of dislocating or dislocated hips may include adductor releases with more extensive reconstruction of femur and/or acetabulum. Painful dislocated hips are the most difficult to manage and require careful assessment. Femoral head resections or fusions often do not relieve the pain, and the residual deformity often limits positioning and function. Knee and ankle surgeries are directed to muscle imbalances. The knee flexion "crouched" gait seen in spastic diplegic CP may be managed with hamstring lengthening or tenotomy procedures. Surgical interventions at the ankle are designed to allow better heel strike at stance and include lengthening and muscle transfer techniques. Postoperative management includes casting for 6 to 8 weeks (knee surgeries usually are not casted), followed by progressive activity. Strengthening can improve outcomes significantly. Care must be taken to avoid overlengthening, which results in improved range of motion but limitation in function that cannot be corrected even with strengthening techniques. Bony surgeries (i.e., arthrodesis, osteotomy) may be considered in fixed or painful deformities, and cautious planning is advised. It is difficult to predict the outcomes of surgeries designed to improve walking. Gait analysis can be helpful; however, the underlying problems with motor control cannot always be factored in successfully. For those with CP with significant deformities limiting sitting, releases may allow better positioning. However, if the deformities are chronic, the rheologic properties of muscles may not allow significantly improved range, even with releases to joint structures.

Scoliosis is commonly seen in persons with CP who use a wheelchair for their functional positioning and as their mobility. Asymmetric muscle balance and control, limited postural control, and biomechanical and structural factors all contribute to the development and progression of scoliosis. Careful monitoring should occur particularly during times of growth. Orthoses may be considered but do not control the rotational component of the scoliosis and may limit function. There may be pain associated with significant curvatures and seating. Surgery is usually indicated with a severe curve of 40 or more degrees. The type of surgery, instrumentation, and approach are dependent on risk factors associated with anesthesia, infection, blood loss, type of deformity, or other features. Postoperative management includes changes to the seating insert and a strengthening or functional program when appropriate.

Upper limb surgeries are not commonly performed. Releases to allow improved positioning of wrist or fingers (i.e., finger flexion, thumb-in-palm) usually do not improve function because of underlying poor motor control and weakness, and contractures often recur. BTX to selected muscle groups, followed by casting and NMES, allows an opportunity to determine possible effectiveness of surgeries but also can be the only intervention required.

Adult Issues

Adults with CP are generally healthy, and there are no known comorbidities associated with the condition. There is a modest change in function noted with aging but no significant change. Change (especially increased use of wheelchair) is usually seen earlier than in the general population, often in the 20s and 30s. The common health conditions noted in adults with CP include pain and musculoskeletal complaints, bladder and bowel issues, and dental health problems. Pain is far and away the most problematic for adults.

Pain is more commonly seen in those who are more functional and have hypertonia. It is commonly seen in lower limbs and back. The pain is often called "arthritis" but in fact it is likely more muscle or soft tissue. Pain complaints require a standard evaluation and treatment program (Table 15.12). Cervical spine stenosis may go unrecognized because of the inaccurate assumption that adults with CP loose considerable function over time. Changes in motor function and control, increased spasticity, change in urinary habits, and pain must alert the physician to the possibility of stenosis. The stenosis can progress and early detection and surgical treatment will avoid permanent loss of function.

Secondary osteoporosis is seen in adults with CP although the specifics of risk factors, diagnosis, and treatment are not clear. The severity seems to relate to level of function and activity, medications, other medical conditions, and nutrition. At least traditional prevention strategies should be employed.

Adults with CP are married and have families; however, society often negates the sexuality and sexual function for them. They are often not provided with preventive health information regarding

**Table 15.12. Pain Etiologies in
Adults with Cerebral Palsy (CP)**

Etiology	Management
Musculoskeletal	Determine position causing discomfort
• Position	Determine task requirements, adjust position for function within capabilities
• Ergonomics	
• Overuse	Adjust position or task
• Weakness	Strengthening program
• Hypertonia	Tone management
• DJD	Standard pain management
	• Manual medicine
	• NSAIDs
	• Trigger point injections
	• Pain medications as appropriate
	• Cognitive coping strategies
	Aquatics therapy
	Joint replacement
Neurologic	Appropriate evaluation
• Radiculopathy	• x-rays and scans
	• Electrodiagnosis
• Peripheral nerve entrapment (CTS, ulnar at elbow or wrist)	Standard nonsurgical management
	Surgical management—requires planning for postop capabilities, possible rehabilitation admission
• Cervical spine stenosis	

CTS, carpal tunnel syndrome; DJD, degenerative joint disease; NSAIDs, nonsteroidal antiinflammatory drugs.

contraception or protection during sex. However, many have little sexual contact throughout life. There are no known differences from aging in sexuality or sexual functioning between adults with and without CP. Women may note an increase in or presence of incontinence at times during the menstrual cycle.

Health promotion should be supported. Because pain is the most common secondary condition, prevention strategies such as exercise should be promoted. Adults with CP do not necessarily require ongoing therapies but rather ongoing and routine exercises through a health club, at home, or through individual recreation choices.

SPINA BIFIDA

Definition

SB is a congenital abnormality of the spinal axis resulting in spinal cord dysfunction and, therefore, encompasses all the typical impairments seen in patients with spinal cord injuries. This dysraphism is subdivided into occulta or cystica lesions, as noted in Fig. 15-3. Along with the neural tube defect, there may also be an associated cephalic anterior neuropore abnormality giving rise to hydrocephalus and possibly resulting in brain dysfunction.

DYSRAPHISM & MYELODYSPLASIA

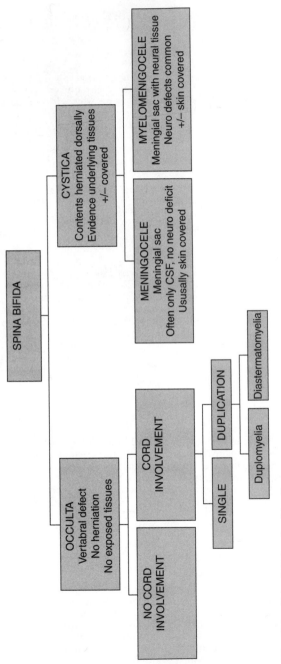

Fig. 15-3. Spina bifida: classification.

Table 15.13. CNS Conditions and Malformations Associated with Spina Bifida

Occulta	Cystica
Found in adulthood incidentally 5%–36%	Meningocele
	• <10%
No hydrocephalus, Arnold Chiari malformations	• No hydrocephalus
	• No neurologic signs
	• Follow for tethering
May be no neurologic symptoms	Myelomeningocele
	• Overwhelming majority
Commonly associated with nevus, dimple, hirsute patch, angioma, sinus tract	• Hydrocephalus 90%
	• Arnold Chiari II usual
	• Motor/sensory deficit; bladder/ bowel involvement
	• 75% at lumbar level
Follow for tethering	• Follow for tethering

CNS, central nervous system.

Other associated CNS conditions and malformations are noted in Table 15.13. The incidence has decreased from 1.31 per 1,000 in 1970 to 0.61 per 1,000 in 1989,

Risk Factors and Etiology

There is a polygenetically inherited predisposition to this malformation. The rate of occurrence is about 1:1,000 when there are no other family members affected, 5.5:100 after one affected child, 13:100 after two affected children, and 20.6:100 after three affected children. The female to male ratio is 1.2:1. Other risk factors are noted in Table 15.14. These factors likely act on the developing embryo until around the twenty-eighth day of gestation when the neural tube closes.

Table 15.14. Risk Factors for Spina Bifida

Genetic
- Familial (higher incidence Irish, German, Hispanic descent; lower incidence Asian and Pacific Islander descent)
- Recurrence rate increases with affected family members
- 1.2:1—female to male

Environment
- Low socioeconomic status
- Maternal obesity
- Heat exposure (maternal febrile illness, high environmental temperature)
- Low folic acid intake
- Anticonvulsants
  - Valproic acid
  - Carbamazepine

Prenatal Diagnosis

Prenatal screening should be completed on pregnant women with positive family history (including having a previous child with SB) or exposure to known teratogenic agents. Alpha-fetoprotein (AFP) and acetylcholinesterase in maternal serum and amniotic fluid can be tested at 16 to 18 weeks; AFP in serum is reliable and in amniotic fluid is reliable at 100% in open tube defects. Addition of elevated acetylcholinesterase confirms the diagnosis. Closed defects are not detected. Fetal ultrasound at 16 to 24 weeks is reliable for detection of malformations. If the pregnancy is not terminated, elective cesarian section has been recommended although there is no evidence that level of paralysis will be affected. In-utero repair is reported but is not standard care.

Neonatal Assessment and Management

The initial management of an infant with SB involves neurosurgical closure of the defect. Nearly all infants with SB cystica have an Arnold Chiari II malformation (caudal displacement of the cerebellum with elongation and kinking of the fourth ventricle), which likely is associated with hydrocephalus. Shunting is performed in most infants; ventriculoperitoneal (VP) shunts are the most common. About half require shunt replacement within the first year.

Urologic evaluation and management also begins neonatally. A small percentage of infants may have vesicoureteral reflux (VUR), and early identification is important. An abdominal examination can demonstrate a distended bladder. Abdominal ultrasound provides information on kidney and bladder size and contour and can provide information regarding postvoid residual (PVR). If the PVR is more than 20 mL, intermittent catheterization should be initiated. Bowel evacuation must be monitored.

The extent of the resulting motor impairment is assessed in the neonatal period with frequent monitoring. There may be spinal shock after delivery or spine closure. Paraplegia with sensory and lower motor neuron involvement is the typical motor impairment. The level and extent of the lesion determines the lower limb function. Activation of major muscle groups is usually apparent in infants through observation of activity and palpation of muscle bulk. Presence of spinal reflexes allows additional information about level of function. Assessment of anal wink may provide information about sacral sparing or functioning. However, these withdrawal or cutaneous reflexes may only be demonstrating an intact reflex arc below the level of function. The functional level usually does not correlate well with the anatomic defect level. Asymmetry in function may also be present. Routine muscle testing through childhood and into adulthood allows assessment of expected function and avoidance of secondary conditions.

Family counseling is an important aspect of early care. Families require information and support. Multiple specialists often provide a variety of needed services, and an organized team approach often allows less confusion with the diversity of specific techniques that can be suggested for management. EI programs can assist families with integrating much of the information they receive and provide needed support and interventions.

Long-Term Medical Management

Because SB is a spinal cord dysfunction, close monitoring of a variety of neurogenically based impairments is required. A coordinated physician and other health professional team approach usually provides the best comprehensive care. Table 15.15 reports commonly noted conditions to be recognized and followed.

General growth and nutrition should be followed closely. Obesity is commonly seen in children with SB, and there may be an association with previous hydrocephalus. It often becomes noted during adolescences and puberty. Precocious puberty is associated with hydrocephalus at 10% to 20%. There is a high incidence of latex allergy.

Vigilance and anticipatory management need to guide the physician in the care of children and adults with SB. Changes in affect, personality, cognition, motor function, and urologic status or the new onset of symptoms such as stridor, aspiration, or pain must be addressed in a timely fashion. Each of these may represent a treatable secondary condition or complication of the underlying CNS malformation and neurologic function, as noted in Table 15.15.

Neurologic bladder and bowel management has significant implications for social integration. Children and adults with SB and their parents report urinary and fecal incontinence as more stressful than mobility impairments. Independence in care as well as continence can limit socialization. There is often poor compliance with programs because of cognitive issues limiting initiation of activities or understanding techniques, poor upper limb and hand function, intolerance of medication side effects, and behavioral manifestations of empowerment and self-determination.

Rehabilitation Management

Therapy Systems and Approaches

Referral to an EI program in infancy is particularly helpful to families of children with SB. The complexity of care is often overwhelming to parents, and the support provided through the EI professionals cannot be overemphasized. A variety of techniques can be considered for treatment programs (Table 15.3), and goals direct the strategies used. Realistic expectations are to be considered in development of therapy and program goals, along with time and financial constraints. General goals are to promote mobility, promote independent self-care (including neurogenic bladder and bowel management at age-appropriate times), prevent secondary conditions, determine adaptations for educational and vocational issues, and advance a positive self-image. No specific therapy approach has been proven more effective than another has. Developmental activities to promote strengthening, flexibility, and range of motion are typical activities. Routine manual muscle testing can be helpful in directing an exercise program and goals of a functional training program. Strengthening may initially require NMES or sEMG to assist with activation and can progress to resistance exercises with typical exercise equipment. Latex-free theraband is also useful. Functional training for self-care tasks is important, and visual motor problems, visual perceptual limitations, and abnormal upper limb and hand function must be factored in to practiced approaches.

**Table 15.15.   Long-Term
Management in Spinal Bifida (SB)**

Body System	Management Issues
Central nervous system	Shunt function • Obstruction • Infection • Length of catheter with growth • Shunt dependency with age Seizures Symptomatic Arnold Chiari II • Central ventilatory dysfunction (CVD) • Brainstem dysfunction Syringomyelia Tethered cord syndrome • Based on progressive symptoms
Urologic	Renal ultrasound every 6 mo for first few years With known reflux, periodic excretory urogram or cystourethrogram Urodynamics first year and periodically to evaluate change or direct management Intermittent cath (IC) for treatment of reflux or to address continence Continence • IC usually with medications • Condom catheters for boys • Surgery (vesicostomy, bladder augmentation, artificial sphincter) • Independence in care Incontinence limiting socialization
Bowel	Regular evacuation with regimen • Impaired rectal sensation • Impaired sphincter function • Decreased motility • Avoid megacolon Continence • Independence • Required for social integration
Growth	Obesity—adolescence especially Precocious puberty—associated with hydrocephalus
Immunologic	High incidence latex allergies • Avoid latex products (catheters, gloves, balloons, theraband) • Negative testing does not rule out future sensitization

continued

Table 15.15. *Continued*

Body System	Management Issues
Sensory	Pressure ulcers • Common sites: perineum, over gibbus deformity in those who do not walk; lower limbs in those with low lumbar area dysfunction • Osteomyelitis • Amputation may result
Cognition	Intellectual function inversely correlated with neurologic level Poor visual perceptual and visual motor skills—limit school performance and self-care tasks (e.g., IC, dressing, hygiene) "Cocktail" personality Concentration/attention deficits likely from hydrocephalus
Musculoskeletal	Limited lower limb growth Abnormal upper limb function secondary to upper motor neuron involvement from anterior neuropore abnormality in SB Monitor strength through adulthood—prognosis and diagnosis Mobility • Rehabilitation • Equipment prescription • Routine exercise program • Appropriately timed surgery • Monitor changes—tethered cord, syringomyelia Contractures/scoliosis • Seating and orthotics • Surgical intervention Osteoporosis/fracture

SB, spina bifida.

Manual muscle testing must be followed throughout life as a mark for functional change from syringomyelia or tethered cord, as well as to identify the focus of a strengthening or functional training program to improve function and to assist with prognostication of walking function. Hip flexion strength at grade 3 or less suggests wheelchair use full or part time. Grade 4 or greater hip extension and ankle dorsiflexion suggests community walking without aids or braces. Manifestation of musculoskeletal complications and possible outcomes are noted in Tables 15.16 and 15.17.

Mobility Aids: Orthotics and Wheelchairs

Use of orthotics is common in children with SB. A variety of orthotics and walking aids may be used and include traditional

Table 15.16.   Typical Motor Presentation in Spinal Bifida (SB) by Motor Level

Motor Neurologic Level	Motor Function	Manifestation
T6–12	Abdominal muscles	Flaccid LL Contractures including scoliosis
L1, L1–2, L2	Hip flex present Hip adduction present	Hip dislocation early Scoliosis common
L3, L3–4, L4	Hip flex, adduction Knee ext Knee flex (med HS) or ankle dorsiflex	Hip dislocation late Scoliosis common
L4–5, L5	Above plus: Hip abduction < antigravity or ankle eversion antigravity Knee flex with med/lat HS Ankle dorsiflex	Contractures from imbalance—common releases proximal and at ankles
L5–S1, S1, S1–2	Above plus: Hip ext just antigravity Plantar flex < antigravity	Equinovarus or cavus foot deformities
S2 and below	Above plus: Hip ext > antigravity Plantar flex antigravity or better ± foot intrinsics	Foot deformities

HS, hamstrings; LL, lower limbs.

orthoses (AFO, floor reaction AFO, KAFO, HKAFO) and aids, the parapodium, the swivel walker, and reciprocal gait orthoses (RGOs). Prognostic indicators and manual muscle testing assist with prescription. Prescription is defined by level of function first, although regional preferences and professional experiences are a part of the decision. Early supported standing is promoted with use of orthotics. However, no studies exist to support the belief that this enhances skeletal alignment; prevents osteoporosis; or improves urinary, gastrointestinal, or pulmonary function. Orthotics are used for scoliosis management.

Wheeled mobility allows the opportunity for early independent environmental interaction. Specifics of patient and family needs and availability and features of components are considered. Figure 15-4 demonstrates changing orthotic needs with development and specific goals.

Table 15.17. Prognosis for Functional Outcome in Spinal Bifida (SB)

Motor Neurologic Level	Functional Outcome
Thoracic	Uses WC Requires assistance for day-to-day care
L1–2	May use RGOs at young age WC in the community 50% independent Rarely employed
L3	May use KAFOs WC in the community 60% independent 20% employed
L4	KAFOs or AFOs used WC for distances Few adults maintain walking
L5	± AFOs 80% independent 30% full time, 20% part-time employed
S1	FOs or no orthotics Independent More commonly employed

Adapted from Hinderer SR, Hinderer KA, Dunne K, et al. Medical and functional status of adults with spina bifida. *Dev Med Child Neurol* 1988;30S:28, with permission.

Orthopedic Surgery Considerations

Orthopedic surgical intervention is common. General indications are to improve muscle imbalance about joints (particularly hip and ankle); to release soft tissue contractures recalcitrant to stretching, which can produce further deformities; to correct congenital deformities; or to improve function, hygiene, or pain complaints.

Muscle imbalance at the hip accounts for hip flexion deformities and hip subluxation or dislocation. Reducing dislocated hips in children who are active and walking may improve function; however, it must be carefully planned and complications considered. Hip flexion contractures postoperatively should be avoided. Repeated procedures are associated with greater joint inflexibility and, therefore, disability. Very late dislocations may represent tethered cord or syringomyelia.

Knee flexion contractures are the most common knee deformities. Patients with L3 or higher levels usually develop contractures by age 8 years. Only about a fourth of those with L4 or L5 levels develop contractures by age 12 years. Releases may be more successful with an active knee extension strengthening program.

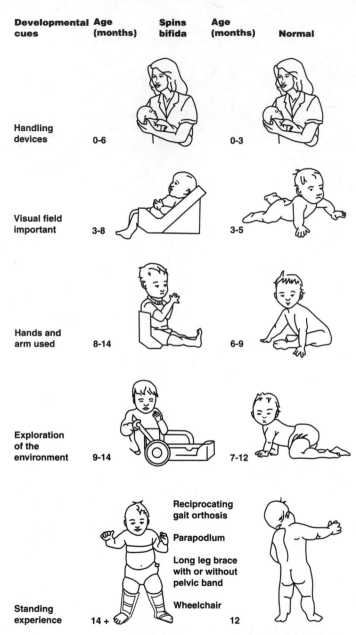

Fig. 15-4. Developmentally appropriate orthotic devices for a child with moderate spina bifida, compared to a normal child. (Adapted from Morloch W. Orthotic philosophies of treatment. *Clin Prosthet Orthot* 1984;8:10.)

Foot deformities are the most common deformity in children with SB, again from muscular imbalance. The goals of surgery and/or orthoses are to achieve balanced muscle control, improve alignment to allow better bracing, and enhance gait. Lack of sensation and autonomic dysfunction account for poor wound healing and secondary skin injury postoperatively. Rigid club foot deformities are associated with higher levels. Later development of neuropathic joints are associated with rigid fusions.

Scoliosis is prevalent in children with SB. Virtually all patients with thoracic level SB develop scoliosis, and about 60% with L4 level develop the deformity. Kyphosis is almost always progressive. Lordotic curves can limit seating and walking. The timing for surgical correction is critical to allow reasonable growth yet not to progress to inability to benefit.

Adult Issues

Adults with SB have more complicated medical care needs because of the multisystem impairment model of spinal cord dysfunction. Ongoing maintenance of neurogenic bladder and bowel needs is important. Although there is better management for neurogenic bladders over a lifetime, vigilance must be practiced. Pressure ulcers continue to be problematic, and secondary osteomyelitis and resulting amputation is common.

Maintenance of motor performance is complicated by the possibility of tethered cord or syringomyelia. Change is status should initiate a workup. Loss of strength, change in motor function, and spasticity are common complaints. Adults often report an antecedent event. Back and leg pain are noted. In adults there is less often an associated progression in deformity. Often MRIs are difficult to obtain because of surgical hardware; CT myelograms may be the only alternative for radiographic assessment. Urodynamics for comparison to previous studies may be helpful. Diagnosis is based on progressive symptoms. There can be complications associated with the surgery. Repeated surgeries are usually associated with poorer outcomes.

Issues of sexuality and sexual functioning need to be addressed. Women can carry pregnancies to term, although high-risk prenatal care is advised. Back pain and deterioration of urologic status have been reported with pregnancies. Men have greater reproductive potential with lower SB levels. Testosterone levels may be normal.

Musculoskeletal issues must be anticipated and addressed. Pain complaints may have a musculoskeletal basis from positioning, overuse, or weakness. Radicular complaints (cervical more common than lumbar) and peripheral nerve entrapments also must be considered. Management to maintain function should ensue. The need for an ongoing exercise program is also important for adults with SB.

SUGGESTED READINGS

Benson MKD, Fixsen JA, Macnicol MF, et al, eds. *Children's orthopaedics and fractures,* 2nd ed. Philadelphia: Elsevier, 2002.

Brin M, ed. Spasticity: etiology, evaluation, management, and the role of botulinum toxin type A. *Muscle Nerve* 1997;(Suppl 6):S1–S232.

Brooke MH, Carroll JE, Ringell SP. Congenital hypotonia revisited. *Muscle Nerve* 1979;2:84–100.

Campbell SK, ed. *Physical therapy for children,* 2nd ed. Philadelphia: WB Saunders, 2000.

DeLisa J, Gans B. *Rehabilitation medicine: principles and practice,* 4th ed. Philadelphia: Lippincott Williams & Wilkins, 2003.

Downey JA, Low NL. *The child with disabling illness,* 2nd ed. New York: Raven Press, 1982.

Jaffe KM. Pediatric rehabilitation. *Phys Med Rehabil Clin North Am* 1991;2:665–970.

Levitt S. *Paediatric developmental therapy.* Boston: Blackwell Scientific Publications, 1984.

Lollar DJ, ed. *Preventing secondary conditions associated with spina bifida or cerebral palsy: proceedings and recommendations of a symposium.* Washington DC: Spina Bifida Association of America, 1994.

McDonald CM, Jaffe KM, Mosca VS, et al. Ambulatory outcome of children with myelomeningocele: effect of lower-extremity muscle strength. *Dev Med Child Neurol* 1991;33:482–490.

Molnar GE, Alexander MA, eds. *Pediatric rehabilitation,* 3rd ed. Baltimore: Williams & Wilkins, 1999.

Turk MA. Disability and health management during childhood. *Phys Med Rehabil Clin North Am* 2002;13;775–1005.

Peripheral Neuropathy and Plexus Injury

Kenneth Kemp, Jr. and Michael J. Vennix

PERIPHERAL NEUROPATHY

Definition

The terms *peripheral neuropathy, polyneuropathy,* or *polyneuritis* refer to an illness marked by disordered function of peripheral nerves.

Etiology and Pathophysiology

Peripheral nerves consist of a bundle of axons; the large- and medium-sized axons are usually covered with a layer of myelin and the small-diameter fibers are often unmyelinated. Most peripheral nerves are mixed nerves carrying both incoming sensory information (afferent fibers) and outgoing motor and autonomic impulses (efferent fibers). Large-diameter afferent fibers convey vibration and position sense; large-diameter efferent fibers innervate the muscles. Pain and temperature sensation and autonomic information are carried by small-diameter unmyelinated fibers.

Peripheral neuropathies result from diseases that affect the axons, their myelin sheaths, or both. Axonal neuropathies are the result of processes that primarily affect the cell body or the axon; demyelinating neuropathies result from involvement of the myelin sheath. Regardless of the initial pathologic process, secondary changes are produced because of the interdependence between myelin and axon. Mixed pathologic changes with evidence of both demyelination and axonal degeneration are seen on biopsy.

The clinical presentation distinguishes the three major types of peripheral nerve diseases: mononeuropathy, mononeuropathy multiplex, and polyneuropathy. Mononeuropathy is a lesion of an individual nerve root or peripheral nerve, usually resulting from local causes such as trauma, entrapment, or compression. Multifocal neuropathy or mononeuritis multiplex refers to involvement of two or more discrete nerves that are usually affected sequentially in different limbs. This is commonly the result of multifocal nerve infarctions resulting from occlusion of the vasa nervorum and is seen in systemic diseases causing vasculitis, such as periarteritis nodosa and diabetes.

Peripheral neuropathy (polyneuropathy) occurs in diseases that affect the peripheral nerves symmetrically, usually distally. The longer and larger axons are affected earlier and more severely than the shorter ones. In the demyelinating type, this occurs because the longer axons have more potential sites for demyelination; in the axonal type, the longer, larger axons do not have adequate nutritional support. Therefore, the symptoms tend to appear in the feet before the hands. Many polyneuropathies affect both the sensory and motor fibers indiscriminately. However, at times either the sensory or motor fibers are primarily affected, either clinically or pathologically.

Pathophysiologically, there are three types of nerve lesions:

Neuropraxia: Both axon and myelin sheath are intact with minimal changes seen in paranodal region. There is physiologic loss of function.

Axonotmesis: There is degeneration of the axon with Schwann's sheath intact.

Neurotmesis: There is complete severance of the nerve.

Assessment and Evaluation

Patients with polyneuropathy often present with complaints of paresthesias, a "pins and needles" sensation, in the feet. Other symptoms are loss of sensation, sometimes accompanied by pain; weakness; muscle cramps; coldness; heaviness; and symptoms of autonomic dysfunction such as impotence, urinary retention or overflow incontinence, diarrhea or constipation, and orthostatic hypotension.

The major signs of peripheral neuropathy are loss of sensation, weakness, muscle atrophy, and loss of tendon reflexes. The most common sensory modalities affected are vibration and pain in a glove and stocking distribution. If position sense or proprioception is markedly affected, the patient may manifest unsteadiness or ataxia. Often the weakness is noted distally, affecting the small intrinsic muscles of the feet. The patient has difficulty spreading the toes and walking on uneven surfaces. With longstanding peripheral neuropathies, imbalance of muscles results in claw toes and high, arched feet. Eventually there is atrophy of the tibialis anterior muscle with prominent tibia. The hands show atrophy of the intrinsics and develop clawing. Tenderness of the soles and palms is typical in neuropathies such as nutritional, alcoholic, arsenic, and porphyric neuropathies, in which pain is a major feature.

There are many causes of peripheral neuropathies. During the patient's examination, distinctive features may suggest a particular diagnosis. When taking the history, include questions regarding alcohol intake, nutritional status, symptoms of diabetes and collagen vascular disease, exposure to toxic substances, and current medications. Try to determine possible patterns of repeated trauma in vulnerable areas (see Table 16.1).

The chronology of presenting symptoms is an important consideration. Mononeuropathies are often acute in onset and sometimes have obvious causes, such as trauma. The most common acute polyneuropathy is Guillain-Barré syndrome. Some other acute polyneuropathies are caused by infections such as diphtheria, toxins, or metabolic processes. Most toxic and metabolic neuropathies develop somewhat slowly, within weeks. Chronic neuropathies are associated with diabetes mellitus and alcoholism and are also found in hereditary disorders such as Charcot-Marie Tooth disease.

Cranial nerve involvement is common in acute idiopathic polyneuropathy and in neuropathies associated with porphyria, diabetes, sarcoidosis, and periarteritis nodosa. It is unusual to find cranial nerve abnormalities in alcoholic, arsenic, and other toxic neuropathies.

On physical examination, note the pattern of involvement. In mononeuropathy, motor and sensory involvement in the

Table 16.1.   Activities and Resulting Nerve Trauma

Activity	Nerve Injury
Scrubbing, vacuuming, typing, sewing, or knitting	Carpal tunnel syndrome
Repetitively resting elbows on hard surfaces, or prolonged positioning with elbows flexed and pronated	Ulnar palsy
Crossing legs while seated or prolonged squatting	Peroneal palsy
Carrying heavy loads on shoulder	Suprascapular palsy

distribution of a single root or peripheral nerve is usually found. Most polyneuropathies produce both motor and sensory involvement. Predominantly motor involvement suggests Guillain-Barré syndrome; recurrent inflammatory polyneuropathy; or porphyritic, lead, diphtheritic, or a hereditary neuropathy. Predominantly sensory involvement is commonly found in diabetic, alcohol, cancer, and nutrition-related neuropathies. Occasionally dissociated sensory losses are seen. The patient has diminished pain and temperature sensation with preservation of other modalities; this is typical in small fiber neuropathies. When pain is preserved but position sense is lost, consider vitamin B_{12} deficiency or the rare Friedreich's ataxia. These neuropathies affect the posterior columns, leading to the involvement of fibers conveying joint position. Predominant autonomic involvement is found in diabetes, amyloidosis, dysproteinemia, and dysautonomia.

Laboratory Investigations

Many common causes of peripheral neuropathy such as diabetes, hypertension, and alcoholism can be evaluated by routine laboratory tests including complete blood count (CBC), erythrocyte sedimentation rate (ESR), serum glucose, blood urea nitrogen (BUN), and thyroid function tests. There are innumerable rare conditions associated with polyneuropathy; an extensive screening process is unnecessary and expensive. History and physical examination can point to an appropriate test, such as that for lead, or a particular toxin, for example, suspected in occupational exposure.

Electrophysiologic Studies

Nerve conduction studies are very helpful in establishing the involvement of peripheral nerves as the site of pathology. Such testing can distinguish a peripheral neuropathy from myopathy or anterior horn cell disease. **Neuropathies can be classified using electrophysiologic data by documenting motor and/or sensory involvement and distinguishing between primary axonal or demyelinating processes (Table 16.2).**

Table 16.2.   Peripheral Neuropathy Classifications Using Electrophysiologic Data

Demyelinating mixed sensory/motor (uniform)
Hereditary sensory motor neuropathy type 1
Hereditary sensory motor neuropathy type 3
Other inherited neuropathies

Demyelinating motor>sensory (segmental)
Acute and chronic inflammatory demyelinating
Polyneuropathy (AIDP and CIDP)
Leprosy
Acute arsenic poisoning
Systemic lupus erythematous
Blood cell dyscrasias
Acquired immune deficiency syndrome
Carcinoma/lymphoma

Axonal motor>sensory
Hereditary sensory motor neuropathy type 2
Axonal Guillain-Barré syndrome
Porphyria
Lead
Vincristine and dapsone
Paraneoplastic
Hypoglycemia

Axonal sensory
Spinocerebellar degeneration
Friedrich ataxia
Paraneoplastic
Pyridoxine toxicity
Fisher variant Guillain-Barré syndrome
Crohn's disease

Axonal mixed sensory/motor
Alcoholism
Sarcoidosis
Chronic liver disease
Nutritional deficiencies
Toxic neuropathies
Connective tissue diseases
Lyme disease
Acquired immune deficiency syndrome
Multiple myeloma
Paraneoplastic

Mixed axonal/demyelinating and mixed sensory/motor
Diabetes mellitus
Uremia

Adapted from Donofrio PD, Albers JW. Polyneuropathy: classification by nerve conduction studies and electromyography. AAEM minimonograph #34. *Muscle Nerve* 1990;889–903, with permission.

The site of involvement in cases of entrapment or compression neuropathies can be revealed in many cases, such as ulnar neuropathy at the elbow or common peroneal neuropathy at the fibular head.

Electromyography (EMG) is useful in detecting or confirming evidence of denervation in distal muscles that can be seen in axonal peripheral neuropathies. Abnormalities on needle examination can also indicate the course of the peripheral neuropathy in the acute period following injury. Amplitude of abnormal spontaneous activity is large and decreases as the process becomes chronic. The configuration of the motor unit also can reflect chronic changes in reinnervation.

Nerve Biopsy

Avoid obtaining a nerve biopsy on a routine basis. It should be done only in cases for which a histologic diagnosis is a possibility, such as vasculitis or amyloidosis.

Treatment

In general, the treatment of neuropathies aims to maintain range of motion (ROM) of the joints, prevent contractures, reeducate the patient in skilled activities, and maximize residual function.

Treatment of mononeuropathies depends on the focal deficit noted. If there is a complete lesion of the nerve, employ techniques to substitute for the loss of musculature. Use orthotic devices to prevent contractures, support weak muscles, or substitute for paralyzed muscles. Educate the patient to prevent complications from the lack of sensation.

Contractures

Peripheral neuropathies cause paralysis of muscles with decrease in, or loss of, muscle tone; therefore, contractures are easily prevented if ROM exercises are performed routinely. Educate the patient in appropriate ROM exercises. If contractures are present, use heat followed by stretching. Try prolonged stretching over 20 minutes. Adequate stretching to increase the ROM means that the joint is taken past the point of pain.

Weakness

Exercising weak muscles with significant denervation must be done in moderation. Experimental evidence suggests that long-duration, low-intensity activity (meaning high-repetition, low-weight) does not damage the muscle. Discourage patients who have significant partial denervation from engaging in moderate to severe intensity, prolonged exercises.

Teach patients with acute polyneuropathy such as Guillain-Barré syndrome to limit their activities in the early recovery period to prevent the possibility of an exacerbation. When recovery has progressed to fair to good muscle strength, patients may resume full activities.

In cases of chronic neuropathy, use maximum isometric or progressive resistive exercises to increase muscle strength.

Orthoses

Orthoses may be used to support an unstable joint, to prevent overstretching of a muscle in an elongated position, or to substitute for the function of paralyzed muscles. Wrist hand orthoses (WHOs) are used commonly for short periods in the upper limbs that do not significantly improve; WHOs actually may interfere with hand function. Orthoses may be used indefinitely for the lower limbs, such as an ankle foot orthosis (AFO).

Temperature

Cold may cause temporary weakness, a heavy feeling, and decreased strength in patients with peripheral neuropathies. Advise patients to wear warm clothes and avoid exposure to cold. Assure them that the weakness is a temporary response to cold.

Electrical Stimulation

Electrical stimulation has not been shown to enhance reinnervation in a denervated muscle. However, electrical stimulation does retard atrophy. It can be used to maintain the contractility and bulk of the muscle, but it is not a very practical treatment because it must be performed intensively for a prolonged period.

Functional Retraining

Teach compensating mechanisms to maximize function. Avoid abnormal habit patterns. Teach substitutions when primary movers are paralyzed, such as using the finger extensors to extend the wrist. Teach the patient to contract isolated muscles to strengthen and prevent disuse atrophy.

Sensory Reeducation

Order sensory reeducation for nerve injuries involving the hand. Initiate therapy when vibratory sensation returns.

Pain

Pain may be present in the distribution of the nerve with mononeuropathy or in a more diffuse manner distally in the hands and feet. The pain is usually a burning type, and the area may be hyperesthetic or dysesthetic. Try small doses of tricyclic antidepressants, such as amitriptyline (Elavil) 50 to 75 mg orally at bedtime, or antiseizure medications such as **gabapentin (Neurontin),** carbamazepine (Tegretol) and phenytoin sodium (Dilantin). Maintain good nutritional status, including vitamin supplementation, especially vitamin B. Use a trial of transcutaneous electric stimulation (TENS) over the proximal location of the offending nerve(s) or over the painful area. Cover the painful area with a light elastic garment or an adhesive plastic such as Op-Site, Tegaderm, or Second Skin. Advise the patient to avoid exposure to cold.

Surgery

Surgical treatment includes nerve suturing following nerve injury; decompression and/or transposition in nerve entrapment; and tendon transfers, if there are muscles of sufficient strength to be used for transfer.

Postoperatively, immobilize the part for 4 to 6 weeks; avoid any tension on the repaired site. Then initiate a gradual stretching and mobilization program. At times, tendon transfers are performed acutely after a complete nerve injury. Usually, however, they are done when the patient's functional recovery has significantly slowed. Preoperatively, strengthen the muscles to be transferred. A transferred muscle looses its strength by one grade. Postoperatively, train the patient to perform the new activity of the transferred muscle. Biofeedback may be useful in retraining. Later, use strengthening exercises.

Complications

Complications are usually due to lack of sensation. Commonly, ulceration of the feet occurs, along with secondary infection. Hand ulcers are rare, but burns occur. Prevent these problems through patient education. Encourage meticulous foot care and use of appropriate shoes. If an ulcer has already formed, prevent further trauma by avoiding weight bearing on the affected foot. A total contact cast may be used until the ulcer heals.

With severe sensory loss, Charcot's joint, a severe form of osteoarthritis with pronounced disruption and disorganization of the midtarsal and tarsometatarsal joints, may develop. This can be associated with loss of pain sensation, proprioception, or a combination of both.

Outcome and Follow-Up

Patients with acute peripheral neuropathy such as Guillain-Barré syndrome usually experience complete recovery in 12 to 18 months.

Chronic neuropathies, for example, diabetic neuropathy, may require periodic evaluation for any deterioration in function and for necessary rehabilitation intervention.

BRACHIAL PLEXUS INJURY

Brachial plexus injury often presents major problems in diagnosis and management. It commonly occurs with trauma to multiple systems, such as from motorcycle accidents, so that concern for preservation of life or limb obscures its presence.

Anatomy

The brachial plexus is usually formed by the union of anterior rami of the last four cervical nerve roots and the first thoracic root. Refer to Fig. 16-1. Often there is contribution from the C4 to C5 root (termed prefixed) or, rarely, from the T2 to T1 root (postfixed). Proceeding distally, the plexus consists of trunks, divisions, cords, and, finally, peripheral nerves. The five segmental roots form three trunks, upper (C5-C6), middle (C7), and lower (C8-T1). Each trunk separates into anterior and posterior divisions. The anterior divisions of the upper and middle trunks unite to form lateral cord, the anterior division of the lower trunk forms the medial cord, and the posterior divisions of all three trunks form the posterior cord. Most of the peripheral nerves originating in the plexus derive from the three cords. Exceptions are the long thoracic and dorsal scapular nerves that arise directly from the spinal roots and innervate muscles around the scapula. The only

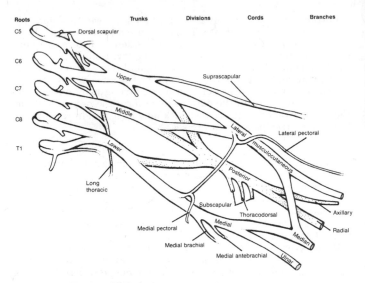

Fig. 16-1. The brachial plexus.

significant nerve that originates from the trunk is the supra-scapular nerve (C5-C6).

Etiology

There are many possible causes of brachial plexus injury. Direct trauma is the most common; others are local compression, tumor, idiopathic, radiation, postoperative, and birth injury.

Direct trauma accounts for more than half of brachial plexus injuries and is usually due to vehicular accidents. The most common mechanism of damage is traction injury. The most frequently seen traction injury is normally produced by a forceful distraction of the head from the shoulder, resulting in Erb's paralysis, as shown in Fig. 16-2. In this injury, C5, C6, and occasionally C7 nerve roots are injured, leaving a nonfunctional shoulder with good distal muscular function of the affected limb. Less commonly, a pull on an abducted arm results in Dejerine-Klumpke's paralysis, in which C8, T1, and occasionally C7 roots are damaged with subsequent loss of hand and forearm function. Refer to Fig. 16-3. Clinical experience shows that multiple level injuries are common; segmental classification is frequently impossible.

Evaluate the patient systematically to make an accurate diagnosis and prognosis for both neurologic and functional recovery.

An accurate history and physical examination is imperative. Record a detailed manual muscle test and sensory examination at the initial evaluation; update it during each subsequent visit.

Review radiographic examinations such as x-ray films of the cervical spine and shoulders, myelogram, computed tomography (CT) scan, and magnetic resonance imaging (MRI) to appreciate the extent of the lesion.

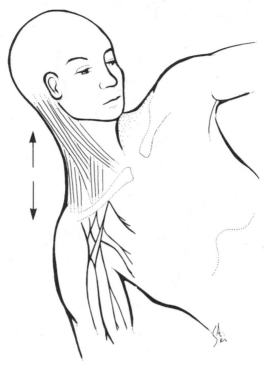

Fig. 16-2. Forces producing injury to the upper portion of the brachial plexus.

Use EMG to demonstrate objectively the extent of the pathologic condition. Serial studies provide a more accurate method of prognosis than does a single study (see Table 16.3).

Sensory nerve action potential (SNAP) is helpful in distinguishing preganglionic (root avulsion) lesions from postganglionic lesions. Refer to Fig. 16-4. SNAP shows a normal response if the lesion is preganglionic, meaning that the sensory ganglion is intact. A positive SNAP in an area of anesthesia or a positive SNAP with a negative sensory evoked potential (SEP) is an almost definite indication of a nerve root avulsion. Distinguish between preganglionic and postganglionic lesions, because prognosis and management are different. Refer to Table 16.4.

Evaluate associated injuries; most patients sustain multisystem trauma, particularly if injured in vehicular accidents.

Recognize social and psychologic problems. Sudden loss of all or part of a limb is psychologically and economically catastrophic.

Address vocational aspects. The largest single group of patients are motorcyclists, who tend to be manual laborers. The alteration in their potential for making a living or simply performing daily activities is dramatic.

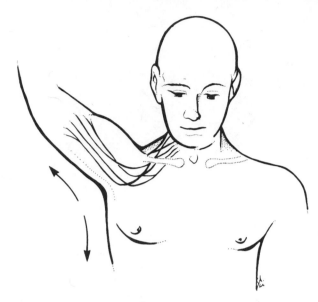

Fig. 16-3.   Forces producing injury to the lower portion of the brachial plexus.

Table 16.3.   Interpretation of Electromyography (EMG)

- Normal muscle
  At rest: electrical silence
  Minimal effort: biphasic and triphasic motor unit potentials
  Maximal effort: complete recruitment pattern
- Denervated muscle
  At rest: spontaneous potentials, i.e., fibrillations and positive sharp waves
  Minimal effort: fast firing motor unit if present
  Maximal effort: incomplete or absent recruitment pattern
- Signs of reinnervation
  At rest: decreasing number of fibrillations and positive sharp waves
  Minimal effort: nascent small polyphasic potentials, increasing number of motor unit potentials
  Maximal effort: increasing recruitment pattern; polyphasic potentials
- Signs of neuropraxia 14–21 days after injury
  At rest: no spontaneous potentials
  Minimal effort: absent or occasional motor unit potentials
  Maximal effort: absent recruitment

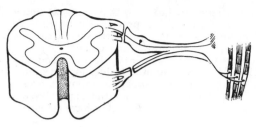

Preganglionic injury

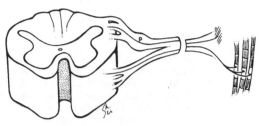

Postganglionic injury

Fig. 16-4. Preganglionic and postganglionic injuries.

Management

From a rehabilitation standpoint, patients with brachial plexus injuries are best managed by a multidisciplinary approach. Physicians, physical and occupational therapists, psychologists, social workers, and vocational counselors all have patient care responsibilities.

Major deficits resulting from brachial plexus injuries include motor paralysis, causing loss of function and secondary deformities such as joint stiffness, muscle contractures, and edema; sensory loss; and pain.

Initiate conservative treatment as soon as possible after injury. Instruct the patient to wear a sling to lessen shoulder subluxation and to decrease the possibility of further traction injury to the neurovascular bundle.

Table 16.4. Signs and Symptoms of Cervical Root Avulsion

Burning pain
Horner's sign
Loss of serratus, rhomboids, and pectorals
Fracture of transverse process
Positive myelogram
Negative SEPs with positive SNAP

Begin physical therapy early for passive range of motion (PROM) to joints of the affected limb to prevent contractures. Also, teach a self-ranging exercise program and active exercises of those muscles that are capable of voluntary movement.

Prevent edema, which can increase stiffness and contractures, by use of PROM and elevation. Consider elastic support of various types, such as Jobs garments and Isotoner gloves, but avoid a tourniquet effect. Electrical stimulation of paralyzed muscle remains controversial; no objective studies have demonstrated that it is effective.

When reinnervation occurs, strengthen the muscles using a full program of resistive exercises.

The occupational therapist trains patients in one-handed activities as well as in use of orthoses. Prevent secondary complications such as injuries or burns that may result in soft tissue infection or osteomyelitis by teaching the patient to protect the anesthetized limb and fingers.

Management of pain in brachial plexus injury patients is difficult. Use a trial of TENS, properly applied, early in treatment. Medication management includes use of **gabapentin (Neurontin),** phenytoin (Dilantin), carbamazepine (Tegretol), amitriptyline (Elavil), and nonsteroidal antiinflammatory medications. (Refer to Chapter 2). Neurosurgical intervention, such as brachial plexus exploration and lysis, is usually not helpful for pain reduction, although nerve blocks may be used in specific cases.

Surgical Management

Although it is generally accepted that neural reconstructive surgery is indicated for brachial plexus injuries, there is controversy about appropriate candidates, timing of surgery, and specific levels of intervention. Commonly used procedures are neurolysis, excision and grafting, and neurotization.

Peripheral reconstructive surgery, such as Steindler flexor plasty and restoration of elbow flexion with pectoral and other muscle transfers, has been used to enhance function. Occasionally, a shoulder fusion with amputation is done in a flail limb and a prosthesis is used.

Following all reconstructive surgeries, intensive rehabilitation for many weeks is necessary to reeducate the muscle.

LUMBOSACRAL PLEXUS INJURY

Anatomy

The lumbosacral plexus originates from all of the nerve roots inferior to and including the T12 nerve root. Refer to Fig. 16-5. The lumbar plexus is formed by the L1-L4 nerve roots with a small communication from the twelfth thoracic nerve root. The L1 root, having received this branch from T12, divides into iliohypogastric and ilioinguinal nerves that travel down the inferior portion of the abdominal wall. Small branches from the L2-L4 nerves merge to form the obturator nerve. Remaining branches exit the ventral rami of the L2-L4 nerves and combine to form the largest peripheral nerve originating from the lumbar portion of the plexus, the femoral nerve. The L4 root usually divides into two parts, one contributing to the obturator and femoral nerves

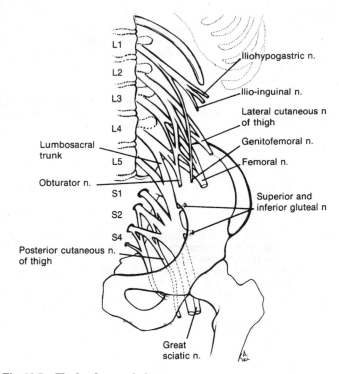

Fig. 16-5. The lumbosacral plexus.

of the lumbar plexus and the other contributing to the sacral portion of the plexus. In the sacral plexus, anterior branches from the L4-S3 roots join to form the tibial nerve, whereas posterior branches from the L4-S2 roots form the peroneal nerve. These two nerves travel together down the thigh within a connective tissue sheath as the sciatic nerve. Other posterior branches from the sacral plexus combine to form the superior and inferior gluteal nerves.

Etiology

As a group, lumbosacral plexus injuries occur much less commonly than injuries to the brachial plexus. As with the brachial plexus, there are many causes for injury to the lumbosacral plexus. Although the term *lumbosacral plexus* is used here, simultaneous injury is less common than involvement of the lumbar plexus or the sacral plexus. Carcinomas of the rectum, prostate, or cervix can, by direct extension, invade the lumbosacral plexus. Metastatic and lymphomatous infiltrates of the plexus can produce a painful paralysis that develops over a long period. Less commonly, a hematoma within the psoas muscle can cause a compression plexopathy.

Diagnosis

Electrodiagnostic studies, imaging studies, and radiographic evaluations are important in differentiating a lumbosacral plexopathy from a radiculopathy, a lesion of the cauda equina, or proximal mononeuropathy.

Treatment

Similar principles of muscle strengthening and pain control are used for lumbosacral plexus injuries as for those already discussed in this chapter in the section on brachial plexus injury.

SUGGESTED READINGS

Brown WF, ed. *The physiological and technological basis of electromyography.* Boston: Butterworth, 1984.

Brown WF, Bolton CF, eds. *Clinical electromyography.* Boston: Butterworth, 1993.

Chaudry V, Glass JD, Griffin JW. Wallerian degeneration in peripheral nerve disease. *Neurol Clin* 1992;19:613–626.

Donofrio PD, Albers JW. Polyneuropathy: classification by nerve conduction studies and electromyography. AAEM Minimonograph #34. *Muscle Nerve* 1990;13:889–903.

Dyck PJ, Thomas PK, eds. *Peripheral neuropathy,* 2nd ed. Philadelphia: WB Saunders, 1993.

Herbison GJ, Jaweed MM, Ditunno JF. Exercise therapies in peripheral neuropathies. *Arch Phys Med Rehab* 1983;64:201–205.

Josifek IF, Bleecker ML. Chapter 84. In: Dyck PJ, Thomas PK, eds. *Peripheral neuropathy,* 2nd ed. Philadelphia: WB Saunders, 1993.

Kimura J. Diseases of the root and plexus. In: Kimura J, ed. *Electrodiagnosis in diseases of nerve and muscle: principles and practice,* 2nd ed. Philadelphia: FA Davis, 1989.

Parry GJ. Mononeuropathy multiplex. *Muscle Nerve* 1985;8:493–498.

Sabin TD. Classification of peripheral neuropathy: the long and the short of it. *Muscle Nerve* 1986;9:711–719.

Sibley W. Polyneuritis—symposium in clinical neurology. *Med Clin North Am* 1972;56:1299–1319.

T'sairis P. Differential diagnosis of peripheral neuropathies. In: Dyck PJ, Thomas PK, eds. *Peripheral neuropathy,* 2nd ed. Philadelphia: WB Saunders, 1993.

Pressure Ulcers

Susan L. Garber and Thomas A. Krouskop

DEFINITION

A pressure ulcer is a localized area of cellular necrosis. In general, it is characterized by an open wound in which tissue necrosis has occurred in response to externally applied pressure. Although the terms pressure ulcer, decubitus ulcer, pressure sore, and bedsore are used interchangeably, *pressure ulcer* is the term currently accepted by the U.S. Department of Health and Human Services, Public Health Service, Agency for Healthcare Research and Quality, the National Pressure Ulcer Advisory Panel; and the Consortium for Spinal Cord Medicine, Clinical Practice Guidelines of the Paralyzed Veterans of America.

ANATOMY

Pressure ulcers usually occur over bony prominences (Fig. 17-1). They are classified by stages according to the degree or extent of tissue damage at the initial assessment (Fig. 17-2).

Stage I. Nonblanchable erythema of intact skin, not to be confused with reactive hyperemia. Indicators of impending pressure ulcers include changes in color (persistent redness in lightly pigmented skin or persistent red, blue, or purple in darkly pigmented skin), skin temperature (warmth or coolness), tissue consistency (firm or boggy feeling), and/or sensation (pain, itching).
Stage II. Partial thickness skin loss involving epidermis and/or dermis. Ulcer is superficial and may present as an abrasion, blister, split in the skin or a shallow crater.
Stage III. Full-thickness skin loss involving damage to or necrosis of subcutaneous tissue that may extend down to, but not through, underlying fascia.
Stage IV. Full-thickness skin loss with extensive destruction, tissue necrosis, or damage to muscle, bone, or supporting structures. May be associated with undermining and sinus tracts.

Some clinicians have described an additional stage as stage V in which the ulcer encompasses large bursae involving joint capsule or body cavities such as the rectum, vagina, and bladder.
Identification of stage I pressure ulcers may be difficult in persons with darkly pigmented skin. Furthermore, when eschar is present, accurate staging of the pressure ulcer is not possible until the eschar has sloughed or the wound has been debrided.

EPIDEMIOLOGY

It is difficult to determine accurately the incidence and prevalence of pressure ulcers because of variations in data gathering from acute care hospitals, rehabilitation centers, long-term facilities, and home care settings. It has been estimated, however, that the incidence of pressure ulcers in hospitals ranges from 3%

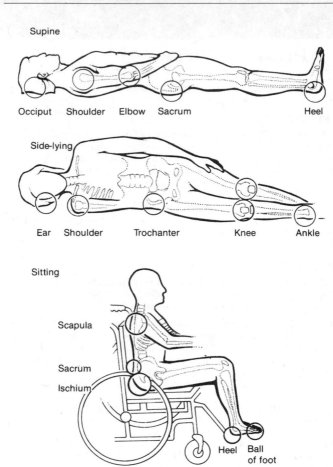

Supine

Occiput   Shoulder   Elbow   Sacrum   Heel

Side-lying

Ear   Shoulder   Trochanter   Knee   Ankle

Sitting

Scapula

Sacrum

Ischium

                                              Heel   Ball
                                                      of foot

Fig. 17-1.   Typical locations of pressure ulcers.

to 29%; in chronic or long-term care facilities, the incidence could be as high as 45%.

Risk factors for the development of pressure ulcers are listed in Table 17.1. Individuals at risk include those with spinal cord injury; the elderly disabled; bed- or chair-bound persons in nursing homes or at home; and persons hospitalized following a stroke, hip fracture, or surgery. Within the population of persons with spinal cord injury, prevalence rates as high as 33% have been reported for individuals residing in the community.

ETIOLOGY/PATHOLOGY

The normal structure of skin and physiologic processes involved in maintaining healthy tissue are fairly well understood. However, the exact causes and mechanisms of soft tissue breakdown

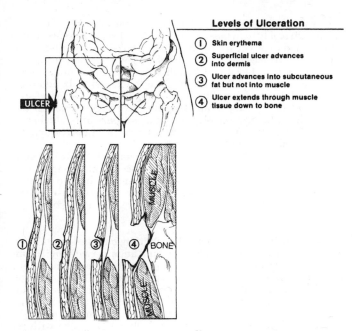

Levels of Ulceration

(1) Skin erythema

(2) Superficial ulcer advances into dermis

(3) Ulcer advances into subcutaneous fat but not into muscle

(4) Ulcer extends through muscle tissue down to bone

Fig. 17-2. Pressure ulcer stage according to depth of tissue involvement. (From Donovan WH. Pressure ulcers. In: DeLisa JA, ed. *Rehabilitation medicine: principles and practice,* 2nd ed. Philadelphia: JB Lippincott, 1993:722, with permission.)

resulting in pressure ulcers are not as clear. Three major factors contribute to the formation of pressure ulcers: biomechanical, biochemical, and medical factors.

Biomechanical Factors

These include pressure, shear, friction, moisture, and temperature. Normal activities such as sitting, lying, and leaning against another surface cause small volumes of flesh to be compressed be-

Table 17.1.   Risk Factors for the Development of Pressure Ulcers

Immobility and altered activity
Incontinence
Nutritional deficiencies
Altered level of consciousness
Altered mental status
Altered or absent sensation
Psychologic stress and depression

tween the internal bony skeleton and an external surface. This results in extremely high tissue stresses. Classically, pressure ulcers are assumed to be caused by pressure-induced vascular ischemia as a result of tissues being deprived of oxygen and nutrients as the nonrigid walls of blood and lymph vessels collapse under pressures that are higher than those of the fluids inside. In addition, mechanical deformation of flesh resulting from high levels of sustained load, or more moderate and repetitive forces, produces tissue damage. Shear forces play a significant part in the occlusion of blood vessels, but large compressive forces must also be applied for suitable shear conditions to develop.

Incontinence and excessive perspiration contribute to skin breakdown. Moist skin is susceptible to maceration through direct trauma or exposure to pressure. Wet skin may adhere to clothing and bed linen, causing shearing. Fecal incontinence causes chemical irritation of the epidermis, which can result in infection.

Biochemical Factors

Associated factors include fat distribution, circulation, collagen metabolism, heterotopic ossification, and anemia (with low serum iron and low serum iron binding). Poor nutrition results in weight loss and reduced padding over bony prominences. Normal tissue integrity is dependent on correct nitrogen balance and vitamin intake. Hypoproteinemia leading to edema causes the skin to become less elastic and more susceptible to inflammation. Slight changes in skin temperature, particularly an elevation with resulting perspiration, can increase metabolic demands of cells in a local region. This is also a potential factor in skin breakdown.

Medical Factors

A large number of diagnostic-specific medical and clinical factors are associated with pressure ulcers. Potential risk factors for an individual with spinal cord injury include level and completeness (motor and sensory) of injury, spasticity, ethnicity, employment, level of education, and socioeconomic factors. Anyone who is immobile as a result of trauma, illness, or disease is at high risk, especially if there is associated malnutrition, anemia, infection, spasticity, contractures, edema, and/or psychologic problems such as depression. The skin of older adults is more fragile, loses its elasticity, and may become drier.

ASSESSMENT/EVALUATION

A key element in maintaining the standard of care for people at risk of developing pressure ulcers is being familiar with three sets of clinical practice guidelines. In 1992, the Agency for Health Care Policy and Research (AHCPR) supported the development of the clinical practice guideline *Pressure Ulcers in Adults: Prediction and Prevention*. In 1994 this agency supported the development of the clinical practice guideline *Treatment of Pressure Ulcers*. These two guidelines presented information about pressure ulcer prevention and treatment for general populations of individuals vulnerable to the effects of pressure on tissue. These include the frail elderly, nursing home residents, and persons who are immobile because of illness or disability. The Paralyzed Veterans of America Consortium for Spinal Cord Medicine sponsored the development of a clinical practice guideline entitled *Pressure Ulcer Prevention and Treatment Following Spinal Cord Injury: A Clinical Practice Guideline for Health-Care Professionals.* This monograph builds on those of the AHCPR but focuses specifically on pressure ulcers in persons with spinal cord injury. Although these documents were developed as clinical guidelines, they often are used to define standards of care. It is important for clinicians to become familiar with them.

It is imperative that skin assessments be performed regularly and that assessments be properly and consistently documented. Patient care plans should address skin issues and refer to the patient's latest risk assessment. Complete and accurate documentation of the skin's condition and any wounds is critical for patient care and to reduce the potential for malpractice suits.

Risk Assessment

1. Use a validated risk assessment tool (such as the Braden scale or the Norton scale) to identify factors predisposing a person to the development of pressure ulcers. Use of these tools ensures systematic evaluation of individual risk factors, primarily mobility and activity levels.
2. Assess skin on admission to the hospital, nursing home, or rehabilitation facility or at home and at regular intervals.
3. Document results of all risk assessments.

Skin Inspection

1. Inspect skin at least twice a day. Pay particular attention to tissue over bony prominences.
2. Document the results of skin inspection.
3. Note potential signs of tissue breakdown. (Table 17.2)

Assess the Person with a Pressure Ulcer

1. Perform a comprehensive assessment of the person with a pressure ulcer including a complete history, physical examination, laboratory tests, behavior, cognitive status, and social and financial resources.
2. Identify the availability and use of personal care assistance.
3. Assess positioning, posture, and related equipment.

Table 17.2. Potential Signs of Tissue Breakdown

Color variation
Blisters
Rashes
Swelling
Temperature variation
Pimples and ingrown hairs
Bruises
Surface breaks
Dry, flaky skin
Treatment

Assess the Pressure Ulcer

1. Describe in detail the anatomic location and general appearance of the pressure ulcer.
2. Describe the size and stage, wound margins, and surrounding tissue.
3. Report on the presence of exudate, odor, necrosis, undermining, sinus tracts, and/or infection.
4. Describe healing (granulation and epithelialization).

TREATMENT

Prevention

Prevention is the most cost-efficient approach to pressure ulcer management. Essential elements of an effective prevention program include an integrated team management approach emphasizing good medical and nursing care; proper training and education of patients, family, and caregivers; encouragement of patient compliance; and the proper prescription of support surfaces.

Skin Inspection

Skin inspection is the basis of prevention. A rigid schedule must become part of the patient's daily routine. Examine the skin regularly each morning and evening and each time the patient is turned or receives a specific treatment. Any sign of redness, skin discoloration, irritation, or abrasion is an indication of impending ulcer formation. Remove all pressure from the area immediately. Teach the patient and family the importance of these skin checks and reinforce these behaviors.

Skin Care and Maintenance

1. Cleanse at time of soiling and at routine intervals.
2. Minimize friction and forces applied to the skin.
3. Individualize the frequency of routine skin cleansing.
4. Use care in positioning, turning, and transferring patients.
5. Avoid massage over bony prominences.
6. Keep the skin clean and dry at all times. Wash areas where perspiration or body fluids collect several times daily with mild soap, rinse with warm water, and pat dry.
7. Apply a lotion or cream after washing. Massage it well into the skin but not over bony prominences.
8. Avoid leaving any moist areas that may result in irritation and maceration.

Pressure Reduction: Turning, Transfers, and Positioning

1. Turn high-risk patients every 2 hours around the clock: 2 hours on the side, 2 hours on the back, and 2 hours on the other side regardless of the type of support surface.
2. Use care in transferring patients. DO NOT drag the patient across the bed. Use a draw sheet under the patient and have two people lift the patient for transfers.
3. Use therapeutic mattress surfaces to minimize pressure on vulnerable areas of the body; use pillows to support extremities so that pressure is reduced where knees and ankles may contact each other.
4. Teach a patient in a wheelchair to shift his or her weight or elevate himself or herself for approximately 15 seconds out of

every 30 minutes. This pressure relief allows the person to continue sitting for several hours at a time without the risk of developing a pressure ulcer.

Pressure Reduction: Support Surfaces

There are more than 150 different support surface products on the market today. Some are recommended for comfort only, some assist with the task of turning patients or reduce the frequency, and some are technologically sophisticated and are intended to reduce significantly the pressure between the body and the support surface. In choosing a support surface for a patient, consider the characteristics listed in Table 17.3 in selecting a product.

Obviously, no one product fulfills all of these requirements all of the time. Support surfaces are rapidly outdated as a result of technologic advances. Choose the appropriate product to meet individual patient needs, recognizing the advantages, disadvantages, and limitations of the different surfaces. Use the most sophisticated technology for the most difficult cases, such as multiple ulcers, severe contractures, and inability to tolerate the prone position.

Categories of Beds and Mattresses

Pressure-reducing devices for beds are categorized as therapeutic mattress surfaces, mattress overlays, or pressure reducing beds. (See Tables 17.4 and 17.5.)

THERAPEUTIC MATTRESS SURFACE OR OVERLAY.   The overlay is placed directly on top of regular mattress; its design and material determine effectiveness in relieving pressure.

REPLACEMENT MATTRESS.   The replacement mattress has an overlay incorporated into it, which must be evaluated over time for effectiveness in relieving pressure. Check the warranty on materials and workmanship.

Table 17.3.   Product Characteristics

Performance Characteristic	Bed/ Mattress	Wheel-chair/ Seating
Minimizes pressure under bony prominences	X	X
Produces low pressure gradient in tissue	X	X
Provides stability		X
Does not interfere with weight shifts	X	X
Does not interfere with transfers	X	X
Controls the temperature at the tissue interface	X	X
Controls moisture at the skin surface	X	X
Lightweight		X
Cost-effective	X	X
Durable	X	X

Table 17.4.   Support Surfaces: Mattresses and Beds

Mattress	Mattress Overlay	Air Flotation Bed
"Replacement"	Convoluted foam	Air-fluidized
Gel and foam	Solid foam	Low-air-loss
Water beds	Alternating air	
Foam	Static air	

AIR FLOTATION BED.   The air flotation bed is used in severe or high-risk cases, when contractures preclude appropriate positioning, and when there is limited access to skilled nursing care. It can be used at home but only after consultation with a physician, therapist, or nurse.

Wheelchair Seating: Pressure Reduction and Positioning

Wheelchair cushions reduce the risk of pressure ulcers in persons with physical disabilities. Cushions function to

- Reduce pressure in vulnerable anatomic areas by providing an additional protective layer between the seating surface and the body
- Distribute the body's weight away from bony prominences
- Stabilize the body for balance and functional positioning

Table 17.5.   Air Flotation Beds

Air-fluidized Bed	Low-air-loss Bed
Description	
A support system in which a high volume of air is forced through a fine granular material so that the material behaves like a liquid with a high density	A support system composed of air-filled pillows that leak air slowly, and a pump that is used to keep the pillows filled to the desired firmness
Advantages	
Ease of operation	Comfortable
Fail-safe	Control of skin maceration
Control of skin maceration	Can change from lying to sitting or semi-Fowler's position without foam components
Disadvantages	
Requires foam for positioning in sitting or semi-Fowler's position	Requires skilled setup
Heavy	Not fail-safe

From Donovan WH, Dinh TA, Garber S et al. Pressure ulcers. In: DeLisa JA, ed. *Rehabilitation medicine: principles and practice,* 2nd ed. Philadelphia: JB Lippincott, 1993:728, with permission.

CATEGORIES OF WHEELCHAIR SEATING.   Wheelchair seating is classified by function: postural control or pressure reduction. Positioning and postural alignment are important considerations during wheelchair sitting. Special back cushions and total seating systems are available to enable a person in a wheelchair to maintain the most functional position while reducing the risk of pressure ulcers.

Seating surfaces for pressure relief are categorized as either dynamic or static devices. Dynamic wheelchair cushions are designed to produce alternating high and low pressures at any point on the sitting surfaces of the body. Dynamic cushions depend on an external power source, such as battery or wall socket, which may limit mobility and interfere with functional independence. In static wheelchair cushions, pressure reduction is determined by the material and/or design of the cushion. There are three major categories of static wheelchair cushions: air-filled, flotation, or foam. Each category has distinct advantages and disadvantages, as described in Table 17.6.

TREATING PREDISPOSING FACTORS

Patients with pressure ulcers often have problems with wound healing because of inadequate nutrition. Evaluate and treat nutritional deficiencies so that underlying tissues receive an adequate supply of amino acids, calories, and other nutrients.

Nutrition

Protein

Ideally, protein is given by mouth in the form of complete food, but oral supplements or even tube feedings may be used. If pressure ulcers are present, the individual's protein requirements may rise to between 1.2 and 2.0 g/kg of ideal body weight to maintain positive nitrogen balance and promote protein synthesis for healing. Fever, infection, and wound drainage all increase protein demands. Protein must be available for wound granulation to occur.

Deficiencies Causing Anemia

Presence of anemia also influences prevention and healing of pressure ulcers. Although not always related to diet, anemia can be caused by various nutritional deficiencies as shown in Table 17.7. Patients with pressure ulcers often have hemoglobin levels of 10 g/100 mL or lower because of decreased appetite, loss of serum and electrolytes from the ulcer, infection, and generalized debilitation. Low hemoglobin levels cause lower blood oxygen content and, therefore, a decrease in oxygen delivered to the tissues. Deficiencies of various nutrients cause malformed red blood cells, which further aggravate the problem.

Other Nutritional Deficiencies

Vitamin C and zinc also have an essential role in wound healing. Vitamin C promotes intracellular "cement," supporting collagen in

Table 17.6. Characteristics of Static Wheelchair Cushions

Category	Definition	Advantages	Disadvantages
Air-filled	An inflatable membrane filled with air	Lightweight Easy to clean Can be customized Can be compartmentalized	Subject to puncture Not easily repaired Must monitor air pressure May cause balance or transfer problems
Flotation-filled	Chemically treated water or rubber or other liquid within plastic membrane	Adjusts to body movement Easy to clean	Heavy May leak if punctured Difficult to transfer
Flotation-gel	Plastic-like material that simulates body fat tissue; ideally, compression of one area of flotation cushion allows liquid or gel to flow into noncompressed areas	Adjusts to body movement Acts as a shock absorber	Same as flotation-filled
Polyurethane foam	Solid blocks or layers of foam Compression of one area has little effect on other areas Pressure distribution depends on design and firmness	Readily available Lightweight Can be cut into any size, shape, or thickness Easy to transfer Provides stability and good balance	Wears out quickly (average 6 months) Cannot be washed or cleaned Should not be exposed to direct sunlight

From Donovan WH, Dinh TA, Garber S et al. Pressure ulcers. In: DeLisa JA, ed. *Rehabilitation medicine: principles and practice*, 2nd ed. Philadelphia: JB Lippincott, 1993:729, with permission.

Table 17.7. Nutritional Deficiencies Relating to Anemia
Iron
Folic acid
Vitamin B_{12}
Vitamin B_6
Some trace minerals, such as copper

capillaries and various connective tissues. Stress conditions and wound healing cause increased loss of body stores of vitamin C. Zinc is recognized as the primary mineral directly involved in wound healing. Twenty percent of the body's zinc is stored in the skin.

WOUND CARE

Cleansing

Preparation of the wound is the first step in wound care. A dressing cannot be applied without first cleansing the wound and removing necrotic tissue; otherwise ineffective and even harmful results, such as infection, can occur. Use normal saline or wound *cleansers* and avoid antiseptic agents. Hydrotherapy is recommended for ulcers with large amounts of exudate and necrotic tissue. Some products may be detrimental side effects. Hydrogen peroxide may be caustic to surrounding skin. Chlorhexidine gluconate and Cetrimide are toxic to fibroblasts, the key cells responsible for laying down the collagen-based scar in soft tissue repair. The debriding action of chlorinated lime and boric acid in water is not specific to necrotic tissue. Furthermore, their use can lead to increased urea and acute oliguric renal failure.

Necrotic Tissue Removal

Necrotic tissue can be removed from a pressure ulcer surgically, mechanically, or chemically. Usually a combination of methods is used.

Surgical Debridement

Surgical debridement is the most efficient method of debridement. It is indicated under the following circumstances:

- Advancing cellulitis with sepsis
- Immunocompromised individuals
- When infection is life threatening
- For clean wounds before surgical closure

Surgical debridement is contraindicated under the following circumstances:

- Cardiac or pulmonary disease
- Uncontrolled diabetes
- Severe spasticity
- Patient who cannot tolerate surgery
- Individuals with a short life expectancy
- Quality of life cannot be improved

Sharp Debridement

Sharp debridement uses sterile instruments (scalpel, scissors, forceps, silver nitrate sticks) that sequentially remove only necrotic wound tissue without anesthesia and with little or no bleeding induced in viable tissue. It is indicated for scoring and/or excision of leathery eschar and for excision of moist necrotic tissue. It is not indicated for clean wounds or advancing cellulitis with sepsis, when infection threatens a person's life, or if the person is on anticoagulant therapy or has coagulopathy.

Mechanical Debridement

Mechanical debridement consists of packing the ulcer with saline-soaked gauze that is allowed to dry for 6 to 8 hours and is then removed. Necrotic tissue adheres to the gauze and is extracted with it. Whirlpool is a useful modality for mechanical debridement. Necrotic tissue is softened, agitated loose, and washed from the area. It is indicated for wounds with moist necrotic tissue or foreign material present. Mechanical debridement is contraindicated for clean, granulated wounds.

Enzymatic Debridement

Enzymatic debridement is a method of chemical debridement that promotes liquefaction of necrotic tissue by applying topical preparations of proteolytic or collagenolytic enzymes to tissues. Proteolytic enzymes loosen and remove slough or eschar while collagenolytic enzymes digest denatured collagen in necrotic tissue. Enzymatic debridement is indicated for the following:

- All moist necrotic wounds
- Eschar after cross-hatching
- Homebound individuals
- People who cannot tolerate surgical debridement

Enzymatic debridement is contraindicated for ischemic wounds unless adequate vascular status has been determined; in the presence of dry gangrene; and for clean, granulated wounds. Enzymatic agents used for debridement of pressure ulcers include collagenase, papain, urea, chlorophyllin, and sutilains. Mixtures that are effective in dissolving fibrin and liquefying pus but have no effect on the dissolution of necrotic tissue include streptokinase, fibrinolysin, and deoxyribonuclease. None of these chemical agents remove large amounts of devitalized collagenous tissue, penetrate thick eschar, affect a well-established bursa or sinus tract, or penetrate a deep wound. Some may actually impair drainage.

Autolytic Debridement

Autolytic debridement is a method of natural debridement promoted under occlusive or semiocclusive moisture-retentive dressings that result in solubilization of necrotic tissue only by phagocytic cells and by proteolytic and collagenolytic enzymes inherent in the tissues. It has the following indications:

- Persons on anticoagulant therapy
- Persons who cannot tolerate other forms of debridement
- All necrotic wounds in persons who are medically stable

Autolytic debridement is contraindicated when wounds are infected, the person is immunosuppressed, and in the presence of dry gangrene or dry ischemia.

Wound Dressings

Use a dressing that keeps the ulcer bed continuously moist and the surrounding intact skin dry. The dressing should control exudates but not desiccate the ulcer bed or macerate surrounding tissue. For most cases, use an occlusive dressing of the clean wound as the primary dressing. These dressings provide an optimal wound environment and protection from outside contamination. The moist environment they create allows epithelial cells to migrate. Occlusive dressings are gas permeable, providing healing tissue an adequate oxygen supply. Many synthetic occlusive dressings are available and can be divided into four groupings, each with its advantages and disadvantages (see Table 17.8).

Topical Antibiotics

There are no conclusive data on the superiority of topical antibiotics over wet-to-dry saline dressings. Topical antibiotics do not penetrate the depths of wounds or affect bacterial growth in granulation tissue. They may cause localized tissue sensitivity and may also have a detrimental effect on healing.

Surgical Management

If surgery is indicated to heal a pressure ulcer, the physiatrist and the plastic surgeon join forces for optimal pressure ulcer management. The patient with a pressure ulcer often has complex medical and disability-specific problems that require input from a functional and rehabilitation perspective throughout the entire course of hospitalization and treatment and includes attention to the following concerns.

Preoperative Care

A number of factors should be addressed before pressure ulcer surgery.

SPASMS. Spasms are short, sudden, involuntary and uncontrollable muscle contractions that often occur in patients with spinal cord or head injuries. Because the spastic movements may rub the body against bed sheets, clothing, bedrails, or adaptive equipment, patients with spasms have a tendency to develop pressure ulcers. The most effective medications for control of spasticity are sodium dantrolene (Dantrium) and baclofen (Lioresal). Before surgery, make every effort to reduce or eliminate spasms or surgery may not be successful.

LOCAL WOUND INFECTION. Prerequisites to achieving successful wound closure include adequate wound debridement and perioperative antibiotics.

NUTRITION. Check serum protein levels, hemoglobin, albumin, transferrin levels, and lymphocyte count.

BOWEL REGULATION. Control fecal incontinence before surgery. A temporary colostomy may be indicated.

COMORBID CONDITIONS. Wound healing may be compromised by cardiac disease, pulmonary disease, and diabetes. All medical comorbid conditions should be stabilized before surgery.

PRESENCE OF SCAR TISSUE FROM PREVIOUS SURGERIES. Flap reconstruction is more difficult (or impossible) if an individual has had multiple previous ulcer surgeries. Scar tissue and lack of remaining flap options may interfere with the surgeon's ability to close the wound.

SMOKING. The reported effects of smoking on wound healing are contradictory. However, as a general rule, patients are discouraged from smoking during their recovery period.

OSTEOMYELITIS. The needle bone biopsy is the most useful single test for osteomyelitis. Osteomyelitis will progress and surgical outcome will be compromised in the presence of inadequate surgical debridement that is followed by attempts to sterilize infected and necrotic bone with prolonged use of antibiotics.

URINARY TRACT INFECTION (UTI). Persons with spinal cord injuries are especially susceptible to UTIs. Therefore, adequate preoperative management is essential due to the risk of sepsis.

HETEROTOPIC OSSIFICATION. Heterotopic ossification of the hips, knees, shoulders, and spine restrict movement and affect seating, positioning, and range of motion. Blood loss may be considerable if extensive bone resection is undertaken.

Surgical Closure

Stage III and IV ulcers heal faster and generate less scar tissue when treated surgically. Surgery for pressure ulcers includes the following:

- Excision of the ulcer, scar tissue, bursa, soft tissue calcification, and underlying necrotic or infected bone
- Filling dead space, enhancing vascularity of healing wound, and distributing pressure off the bone
- Resurfacing with a large regional pedicle flap with suture line away from pressure areas
- Preserving options for future breakdowns

The major procedures for closure are standard, safe, time-tested techniques that are used the first time a pressure ulcer develops and while there is still adequate skin, subcutaneous tissue, and muscle in the adjacent area. They include primary closure, skin grafts, skin flaps, and skin flaps plus muscle interposition.

PRIMARY CLOSURE. Primary closure consists of excision of the ulcer margin and conversion of the wound into an ellipse. The wound is then closed in layers to obliterate the dead space. The skin margins are opposed and sutured. Occasionally, a drain is required. Primary closure can usually be completed as an outpatient procedure in a day surgery unit. Keep pressure off the area for 2 weeks following the closure; begin sitting after the second week, depending on the case. Remove sutures in the third week. With this form of treatment, the patient loses a minimum of time and can remain reasonably active.

SKIN GRAFT. A skin graft is a segment of dermis and epidermis that is completely separated from its blood supply at the donor site and transferred to the surface of a wound. There are two kinds of skin grafts: full-thickness skin grafts (FTSGs) containing the epidermis and all of the dermis and partial-thickness or split-thickness skin grafts (STSGs), which consist of the epidermis and only

(text continues on page 258)

Table 17.8. Characteristics of Dressing Categories[a]

Category and Definition	Indications	Advantages	Limitations
Transparent films Clear, adhesive, semipermeable membrane dressing	• Stage I and II pressure ulcers • Autolytic Debridement • Skin donor sites	• Wound is visible • Impermeable to external fluids and bacteria • Promote autolytic debridement • Minimize friction	• Nonabsorptive • Wrinkle • Do not use on ulcers with fragile surrounding skin, copious drainage, or infection
Hydrocolloids Occlusive or semiocclusive adhesive wafers containing hydroactive/absorptive particles that interact with wound fluid to form gelatinous mass over wound bed	• Protects partial-thickness wounds • Autolytic debridement of necrosis • Wounds with mild exudate	• Maintain moist environment • Nonadhesive to healing tissue • Impermeable to external bacteria • Support autolytic Debridement • Absorbant • Waterproof • Reduce pain • Easy to apply • Thin forms diminish friction	• Nontransparent • Soften and change shape with heat or friction • Edges may curl • Odor and yellow drainage on removal (melted dressing material) • Not for wounds with heavy exudates, sinus tracts, infections • Not for wounds with exposed bone or tendon • Not for wounds with fragile surrounding skin

continued

Table 17.8. *Continued*

Category and Definition	Indications	Advantages	Limitations
Hydrogels Water or glycerin-based gels, insoluble in water, available in solid sheets, amorphous gels, or impregnated gauze	• Partial or full-thickness wounds • Wounds with necrosis and slough • Burns and tissue damaged by radiation	• Soothing and cooling • Fill dead space • Rehydrate dry wound beds • Promote autolytic debridement • Provide minimal to moderate absorption • Conform to wound bed • Transparent to translucent • Use amorphous form with infection	• Require secondary dressing • Not for wounds with heavy exudates • May dry out and adhere to wound bed • May macerate surrounding skin
Foams Semipermeable membranes that are either hydrophilic or hydrophobic; vary in thickness, absorptive capacity, and adhesive properties	• Partial and full-thickness wounds with minimal to moderate exudates • Secondary dressing to provide additional absorption • Provide protection	• Insulate wounds • Provide some padding • Most are nonadherent • Conformable • Manage light or moderate exudates • Easy to use • Some are designed for deep cavities	• Nontransparent • Nonadherent foams require secondary dressing, tape, or net • Some newer foams have tape on edges • Poor conformability to deep wounds • Not for use with dry eschar or wounds with no exudate

Alginates Soft, absorbent, nonwoven dressings derived from seaweed that have a fluffy cottonlike appearance; react with wound exudates to form a viscous hydrophilic gel mass over wound; available in ropes or pads	• Wounds with moderate to large amounts of exudates • Wounds with combination exudates and necrosis • Wounds that require packing and absorption • Infected and noninfected exuding wounds	• Absorb up to 20 times their weight in drainage • Fill dead space • Support debridement in presence of exudates • Easy to apply	• Require secondary dressing • Not recommended for dry or lightly exudating wounds • Can dry wound bed
Gauze dressings Cotton or synthetic fabric, absorptive and permeable to water and oxygen; may be used wet, moist, dry, or impregnated with petrolatum, antiseptics, or other agents; come in various weaves. Includes: Wet to dry Continuous dry Continuous moist	• Exudative wounds • Wounds with dead space, tunneling, or sinus tracts • Wounds with combination exudates or necrotic tissue	• Readily available • Can be used with gels, normal saline, or topical antimicrobials • Can be used on infected wounds • Good mechanical debridement if properly used • Cost-effective filler for large wounds • Effective delivery of topicals if kept moist	• Delays healing if improperly used • Pain on removal, especially wet to dry • Labor intensive • Require secondary dressing

[a]Adapted from *Pressure ulcer prevention and treatment following spinal cord injury: a clinical practice guideline for health-care professionals*. Consortium for Spinal Cord Medicine, Paralyzed Veterans of America, Washington, DC: 2000, with permission.

a portion of the underlying dermis. The STSG is the more likely of the two to survive on the recipient site because it accepts a longer phase of plasmatic absorption and, therefore, can survive longer before vascularization occurs. STSGs do not contain dermal appendages (sweat glands and hair follicles) and, therefore, need continuous lubrication.

FLAP CLOSURES. Muscle and musculocutaneous flaps, the mainstay of pressure ulcer surgery, are used when wounds are too extensive for primary closure and loss of tissue mass precludes grafting. A flap is a "tongue" of tissue detached from surrounding tissue except for a pedicle or base, through which blood supply is maintained. It consists of full thickness of skin and underlying subcutaneous tissue and can be elevated and moved to another area of the body within the limits of its vascular pedicle. If a defect requires a flap, the patient must be prepared for a major operative procedure and anticipate 4 to 6 weeks of hospitalization. Usually, only ischial, trochanteric, or sacral ulcers necessitate flaps. The musculocutaneous flap is the most commonly used. A composite of skin, subcutaneous tissue, and underlying muscle, its blood supply derives from the major vascular leash (artery and veins), which enters the proximal undersurface of the muscle and is elevated along with the muscle. To mobilize the flap, the fascia and subcutaneous tissue are sutured together to avoid disrupting the perforating vessels in the loose, gossamer-like, and areolar tissue at the interface of these two layers. Transfer of a musculocutaneous flap leaves a deep donor site that must be covered by a skin graft in most cases. Occasionally, it can be closed primarily.

COMPLICATIONS

There are different types of medical complications that can result from the development of pressure ulcers and subsequent treatment.

Use of Air-fluidized Beds

Use of an air-fluidized bed can cause multiple problems, which can usually be avoided. Severe dehydration occurs in 3% to 4% of patients because of increased insensible fluid loss caused by the continuous flow of warm, dry air through the filter sheet. Extra fluid intake is necessary. Dry scaly skin may develop, especially in older adults. The low relative humidity of the bed environment causes drying of the nasal mucosa, potentially resulting in epistaxis. Hypernatremia may occur, as well as hypophosphatemia and hypocalcemia with chronic use, because of prolonged periods in a weightless environment. The sensation of floating can lead to confusion and disorientation. New pressure ulcers may develop, especially at the heels. One should turn the patient and perform frequent skin checks. The patient's cough mechanism may be rendered ineffective because of the lack of a firm back support; therefore, pulmonary hygiene is an essential measure in patients with restricted mobility. Leakage of particles may cause eye injury to the patient and caregivers. Inspect the filter sheet frequently for tears; replace as necessary.

Osteomyelitis

There is a 10% incidence of osteomyelitis related to pressure ulcers. In addition, sepsis secondary to pressure ulcers can be a serious and sometimes fatal complication. There may be difficulty differentiating osteomyelitis underlying the pressure ulcer from soft tissue infection. Surgical debridement of the ulcer combined with broad-spectrum antibiotics is needed in soft tissue infection. The presence of osteomyelitis will indicate the extent of ostectomy and can modify the length of antibiotic treatment. Radionuclide bone scanning has been proposed as a sensitive diagnostic tool for osteomyelitis. However, a significant problem with false-positive results has been recognized. Needle biopsy of the underlying bone is the most accurate method for diagnosis of osteomyelitis. However, if any test is positive, recent studies have advocated use of a plain x-ray film, white blood cell count ($15,000/mm^3$), and erythrocyte sedimentation rate (120 mm/hour) as the most sensitive, specific, and cost-effective workup for osteomyelitis.

Amputation

Amputation and the fillet procedure are reserved for those patients who have extensive ulceration, with or without underlying osteomyelitis, and cannot be treated successfully with any of the procedures previously described. The procedure can consist of an above-knee amputation, fillet (removal of the femur), and use of the entire thigh for flap coverage. A more extensive and formidable technical procedure comprises amputation at the level of the ankle and fillet of the entire leg. This provides the largest possible amount of muscle and subcutaneous tissue to cover the defects. This technique must be classified as a tertiary procedure and performed only when all other procedures are unsuccessful. The psychologic consequences of amputation compound those of the primary disability.

SUMMARY

There are no ideal or universal methods for preventing and managing pressure ulcers. However, awareness of risk factors, preventive interventions, and the latest technology in support surfaces and dressings enable clinicians to select the most effective and economical approaches that meet individual patient needs.

SUGGESTED READINGS

Agris J, Spira M. Pressure ulcers: prevention and treatment. *Clin Symp* 1979;31:2–32.

Allman RM, Walker JM, Hart MK, et al. Air-fluidized beds or conventional therapy for pressure sores: a randomized trial. *Ann Intern Med* 1987;107:641–648.

Alpert SH. The psychological aspects of amputation surgery. *Orth Prosth* 1982;36:50–56.

American Academy of Physical Medicine & Rehabilitation handbook. Chicago: American Academy of Physical Medicine & Rehabilitation, 1989:Appendix 7–10.

Bergstrom N, Allman RM, Alvarez OM, et al. Treatment of pressure ulcers. Clinical Practice Guideline, No 15, AHCPR Publication No. 95-0652. Rockville, MD: U.S. Department of Health and Human Services, Public Health Service, Agency for Health Care Policy and Research, December 1994.

Bergstrom N, Braden BJ, Laguzza A, et al. The Braden scale for predicting pressure sore risk. *Nurs Res* 1987;36:205–210.

Constantian MB. *Pressure ulcers: principles and techniques of management.* Boston: Little, Brown and Company, 1980:146.

Donovan WH, Dinh TA, Garber SL et al. Pressure ulcers. In: DeLisa JA, ed. *Rehabilitation medicine,* 2nd ed. Philadelphia: JB Lippincott, 1993:716–732.

Garber SL, Biddle AK, Click CN, et al. Pressure ulcer prevention and treatment following spinal cord injury: a clinical practice guideline for health-care professionals. Consortium for Spinal Cord Medicine Clinical Practice Guidelines. Washington, DC: Paralyzed Veterans of America, 2000.

Kosiak M. Etiology of decubitus ulcers. *Arch Phys Med Rehabil* 1961; 42:19–28.

Krasner D. *Chronic wound care: a clinical source book for health care professional.* King of Prussia, PA: Health Management Publications, 1990:74–77, 152–156.

Krouskop TA. Selecting a support surface. *CAET J* 1990;9:5–10.

Krouskop TA, Noble PC, Garber SL, et al. The effectiveness of preventive management in reducing the occurrence of pressure sores. *J Rehabil Res Dev* 1983;20:74–83.

Lewis VL, Baily MH, Pulawski G, et al. The diagnosis of osteomyelitis in patients with pressure sores. *Plast Reconst Surg* 1988; 81:229–232.

Nimit K. Guidelines for home air-fluidized bed therapy. *Health Technol Assess Rep* 1989;5:1–11.

Panel for the Prediction and Prevention of Pressure Ulcers in Adults. Pressure ulcers in adults: prediction and prevention. Clinical Practice Guideline, Number 3. AHCPR Publication No. 92-0047. Rockville, MD: Agency for Health Care Policy and Research, Public Health Service, U.S. Department of Health and Human Services, May 1992.

Seiler WO, Stahelin HB. Recent findings on decubitus ulcer pathology: implications for care. *Geriatrics* 1986;41:47–57.

Webster JG. *Prevention of pressure sores: engineering and clinical aspects.* Bristol, Philadelphia, and New York: Adam Hilger, 1991: 208–212.

Woolsey RM, McGarry JD. The cause, prevention, and treatment of pressure sores. *Neurol Clin* 1991;9:797–808.

Pulmonary Rehabilitation

Sally Ann Holmes

DEFINITION

According to the American College of Chest Physicians, pulmonary rehabilitation is "the art of medical practice wherein an individually tailored, multi-disciplinary program is formulated which, through accurate diagnosis, therapy, emotional support, and education, stabilizes or reverses both the physical and psychopathological aspects of pulmonary diseases." Although a comprehensive rehabilitation program may have little effect on the rate of progress of the underlying disease, a number of beneficial effects have been documented, including reduction in the average number of hospitalization days per year and subjective improvement in symptoms and quality of life. The primary goal is to return the patient to the highest possible functional capacity despite the pulmonary disease.

EPIDEMIOLOGY

Chronic respiratory diseases are a leading cause of major limitation in activity, loss of work days, and premature retirement resulting from disability and hospitalizations. In the United States, chronic obstructive pulmonary disease (COPD) is the third leading cause of death among men and the fourth leading cause of death among women aged 55 to 74. Cigarette smoking is the major risk factor in the development and clinical course of COPD. Studies indicate that physician-delivered smoking intervention can be effective and that smoking cessation results in lowering the excessive rates of lung functional loss associated with smoking. Therefore, healthcare providers should provide education and encourage smoking cessation.

Pulmonary disease is the most common cause of early death in traumatic quadriplegia and neuromuscular disorders.

ANATOMY AND PHYSIOLOGY

There are four groups of muscles of respiration. The diaphragm, which is innervated by the phrenic nerve (C3, C4, and C5), is the principal muscle of respiration. The chest wall muscles include the internal and external intercostals, the scalenes, and the accessory muscles of respiration (sternocleidomastoid, trapezius, and pectoralis major). The abdominal muscles enhance the mechanical advantage of the diaphragm during inspiration and are the primary expiratory muscles. The muscles of the upper airway are important for keeping the upper airway open; they include the muscles of the mouth, tongue, uvula, palate, and larynx.

During quiet breathing, diaphragmatic contraction forces the abdominal contents away from the thorax and elevates the ribs in a bucket-handle fashion resulting in inspiration. Subsequently, the elastic recoil of the thoracic and abdominal wall produces expiration, a passive process in normal quiet breathing. With increased ventilatory demand the chest wall, abdominal, and accessory muscles actively contribute to the respiratory effort. Expiratory muscles participate in the mobilization of secretions during coughing and sneezing. Chest wall structure and compliance, as well as airway resistance, are important determinants of respiratory function.

CONTROL OF RESPIRATION

The respiratory center in the medulla receives input from the central chemoreceptors (stimulated by hypercarbia) and from the peripheral chemoreceptors in the carotid and aortic bodies (stimulated by hypoxia) to maintain normal blood gas levels under great variations in metabolic demand and carbon dioxide production. Voluntary control of respiration originates in the cortex and descends in the spinal cord to the respiratory muscles. With respiratory dysfunction the demand for work may exceed the ability to supply energy; thus, respiratory muscle fatigue occurs with resulting hypoxia and hypercarbia or respiratory acidosis. With chronic respiratory acidosis, bicarbonate concentration increases to maintain near-normal pH, altering the "set point" of the control of respiration. Chronic hypoxia can lead to pulmonary hypertension and cor pulmonale and death if left untreated.

ETIOLOGY

Causes of COPD include the following:

Emphysema
Chronic bronchitis
Bronchiectasis
Asthma

Causes of chronic restrictive pulmonary disease include the following:

Neuromuscular diseases with respiratory muscle weakness
Duchenne muscular dystrophy
Postpoliomyelitis syndrome
Spinal muscular atrophy
Congenital myopathies
Amyotrophic lateral sclerosis (ALS)
Myasthenia gravis
Eaton-Lambert syndrome
Distortion of the thoracic cage
Kyphoscoliosis
Ankylosing spondylitis
Postthoracotomy
Paralysis of respiratory muscles
Traumatic tetraplegia
Guillain-Barré syndrome

LUNG VOLUME DEFINITIONS (FIG. 18-1 AND TABLE 18.1).

Forced vital capacity (FVC): amount of air moved when lungs are
    forcefully expanded after maximal expiration
Total lung capacity (TLC): amount of gas contained within the
    lungs at the end of maximal inspiration

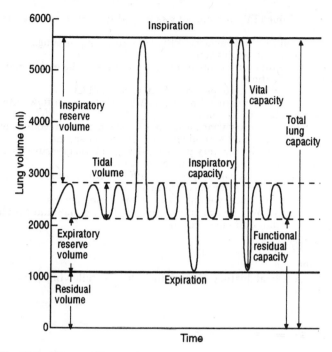

Fig. 18-1. Diagram illustrating respiratory excursions during normal breathing and during maximal inspiration and maximal expiration. (From Guyton AC. *Textbook of medical physiology*, 7th ed. WB Saunders, 1986:470, with permission.)

	Table 18.1. Characteristic Alterations in Pulmonary Function Tests	
	Obstructive Pattern	**Restrictive Pattern**
FEV1	↓	↓
FVC	↓	↓
Airflow (FEV1/FVC, %)	↓	←→/↑
Airflow response to bronchodilators	↑/←→	←→
TLC	↑/←→	↓
FRC	↑	↓/←→
RV	↑/←→	↓/←→
MVV	↓	↓
Lung compliance	←→/↓	↓

Tidal volume (TV): amount of gas moved in normal inspiratory effort

Functional residual capacity (FRC): amount of gas in lungs at the end of normal expiration

Residual volume (RV): amount of gas in lungs at the end of maximal expiration

FEV_1: amount of air expelled in first second of FVC

Maximal midexpiratory flow rate (MMEF): average flow rate, between 25% to 50% of FVC

Maximum voluntary ventilation (MVV): the maximum volume of air exhaled in a 12-second period in liters per second

Maximal static inspiratory pressure (PI_{max}): static pressure measured near RV after maximal expiration

Maximal static expiratory pressure (PE_{max}): static pressure measured near TLC after maximal inspiration

Minute volume: tidal volume × rate of breathing per minute

Peak cough flow: the amount of airflow during maximal cough expressed in liters per second

EVALUATION

History

The medical history should include the following possible symptoms:

Dyspnea
Fatigue
Orthopnea
Decreased activity
Morning headache
Anorexia
Dysphoria
Poor sleep/vivid nightmares

Physical Examination

The physical examination should document the following conditions:

Tachypnea
Shallow breathing pattern
Inward (paradoxical) motion of abdomen with inspiration
Accessory muscle activity during quiet breathing
Prolongation of audible expiratory sounds
Increased intensity of pulmonic second sound
Tachycardia
Dependent edema
Clubbing
Cyanosis

Diagnostic Tests

The following diagnostic tests should be considered:

Chest x-ray
Electrocardiogram
Hemoglobin and hematocrit
Pulmonary function tests
Pulse oximetry and end-tidal CO_2 monitors

Arterial blood gas
Serum protein electrophoresis for alpha$_1$-antitrypsin
Echocardiogram
Sleep studies
Others as indicated by underlying disease process

Functional Evaluation

Evaluate effect of pulmonary disease on morbidity, self-care, and vocational and recreational activities. Symptoms are classified according to functional impairment. See Table 18.2.

MANAGEMENT

Medical Management

Preventive care plays an important role in stabilizing and preventing complications in chronic pulmonary disorders. Smoking cessation is by far the most important component of preventive care for these patients. Influenza and pneumococcal vaccines have been shown to reduce the incidence of infectious respiratory illnesses in this at-risk population. These patients should avoid exposure to irritants such as dust and chemicals at home and at the workplace. Treatment of other medical conditions, as well as aggressive treatment of pulmonary infections, is important in the medical management of patients with chronic respiratory disorders. Patients with COPD may benefit from the use of bronchodilators and corticosteroids delivered by metered dose inhalers or hand-held nebulizers or orally. Commonly used bronchodilators include beta$_2$-agonists (Albuterol, Metaproterenol), theophylline, and anticholinergics (Ipratropium).

Oxygen therapy should be used with caution in patients with chronic respiratory failure. Because hypoxic ventilatory drive predominates in these patients, oxygen therapy may exacerbate hypoventilation and place the patient in danger of respiratory arrest.

Table 18.2.   Moser Classification of Functional Pulmonary Disability

Class	Assessment
Class 1	Dyspnea with strenuous activity
Class 2	Dyspnea on climbing stairs, but not with essential activities of daily living
Class 3	Dyspnea with some activities of daily living, but able to walk one block at a slow pace
Class 4	Dyspnea with minimal exertion; dependent on others for some activities of daily living
Class 5	Dyspnea at rest; requires assistance for most activities of daily living; essentially housebound

Adapted from Rondinelli RD, Hill NS. Rehabilitation of the patient with pulmonary disease. In: DeLisa JA, ed. *Rehabilitation medicine principles and practice.* Philadelphia: JB Lippincott, 1988:691, with permission.

Assisted ventilation can provide respiratory muscle rest, thus decreasing the energy expenditure of ventilatory muscles. Weaning protocols should include progressively increasing time off the ventilator with complete rest between work periods.

Forms of assisted ventilation include the following:

Negative pressure ventilators exert negative pressure on the chest wall, resulting in inspiration (iron lung, chest cuirass).

Positive pressure ventilators displace the abdominal contents, assisting diaphragm movement (rocking bed, pneumobelt).

Pressure-limited positive pressure ventilators deliver air via a nose mask until a preset amount of pressure is reached; thus, the tidal volume varies with airway resistance (CPAP, BiPAP).

Volume-limited positive pressure ventilators deliver a preset volume of air with each breath; thus, constant ventilation is maintained by the minute. Portable models are available for home use. Air may be delivered via mouthpiece, nose mask, strapless oralnasal interface (SONI), or tracheostomy.

Surgical Management

Tracheostomy may be indicated for chronic positive pressure ventilation. Electrophrenic nerve pacing may be appropriate for high cervical spinal cord injury (the patient must have intact phrenic nerves for pacing).

Rehabilitative Management

A multidisciplinary team including a physiatrist, social worker, physical therapist, occupational therapist, respiratory therapist, dietician, psychologist, and nurse work with the patient to optimize medical management, functional independence, and quality of life.

Chest Physical Therapy

Breathing techniques are as follows:

Diaphragmatic breathing. This technique involves retraining the patient to use the diaphragm while relaxing abdominal muscles during inspiration. The patient can feel the abdomen rise, while the chest wall remains stationary (Fig. 18-2).

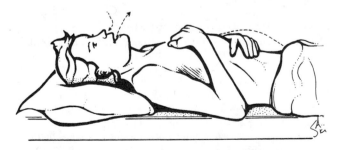

Fig. 18-2. **Diaphragmatic breathing technique. (Adapted from Rondinelli RD, Hill NS. Rehabilitation of the patient with pulmonary disease. In: DeLisa JA, ed.** *Rehabilitation medicine: principles and practice.* **Philadelphia: JB Lippincott, 1988:696, with permission.)**

Pursed lip breathing. The patient's lips are pursed during expiration to prevent air trapping resulting from small airway collapse.

Glossopharyngeal breathing. The patient uses a pistoning action of the tongue to project boluses of air into the lungs after taking a maximum breath.

Postural drainage. The use of gravity-assisted positioning can improve the mobilization of secretions. There are a variety of positions, designed for maximum drainage of each lung segment.

Manual percussion. Percussion or vibration of the chest wall can assist in the mobilization of secretions.

Controlled coughing. The patient sits leaning forward and initiates a timed, deliberate cough with enough force to mobilize mucus without causing airway collapse.

Assisted coughing. In this technique, upward pressure is applied to the abdomen during exhalation.

Physical Therapy

Assess endurance and provide an exercise program to progressively increase endurance while encouraging proper breathing techniques and body mechanics. Pulse oximetry monitoring may be indicated. Exercise is controversial in disorders such as post-poliomyelitis and muscular dystrophy; with these disorders, avoid exercise to the point of fatigue.

Provide an appropriate home exercise program.

Instruct patient and family or caretakers in chest physical therapy and postural drainage techniques.

Provide and train patient to use assistive devices as needed for mobility and functional independence.

Occupational Therapy

Assess and provide an exercise program for upper extremity range of motion and strengthening.

Assess self-care activities and provide training.

Recommend adaptive equipment to increase independence and minimize energy expenditure.

Evaluate home and work environment.

Give suggestions to increase independence and energy conservation.

Respiratory Therapy

Instruct patient and caregivers in the use of metered dose inhalers, nebulizers, supplemental oxygen, and home ventilator as needed.

Equipment

Nebulizer. The nebulizer delivers medication suspended in liquid particles to lower airways and loosens secretions.

In-exsufflator (noninvasive) or suctioning. Devices (invasive) assist with clearing tracheal secretions.

Intermittent positive pressure breathing (IPPB). IPPB device provides positive airway pressure to augment inspiration and expand the lungs; these may be used with a nebulizer to deliver medication or saline solution.

Supplemental oxygen. Supplemental oxygen is provided via nasal cannula, facemask, or transtracheal cannula.

Ventilator. See previous descriptions of positive and negative pressure ventilators.

Wheelchair or walker. A wheelchair or walker can be modified if needed for supplemental oxygen or portable ventilator.

Tracheostomy tubes are classified as follows:

Cuffed portex. This plastic tube is pliable with an inflatable cuff to prevent air leaking.

Shiley fenestrated or nonfenestrated. This plastic tube has a removable inner cannula; the fenestrated tube allows vocalization while off the ventilator.

Jackson metal (fenestrated). This tube is for long-term use.

Passy-Muir valve. This one-way valve used with the tracheostomy tube cuff deflated allows vocalization on or off the ventilator.

Bavona (Fome-cuff). This high-volume/low-pressure cuff protects the airway with minimal trauma to mucosa; vocalization is not possible.

COMPLICATIONS

Complications include the following:

Decreased ventilatory capacity with resulting activity limitations and decreased functional independence.

Increased risk of infection secondary to decreased ability to clear secretions. There is a high risk of acute respiratory failure even with mild pulmonary infections because of low respiratory reserve.

Respiratory arrest secondary to use of supplemental oxygen, as a result of suppression of hypoxic ventilatory drive in patients with chronic carbon dioxide retention.

Pulmonary hypertension and cor pulmonale secondary to chronic hypoxia.

Tracheostomy risks. Refer to Table 18.3.

OUTCOME

Documented benefits of a comprehensive pulmonary rehabilitation program include a reduction in the average number of hospitalization days per year and subjective improvement in symptoms and quality of life. Rehabilitation goals and prognosis are determined by the underlying disease process, the psychologic adjustment of the patient and family, and available financial resources.

Table 18.3. Risks with Tracheostomy

Hemorrhage
Infection
Increased secretions
Lesions of tracheal mucosa from cuff or suction catheter
Thickening or mucus from inflow of dry air (always humidify air)
Stoma stenosis
Tracheomalacia
Tracheoesophageal fistula
Tracheal granulations

SUGGESTED READINGS

Bach JR. Alternative methods of ventilatory support for the patient with ventilatory failure due to spinal cord injury. *J Am Paraplegia Soc* 1991;14:158–174.

Bach JR, Alba A. Management of chronic alveolar hypoventilation by nasal ventilation. *Chest* 1990;97:52–57.

Bach JR, et al. The ventilator assisted individual: cost analysis of institutionalism vs. rehabilitation and in-home management. *Chest* 1992; 101:26–30.

Coultas DB. The physician's role in smoking cessation. *Clin Chest Med* 1991;12:755–768.

Curran FJ, Colbert A. Ventilator management in Duchenne muscular dystrophy and post poliomyelitis syndrome: twelve years experience. *Arch Phys Med Rehabil* 1989;70:180–185.

DeTroyer A, Estenne M. Functional anatomy of the respiratory muscles. *Clin Chest Med* 1988;9:175–193.

Dingemans LM, Hawn JM. Mobility and equipment for the ventilator-dependent tetraplegic. *Paraplegia* 1978;16:175–183.

Holmes SA. Muscles of respiration. In: Cutter NC, Kevorkian CG, eds. *Handbook of manual muscle testing.* McGraw-Hill, 1999:259–268.

Kelly BJ, Luce JM. The diagnosis and management of neuromuscular diseases causing respiratory failure. *Chest* 1991;99:1485–1494.

Nosek MA, Holmes SA. Independent living and quality of life among persons who use ventilators. *Phys Med Rehabil Clin North Am* 1996; 7:445–456.

Stewart DG, et al. Benefits of an inpatient pulmonary rehabilitation program: a prospective analysis. *Arch Phys Med Rehabil* 2001;82: 347–352.

Tobin M. Respiratory muscles in disease. *Clin Chest Med* 1988;9: 263–285.

Tobin MJ. Advances in mechanical ventilation. *N Engl J Med* 2001; 344:1986–1996.

19

Spinal Cord Injury

Jennifer J. James and Diana D. Cardenas

DEFINITION

A spinal cord injury (SCI) is a disruption to the spinal cord or, in the case of the cauda equina injury, a disruption to the nerve roots at the lowest end of the cord that lie within the bony canal. The term *spinal cord injury* is often reserved for injuries caused by trauma, but there are other causes. For purposes of this discussion, SCI refers to injury caused by trauma. A discussion of diseases that may affect the spinal cord such as tumors, transverse myelitis, and multiple sclerosis is beyond the scope of this chapter.

ANATOMY

This section is divided into neuroanatomy and skeletal anatomy.

Neuroanatomy

The spinal cord is a complex but highly organized mass of nerve tissues that extends from the medulla of the brainstem, just below the foramen magnum, to taper to an end approximately adjacent to the L1 or the L2 vertebra. The nerve roots extend beyond the end of the cord, the conus medullaris, to form a network of nerve roots called the cauda equina, which means "horse's tail." There are 31 pairs of nerve roots: 8 cervical, 12 thoracic, 5 lumbar, 5 sacral, and 1 coccygeal. All cervical nerve roots exit through bony foramina above their corresponding vertebral level, until the C8 nerve root exits between the C8 and the T1 vertebra, then the roots exit below their corresponding vertebra. Because the spinal cord is shorter than its bony housing, the T12 nerve root is actually located at the level of the tenth thoracic vertebral body. The spinal cord is very short below the L1 vertebral body; therefore, it is not practical to attempt correlation (Fig. 19-1).

In the sagittal plane, there are two enlargements of the cord, one between C2 and T2 and the other between T10 and T12, with the largest diameter at C5-6. The average spinal cord diameter is 17 mm.

A cross-sectional axial plane reveals the butterfly-shaped gray matter surrounded by white matter, with a central canal containing cerebrospinal fluid. A detailed discussion of somatotopic organization of the cord is beyond the scope of this chapter. The gray matter is comprised of neuron cell bodies and is divided into horns. The posterior horn contains projections of cell bodies of sensory fibers from the dorsal root ganglion, the lateral horn contains preganglionic neurons of the sympathetic nervous system, and the anterior horn contains motor neuron cell bodies.

The white matter is composed of ascending and descending, myelinated and unmyelinated, longitudinal nerve fiber tracts. It is important to know the location, function, and decussation of these tracts to understand different SCI syndromes. There are basically four important tracts: three ascending sensory and one descending motor tract (Fig. 19-2).

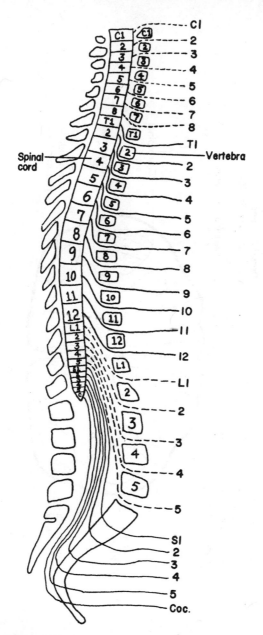

Fig. 19-1. The spinal nerves. C, cervical; T, thoracic; L, lumbar; S, sacral; Coc, coccygeal.

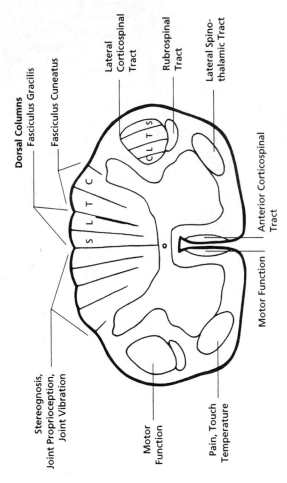

Fig. 19-2.   Cross section of spinal cord showing major ascending and descending tracts.

Sensory Tracts

1. Dorsal column medial lemniscus tract resides in the posterior columns; it is somatotopically organized into a medial portion carrying messages about light touch and proprioception from lower extremities and a lateral portion with messages from upper extremities. It ascends and then decussates in the medial lemniscus of the medulla.
2. Anterolateral spinothalamic tract (ALST) resides in the lateral and anterior white matter, conveying pain and temperature sensation. It decussates within the anterior commissure of the spinal cord, approximately two segments cephalad after entry of the fibers.
3. Dorsal spinocerebellar tract resides in the far lateral white matter, remains ipsilateral, and conveys information to the cerebellum about quality of movement.

Motor Tract

The descending corticospinal pyramidal tract carries volitional motor innervation from the opposite cerebral cortex, through the internal capsule, decussating in the pyramidal tract of the medulla and terminating in the midlateral white matter of the spinal cord. It is thought to be somatotopically organized, with the medial portion governing upper extremities and the lateral portion governing the lower extremities.

The principle vascular supply to the spinal cord is via the single anterior spinal artery and the two posterior spinal arteries supplying the posterior third of the cord. There is a vulnerable watershed area located in the anastomosis. In the sagittal plane, the midthoracic area supplied by the artery of Adamkiewicz radicular artery from the aorta is the area vulnerable to watershed ischemic injury.

Upper and Lower Motor Neuron Tracts

It is important to fully understand the concept of upper and lower motor neuron injury not only for accurate assessment of SCI but also for ongoing treatment and for management of neurogenic bowel and bladder. The upper motor neuron (UMN) tract is also known as the pyramidal or corticospinal tract, and its course is described previously. The lower motor neuron (LMN) supply originates in the anterior horn cells of the spinal cord and terminates in the peripheral nerve supply. Most cervical and thoracic cord lesions involve the UMN tract; however, there may be limited damage to the anterior horn cells resulting in LMN damage at the lesion level. Injuries below the conus medullaris result in LMN sequelae. Table 19.1 shows the important differences between the two systems.

Skeletal Anatomy

The spine has 7 cervical, 12 thoracic, 5 lumbar, and 5 sacral (fused) vertebrae. Spine stability is determined according to the location of the injury.

Upper cervical: The stability of injuries to the occipital condyle, atlas (C1) and axis (C2) are determined by fracture pattern. The atlas, or first cervical vertebra, is a ring structure. The odontoid

Table 19.1.   Difference Between Upper and Lower Motor Neuron Injuries

	UMN	LMN
Deep tendon reflexes	Increased	Decreased
Muscle tone	Spastic	Flaccid
Babinski reflex	Present	Absent
Bowel/bladder	Spastic	Flaccid

LMN, lower motor neuron; UMN, upper motor neuron.

process is the bony projection of the axis, the second cervical vertebra. A strong ligament holds the odontoid against the anterior part of the atlas ring, keeping if from compressing posteriorly against the spinal cord (Fig. 19-3).

Lower cervical: Assessment of C3 through C7 requires determination of translation and angulation in cervical flexion and extension films. Sagittal plane translation greater than 3.5 mm or angulation greater than 11 degrees is considered unstable.

Thoracolumbar: Evaluation uses the three-column model. Fractures are stable if only one column is involved. If fractures, displacement, or ligamentous injury involves two columns, the spine is considered unstable (Fig. 19-4).

Anterior column: Anterior longitudinal ligament, anterior vertebral body, and anterior annulus fibrosis.

Middle column: Posterior vertebral body, posterior annulus, and posterior longitudinal ligament.

Posterior column: Spinous processes, laminae, facets, pedicles, and posterior ligamentous structures (ligamentum flavum, intraspinous/supraspinous ligaments).

EPIDEMIOLOGY

The incidence of SCI in the United States is estimated to be about 40 cases per million population per year or approximately 11,000 new cases per year. Because there is no mandatory national surveillance system, the true incidence is unknown. The estimated prevalence in the United States is given as between 183,000 and 230,000 persons or between 721 and 906 per million population. Recent data suggest that the age at injury is correlated to survival, with a markedly decreased life expectancy in older persons, especially with cervical injuries and complete injuries as compared with age-matched controls. The average age at injury for those injured after 1990 is 35.3 years, which is higher than in past decades. Another trend is an increase in the proportion of those who were at least 61 years of age at injury, which has increased to 10% since 1990. Males comprise about 80% of all those who are injured.

Although the incidence is low compared with other diseases, the economic consequences are disproportionally high. The annual cost of SCI to society is about $7.3 to $8.3 billion. The average yearly costs after initial rehabilitation average between $24,000 and $28,000. The lifetime costs of paraplegia for someone injured at 50 has been estimated as $873,000.

C1 and C2 Vertebrae

Atlas

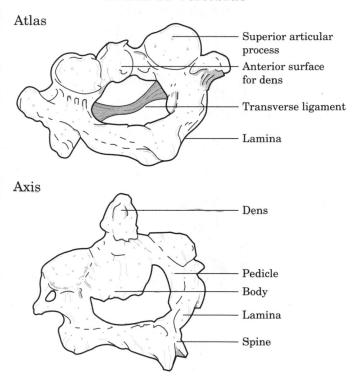

Superior articular process

Anterior surface for dens

Transverse ligament

Lamina

Axis

Dens

Pedicle

Body

Lamina

Spine

Fig. 19-3. C1 and C2 vertebra.

ETIOLOGY AND PATHOPHYSIOLOGY

The most common etiology of SCI since 1990 is motor vehicle accidents (38.5%) followed by acts of violence (24.5%), falls (21.8%), and sports injuries (7.2%). The proportion of spinal cord injuries from acts of violence, which are primarily gunshot wounds, and falls have increased steadily since 1973. The most frequent neurologic category is incomplete tetraplegia (29.1%), followed by complete paraplegia (27.3%), incomplete paraplegia (20.6%), and complete tetraplegia (18.6%). Rarely is there a complete transection of the spinal cord; however, complete transection is not necessary for a complete lesion. Rarely a patient who may seem to have a complete injury goes on to develop some further recovery below the neurologic level. Most recovery begins in the first few days to weeks, but there are cases in which recovery does not seem to begin until weeks to months after injury. Serial examinations are, therefore, important. To date there remains only one acute pharmacologic intervention, intravenous methylprednisolone, that has been shown to have a

Three Column Model
of Spine Stability

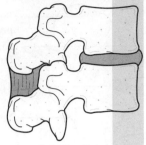

Anterior Column

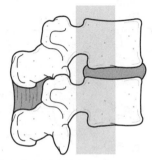

Middle Column

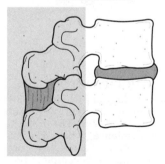

Posterior Column

Fig. 19-4. Three-column model of spine stability.

beneficial effect on recovery after acute SCI. This steroid helps reduce free radical damage and lipid peroxidation when given within the first few hours of injury.

ASSESSMENT AND EVALUATION

A comprehensive systematic approach is imperative to complete assessment. This includes evaluation of spinal stability, as well as assessment of neurologic, musculoskeletal, pulmonary, cardiovascular, gastrointestinal, genitourinary (GU), and integumentary systems. Treatment is thoroughly discussed in another section.

Evaluation of Spinal Stability

Skeletal spinal stability evaluation is based on a division of upper cervical, lower cervical, and thoracolumbar injuries (see section on spinal anatomy). Radiographic studies must visualize all components of the spine. A cervical spine x-ray series must include an open-mouth odontoid view, swimmer's view (to visualize C7), anterior-posterior, lateral, and bilateral oblique views. A computed tomography (CT) scan may also be needed to identify fractures, and a magnetic resonance imaging (MRI) to determine ligamentous injury affecting stability. Based on the type and extent of injury, it is determined if the injury requires surgery versus external orthotic intervention. Postoperatively the injury requires an additional 10 to 12 weeks for complete healing; therefore, an external orthotic device must be used to decrease stress forces across the site. The choice of orthotic device depends on the degree and type of stabilizing force required. The halo vest provides the most stability for cervical fractures. There are many different types of cervical orthoses, which include the SOMI, Minerva, Miami J, and Philadelphia collar. Thoracolumbar sacral orthoses (known as TLSO braces) are also available in a variety of brands; however, a custom-molded TLSO is usually the most ideal choice for optimal stability. After the appropriate period of time, flexion and extension films in an upright position with external support removed must be obtained to determine complete healing and to evaluate for instability. The individual is usually weaned out of a brace, because the muscles are initially weakened.

Neurologic Assessment

Determination of the neurologic level of injury must be made, based on the results of precise motor and sensory examination. Standard dermatome and myotome references have been established by the American Spinal Injury Association (ASIA). The level of injury is defined as the last caudal segment with intact motor and sensory innervation. The initial examination should occur within 72 hours of the injury. Interval changes in the neuromuscular examination can be an indication of functional return or portend subsequent loss of function because of numerous causes including posttraumatic syringomyelia or spinal instability. Classification of the injury is made by sensory and motor levels, as well as by the pattern of injury. Comprehensive clinical examination of the SCI individual, with correct ASIA classification, is imperative not only for documenting clinical changes but also for determining functional prognosis. Practitioners should refer to the *International Standards for Neurological*

MOTOR

	R	L	KEY MUSCLES
C2			
C3			
C4			
C5			Elbow flexors
C6			Wrist extensors
C7			Elbow extensors
C8			Finger flexors (distal phalanx of middle finger)
T1			Finger abductors (little finger)
T2			
T3			
T4			
T5			
T6			
T7			
T8			
T9			
T10			
T11			
T12			
L1			
L2			Hip flexors
L3			Knee extensors
L4			Ankle dorsiflexors
L5			Long toe extensors
S1			Ankle plantar flexors
S2			
S3			
S4-5			Voluntary anal contraction (Yes/No)

0 = total paralysis
1 = palpable or visible contraction
2 = active movement, gravity eliminated
3 = active movement, against gravity
4 = active movement, against some resistance
5 = active movement, against full resistance
NT = not testable

TOTALS ☐ + ☐ = ☐ **MOTOR SCORE**
(MAXIMUM) (50) (50) (100)

LIGHT TOUCH

	R	L
C2		
C3		
C4		
C5		
C6		
C7		
C8		
T1		
T2		
T3		
T4		
T5		
T6		
T7		
T8		
T9		
T10		
T11		
T12		
L1		
L2		
L3		
L4		
L5		
S1		
S2		
S3		
S4-5		

TOTALS ☐ + ☐ –
(MAXIMUM) (56) (56)

NEUROLOGICAL LEVEL
The most caudal segment with normal function

	R	L
SENSORY		
MOTOR		

COMPLETE OR INCOMPLETE? ☐
Incomplete = Any sensory or motor function in S4-S5

This form may be copied freely but should not be altered without permission from the American Spinal Injury Association.

Fig. 19-5. Standard neurologic classification of spinal cord injury.

SENSORY

KEY SENSORY POINTS

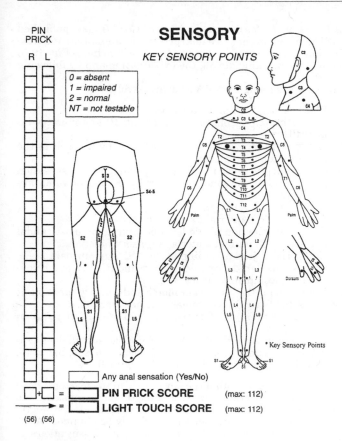

PIN
PRICK

R L

0 = absent
1 = impaired
2 = normal
NT = not testable

* Key Sensory Points

Any anal sensation (Yes/No)

☐ + ☐ = ☐ **PIN PRICK SCORE** (max: 112)

→ = ☐ **LIGHT TOUCH SCORE** (max: 112)

(56) (56)

ASIA IMPAIRMENT SCALE ☐

**ZONE OF PARTIAL
PRESERVATION**
Partially innervated segments

R L

SENSORY ☐ ☐
MOTOR ☐ ☐

Version 4p
GHC 1996

and Functional Classification of Spinal Cord Injury, published by ASIA, for comprehensive instructions. Examination and classification is facilitated by having the scoring chart (Fig. 19-5) available for marking during the examination and by following these steps.

Steps for assigning an ASIA level are as follows:

1. Place patient in supine position
2. Assign muscle strength scores to the 10 key muscles bilaterally
3. Assign sensory scores for pinprick and light touch to the 28 dermatomes bilaterally
4. Determine the presence of sacral sparing: normal sensation in the S4-5 dermatome, deep rectal pressure, or voluntary anal contraction
5. Determine left and right motor levels
6. Determine left and right sensory levels
7. Determine the neurologic level of injury, the most caudal segment with normal motor and sensory function
8. Categorize injury according to the ASIA impairment scale, with A considered a complete injury and B, C, D, and E considered incomplete injuries (Fig. 19-6)
9. Determine if the pattern of motor and sensory function fit one of the five SCI syndromes (See next section.)
10. Determine presence of a zone of partial preservation if complete injury
11. Although it is not used in ASIA classification, all deep tendon reflexes and the presence of bulbocavernosus, Babinski, and Hoffman reflexes should be determined

ASIA scoring requires that the key muscle in the myotome have at least antigravity grade 3 muscle strength and is considered to have intact innervation if the segment above has grade 5 strength. A left and right motor and sensory level may be obtained. ASIA standards have been revised three times since the classification system was established in 1992. Refer to Table 19.1 for the 10 key muscles, which are examined by convention in the supine position. It is also important to know the concept of upper and LMN injury. Volitional, controlled muscle movement requires both upper and LMN innervation. Assessment of UMN versus LMN injury must be made after the period of spinal shock resolves after the initial injury.

ASIA also describes five different syndromes that can result from SCI, which depend on the characteristics of the injury. Each syndrome carries its own set of prognostic indications and affect treatment. These syndromes are as follows:

Anterior cord syndrome: Results from vascular injury to the anterior spinal artery, thus causing bilateral weakness, spasticity, and loss of pain/temperature sensation with sparing of bilateral proprioception and light touch sensation associated with the posterior columns (Fig. 19-7).

Brown-Séquard syndrome: Occurs from a lesion to half of the spinal cord in the axial plane, resulting in weakness, spasticity, and alteration of light touch on one side of the body, with decreased pain/temperature sensation on the opposite side (resulting from the decussation of the ALST within the cord) (Fig. 19-7).

ASIA IMPAIRMENT SCALE

☐ **A = Complete:** No motor or sensory function is preserved in the sacral segments S4-S5.

☐ **B = Incomplete:** Sensory but not motor function is preserved below the neurological level and includes the sacral segments S4-S5.

☐ **C = Incomplete:** Motor function is preserved below the neurological level, and more than half of key muscles below the neurological level have a muscle grade less than 3.

☐ **D = Incomplete:** Motor function is preserved below the neurological level, and at least half of key muscles below the neurological level have a muscle grade of 3 or more.
☐

E = Normal: motor and sensory function are normal

CLINICAL SYNDROMES

☐ Central Cord
☐ Brown-Sequard
☐ Anterior Cord
☐ Conus Medullaris
☐ Cauda Equina

Fig. 19-6. Asia Impairment Scale.

Central cord syndrome: Usually resulting from a cervical level hyperextension injury, this results in weaker upper extremities compared with lower extremities (Fig. 19-7).

Cauda equina syndrome: Lesions below the conus medullaris result in LMN type of symptoms, with flaccid lower extremities, bowel, and bladder (Fig. 19-8).

Conus medullaris syndrome: Lesions at the level of the conus usually have a mixture of UMN and LMN characteristics (Fig. 19-8).

Musculoskeletal Assessment

Determination of muscle strength and innervation is described previously. Clinicians may choose to perform serial myometry, for a more objective measurement of muscle strength. A myometer is a handheld device that the clinician holds against the patient's limbs during muscle testing. When instructed to volitionally contract the

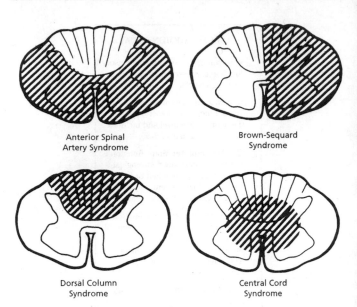

Anterior Spinal
Artery Syndrome

Brown-Sequard
Syndrome

Dorsal Column
Syndrome

Central Cord
Syndrome

Fig. 19-7.   Clinical syndromes.

muscle against resistance, the myometer provides a measurement of strength in kilograms of force.

Following the period of spinal shock, patients with UMN lesions begin developing spasticity. Spasticity is a velocity-dependent phenomenon and may be induced by using a reflex hammer on tendons or by quick stretch to the muscle. Most SCI patients develop a primarily extensor pattern of lower extremity spasticity. Spasticity can also be increased or "set off" by a variety of medical complications such as urinary tract infections (UTIs), heterotopic ossification (HO), pressure ulcers, or a noxious stimulus such as an ingrown toenail. Assessment of spasticity should be performed in different positions, because an extended posture usually enhances spasticity and components of postural flexion tend to diminish spasticity. The patient may complain of increased spasticity at night when in a recumbent extended position. Objective scoring of spasticity may be accomplished by the Ashworth scale, the modified Ashworth scale, the spasm frequency scale, or by the pendulum test (Fig. 19-9 and Table 19.2).

Assessment of musculoskeletal pain after SCI is complex and must be distinguished from neuropathic pain caused from abnormal neural signals from the nerve damage. This distinction is important because the pharmacologic and nonpharmacologic treatment is dependent on the cause of the pain. Treatment is discussed in the next section. Clinicians should perform a comprehensive pain assessment, using an objective scale when possible. The visual analog scale is frequently and easily used (requesting the patient to rate the degree of pain on a 10-point scale of intensity)

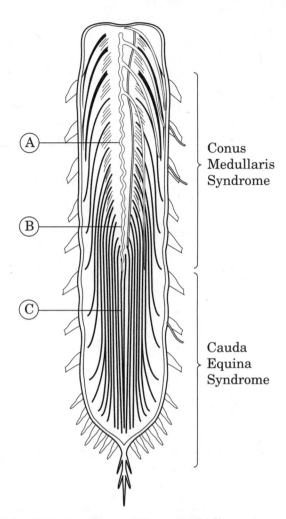

Conus
Medullaris
Syndrome

Cauda
Equina
Syndrome

Fig. 19-8.   Clinical syndromes. A: Represents higher conus medullaris syndrome. B: Represents a lower conus medullaris syndrome. C: Represents the cauda equina syndrome.

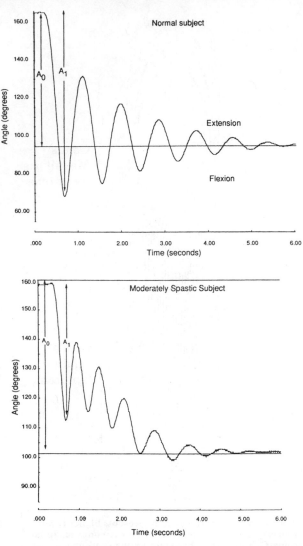

Fig. 19-9. Pendulum test for spastic hypertonia used to assess spastic hypertonia of the quadriceps and hamstring muscle groups. Stiffness of the limb is assessed by placing the patient in a supine position with both legs extending over the edge of a table that supports the patient only as far as the distal thigh. A_0 represents the amplitude of the plotted waveform from full extension to its first absolute minimum. The upper tracing depicts a normal subject. The lower tracing depicts a moderately spastic subject. Notice that the initial swing from full extension (A_1) does not reach the vertical, whereas the normal subject obtains 27 degrees of flexion beyond the vertical. The marked damping of the altered sinusoidal curve is evident in the spastic subject. (From Katz RT, Rovai G, Brait C et al. Quantification of hypertonia. *Arch Phys Med Rehabil* 1992;73:343, with permission.)

Table 19.2.   Clinical Scale for Spastic Hypertonia

0	No increase in tone
1	Slight increase in muscle tone, manifested by a catch and release or by minimal resistance at the end of the range of motion when the affected part(s) is moved in flexion or extension
1+	Slight increase in muscle tone, manifested by a catch, followed by minimal resistance throughout the remainder (less than half) of the range of motion
2	More marked increase in muscle tone through most of the range of motion, but affected part(s) easily moved
3	Considerable increase in muscle tone, passive movement difficult
4	Affected part(s) rigid in flexion or extension

From Bohannon RW, Smith MB. Interrater reliability on a modified Ashworth scale of muscle spasticity. *Phys Ther* 1987;67:206–207, with permission.

with a score of 1 as the least noxious, and the score of 10 as most intense. Pain assessment should include questions about traumatic versus nontraumatic sources of the pain and situations that cause the pain to be better or worse. The character of the pain is important in distinguishing neuropathic from musculoskeletal pain. SCI individuals usually describe neuropathic pain as burning, tingling, radiating, hypersensitive, or as a pressure sensation. Discrete skeletal pain following trauma should be radiographically studied, because fractures are often missed on initial examination. SCI individuals are prone to develop overuse, entrapment neuropathies such as carpal tunnel syndrome or ulnar neuropathies, as well as nerve root radiculopathies. These may develop acutely, or after chronic injury, and should be evaluated by electrodiagnostic testing based on clinical presentation.

Pulmonary Assessment

Respiratory compromise after SCI is due to impairment of both ventilation and the coughing mechanism. The higher the level of SCI, the more severe are the impairments. Injuries caudal to T12 are generally spared pulmonary dysfunction. T12 to T5 lesion levels show progressive loss of abdominal and intercostal muscle function that impairs the force of coughing and expiration. T5 to T1 lesion levels have further impairment of intercostal musculature. Cough is further compromised in C8 to C4 lesion levels. At and above the C3 level, diaphragmatic innervation is disrupted, necessitating mechanical ventilation. Initial cervical injuries experience a forced vital capacity (FVC) reduction between 24% and 31% of predicted normal FVC because of paradoxical breathing patterns. Following the development of intercostals and abdominal spasticity, FVC can improve up to 50% to 60% of the predicted normal. Initial assessment should include possible trauma-associated injuries such as hemothorax or lung contusions. Concomitant head injury increases the chance of

aspiration or the development of neurogenic pulmonary edem.
Acute assessment should include bedside pulmonary functio
testing (PFTs) with FVC, tidal volume, negative inspiratory pressure, and arterial blood gases.

Cardiovascular Evaluation

Early detection of deep venous thrombosis (DVT) and the
associated risk of pulmonary embolism (PE) should be given
careful consideration, even with prophylaxis. In some centers
patients undergo daily leg and thigh measurements, and a unilateral discrepancy greater than 1 cm is considered clinically
significant. Assessment for DVT is usually by a venous Doppler
(Duplex Scan) and a laboratory D-dimer study may be of value.
A ventilation-perfusion scan is usually the preliminary study to
rule out PE; however, a pulmonary arteriogram or spiral CT may
be more definitive.

Orthostatic hypotension is a common occurrence immediately
after SCI, because of the loss of the sympathetic peripheral vasoconstriction. Sympathetically mediated hypotension should be distinguished from a lack of hydration or intravascular volume.
Treatment of neurogenic orthostatic hypotension is addressed in
the treatment section.

Genitourinary Evaluation

During the period of spinal shock, the bladder is usually are-
flexic, and an indwelling catheter should be placed to allow
drainage. Assessment of the GU system after spinal shock is based
on whether the individual has sustained a UMN versus a LMN
(cauda equina) injury and the presence of detrusor sphincter
dyssynergia (DSD). Baseline evaluation of the function of the GU
system during the first weeks postinjury should include a renal
ultrasound and urodynamic studies. The choice and timing of urodynamic studies depends on the level and type of SCI, pattern
of neurologic return, and degree of spasticity. Urodynamic studies
may include a voiding cystourethrogram and pressure flow studies
to evaluate bladder compliance, resting and voiding intravesicular
pressures, detrusor activity, and voiding flow rates. Urodynamic
studies assist in determination of the functional classification of
neurogenic bladder, as well as assist in clinical recommendations
for type of bladder management. Patients with spastic tetraplegia
and insufficient hand function (even with splints) may wish to continue with an indwelling Foley catheter, because intermittent
catheterization procedure (ICP) every 4 to 6 hours may make the
individual dependent on an attendant to perform ICP. SCI males
with DSD cannot adequately drain the bladder without a sphinc-
terotomy, if a condom catheter bladder management method is
chosen. There are many considerations for bladder management
that include prognosis for bladder recovery, prognosis for recovery of hand function, type of neurogenic bladder, presence of DSD,
sexual activity, and lifestyle. The goals of bladder management
are to maintain continence, allow adequate emptying of the
bladder, prevent accumulation of postvoid residual volumes
above 150 to 200 mL, and enable the individual to be as functionally independent as possible. See the treatment section of
this chapter.

Gastrointestinal Evaluation

During the period of spinal shock immediately after SCI, a paralytic ileus is usually present; therefore, management should focus on rapid assessment of potential secondary complications. Complications of the ileus may include nausea, vomiting, stress-induced hypercatabolic state and nutritional compromise, reflux, stress-induced gastric ulcerations, and diminished diaphragm excursion and thus vital capacity from accumulation of intestinal contents.

During the transitional and chronic phases, assessment of neurogenic bowel is similar to that of the neurogenic bladder. A scheduled bowel program should be established as soon as possible and will depend on the type of injury. If the individual has the presence of limb spasticity and a spastic external anal sphincter, it is likely that UMN-type of bowel exists. The UMN bowel program consists of judicious use of stool softener medications and insertion of an enema, followed by digital stimulation of the rectum until the bowels have reflexively evacuated stool. This should be performed daily or on an every-other-day basis. Lack of limb spasticity and a flaccid external anal sphincter indicates a LMN-type of bowel. The LMN bowel program consists of judicious use of stool-bulking agents and manual disimpaction of stool. Individuals may require daily or twice-daily disimpaction to maintain continence, because of the flaccid characteristic of the bowel and sphincter.

Integument Evaluation

Neurogenic skin is at significant risk for pressure and shear injury, especially over bony prominences. SCI individuals must immediately be placed on a special mattress that allows for enhanced equal distribution of pressure and turned at least every 2 hours. Before sitting in a wheelchair, the wheelchair must be fitted with a special cushion, and the individual's weight must be shifted every 15 minutes. The transition of responsibility for maintaining skin integrity and prevention of pressure and shear injury, from caregivers to the patient, is an interdisciplinary rehabilitation team effort. Prevention and comprehensive management of pressure ulcers is a multifaceted effort and is addressed in the treatment section.

COMPLICATIONS

There are a number of potential complications that may occur as result of a SCI. These include respiratory complications, DVT and PE, pressure ulcers, autonomic dysreflexia (AD), HO, UTIs, calculi, gastrointestinal complications, spasticity, depression, and pain. Some of these complications, that is, DVT and PE, are much more common during the acute stage after SCI. Others may occur anytime after SCI, that is, UTIs and pain; and they may become lifelong problems. Still other complications such as AD and spasticity do not occur until after the period of spinal shock wears off. The following is a discussion of some of these more common complications.

Respiratory Complications

The patient with a complete SCI is at a greater risk for atelectasis and pneumonia than those with incomplete injuries. Atelectasis and pneumonia are more common during the first 3 weeks after injury. Prevention includes deep breathing exercises, changes in bed position, incentive spirometry, and "quad" coughing for those who do not have adequate abdominal strength. Vigorous pulmonary toilet can decrease the incidence of pulmonary complications. A useful alternative to tracheal suctioning is the intervention provided by the mechanical in-exsufflator (MI-E). The MI-E is a device that provides deep insufflation followed by an immediate decrease in pressure to create a forced exsufflation. It may be applied via endotracheal or tracheostomy tubes or via oral-nasal interfaces. It is recommended to immediately follow the MI-E with assisted coughing. MI-E is usually well tolerated by patients and can be an effective method for clearing mucous plugs, attenuating atelectasis, and increasing vital capacity. Weaning from a ventilator in the SCI patient may proceed more slowly than in patients with strictly pulmonary problems, because SCI may impair the function of intercostal and abdominal muscles. Often the patient who is weaned during the day has more difficulties at night and may benefit from continued ventilation at night or the use of BiPAP or CPAP. The patient with a complete C1 or C2 tetraplegia may be an appropriate candidate for phrenic nerve stimulators, also called diaphragm pacing. If the patient has an incomplete injury, even if only sensory examination, weaning may still be possible many months post-injury. Implanting phrenic nerve stimulators has the potential to damage the phrenic nerves and should, therefore, be avoided in sensory-incomplete patients in the first year or two postinjury. Damage to the nerves in the incomplete patients would risk needing to use a ventilator on a permanent basis.

Deep Venous Thrombosis and Pulmonary Embolism

The highest risk from DVT is in the first few weeks after injury. The reported incidence of DVT has ranged from 47% to 100%. One study reported that 62% of patients had a positive venogram 6 to 8 days after injury. Current published clinical practice guidelines recommend DVT prophylaxis for 8 to 12 weeks after acute SCI depending on risk factors. It is important to attempt to prevent lower-extremity DVTs with compression stockings, sequential-compression devices (SCDs) or pumps, and either adjusted-dose heparin or low molecular weight heparin. The SCDs usually lose value quickly once the patient becomes wheelchair mobile and can be discontinued. In our experience a single DVT confined to the calf often becomes multiple DVTs or may extend above the knee; thus, it may be better for the patient with SCI who develops a DVT in the calf to institute full anticoagulation. Even patients with the ability to ambulate in a few days after SCI appear at greater risk for DVT and require the same degree of prophylaxis and vigilance. Duplex ultrasonography is a useful noninvasive tool for the detection of DVT. Because DVT may lead to PE, it is important to ask the patient with or without DVT regarding chest or shoulder pain or discomfort, cough, or shortness of breath and to report any such symptoms anytime during the course of treatment. Although a PE may be fatal or cause severe respiratory compromise, sometimes the signs and symptoms are minimal.

Pressure Ulcers

Pressure ulcers may develop anytime after SCI and are one of the costliest complications that can occur. Ulcers develop in ependent areas of the body, usually over bony prominences. The terms decubitus ulcers and pressure ulcers are usually used interchangeably. Sacral ulcers are the most common type during initial hospitalization and ischial ulcers in chronic SCI. Unrelieved pressure and shear injury are usually causes of skin breakdown and require multidisciplinary team assessment and intervention, as well as patient vigilance, for acute and chronic management. Patients are instructed in methods of weight shifting while in the manual wheelchair, and patients with quadriplegia above the C5-6 level of injury will likely require a power-tilting mechanism to enable weight shifting. Pressure support surfaces such as mattresses and wheelchair cushions must be carefully assessed, based on the individuals body habitus and functional level. Once a pressure ulcer develops, the pressure must be alleviated to heal the wound, which may entail bedrest on a dynamic mattress. In extreme cases with deep ulcers, a myocutaneous flap surgery may be required for healing. Comprehensive assessment and management of pressure ulcers is beyond the scope of this chapter.

There are other comorbid medical complications that predispose to poor skin integrity and the development of pressure ulcers, as well as the perpetuation of a systemic environment that makes healing difficult for the SCI individual. These conditions can include low levels of testosterone (endogenous anabolic protein synthesis stimulus), hypoalbuminemia from nutritional depletion, poorly controlled diabetes, and peripheral vascular disease. Poor nutrition complicates the healing of ulcers. The patient with multiple medical complications during the acute stage is at risk unless caloric needs are met. There is a tendency for physicians to accept great loss of body mass as part of the paralysis without regard for the nutritional status of the patients. Once an individual develops an open wound, the body develops a state of catabolism, which causes lean body weight loss and perpetuates healing difficulty. Many studies show a direct correlation between low albumin levels and the presence, severity, and duration of pressure ulcers. Studies also show that SCI patients with pressure ulcers may have almost twice as much nutritional intake as control-matched individuals without ulcers and still be unable to take in enough substrate for protein synthesis that is required to heal a wound. Patients with open wounds, weight loss, and low albumin should be considered for short-term treatment with an anabolic medication to attenuate the catabolic state. Oxandrolone is the only Food and Drug Administration (FDA)-approved medication for complications associated with weight loss.

Autonomic Dysreflexia

The signs and symptoms of AD include an acute elevation of blood pressure associated with headache, sweating above the lesions, nasal congestion, piloerection, and, sometimes, bradycardia. AD may occur in the patient with a SCI at or above the T6 level after the period of spinal shock. The most common causative agent is bladder distention followed by bowel distention. However, any noxious stimulus below the level of the lesion may lead to AD. The treatment is directed to removing the stimulus, for example, checking the catheter for kinks if the catheter is indwelling or catheterizing the bladder if the patient is on intermittent catheterization (IC). Sometimes the blood pressure requires immediate treatment often using nitro-paste, nitroglycerin 1/150 sublingually, or an agent such as hydralazine. Refractory cases may require a labetalol drip for acute treatment, and the patient may need chronic prophylaxis with an alpha-blocker. Clinical practice guidelines for detection and treatment of AD have been published by the Consortium for Spinal Cord Medicine. The use of sublingual nifedipine has been discouraged by a FDA moratorium.

Heterotopic Ossification

The cause of HO is unknown but is likely related to a combination of immobility and neurogenic and traumatic factors because it also may be seen after traumatic brain injury, burns, and total hip replacement. HO is the abnormal development of bone in the soft tissues surrounding a joint and occurs in about 16% to 53% of patients with SCI. A triple bone scan is abnormal before calcification appears in x-ray films. Elevation of serum alkaline phosphatase is helpful in diagnosis and response to treatment, which may consist of disodium etidronate or indomethacin. In refractory cases, surgery and radiation therapy may be necessary. The most common location for HO to develop is at the hips, but HO has been found in many different locations. HO develops only below the level of the lesion in persons with SCI. HO may also be associated with a state of hypercoagulability, requiring anticoagulation.

Spasticity

Spasticity may not always be a problem to the patient and need not always be treated. However, severe spasticity may interfere with function and self-care or lead to contractures and even pain. By 1 year after SCI, 78% of patients with SCI and 91% of those with tetraplegia develop spasticity. The most basic form of treatment is stretching, but this may only provide very temporary relief of spasms. Several medications are available including baclofen, tizanidine, and sodium dantrolene. Diazepam may provide quick relief of spasticity, but it is addicting and, therefore, not a first-line drug. Common antispasticity medications are shown in Table 19.3. Blocks using phenol or botulinum toxin may be beneficial. Some patients may not obtain enough relief of spasticity with medications or blocks and benefit from the use of intrathecal baclofen. The choice of treatment should proceed from the least invasive to the more invasive treatments. Common infections such as UTIs may aggravate spasticity and should be treated. Of note, the newer selective serotonin reuptake inhibitors (SSRIs) used for depression may increase spasticity.

Urinary Tract Infections

UTIs are common in patients with SCI during the initial hospitalization and in many persons throughout the remainder of life. The signs and symptoms of UTI may include increased spasticity, cloudy and odorous urine, urinary incontinence, AD, general malaise, fever, and chills. Patients with complete injuries do not sense dysuria. IC is less likely to lead to recurrent UTIs; however, this applies only to those who perform self-catheterization because having a caregiver perform IC is more likely to be associated with

Table 19.3.   Common Antispasticity Medications

1. **Tizanidine** is an α_2-agonist similar to clonidine, but it is formulated to produce negligible effects on lowering blood pressure. It has a short half-life and therefore should be dosed four times a day. Side effects may include sedation and headache.
2. **Gabapentin**, a GABA analog, is FDA-approved as an adjunct for partial seizures, but it is also used for neuropathic pain. It should be considered when a patient has neuropathic pain as well as spasticity. Because it is excreted unchanged in the urine, the side-effect profile is minimal and it has no known drug interactions.
3. **Baclofen** is also a GABA analog, dosed four times a day, and is usually the first choice for both spinal and centrally mediated spasticity. Although many clinicians prescribe more than the 80 mg/day recommended maximum, this is not without precautions. Higher doses may actually cause receptor upregulation, creating the need for more baclofen to achieve the same effect. Recent literature also suggests that higher doses may exacerbate sleep apnea and respiratory depression. Baclofen side effects also include fatigue and clouded mental status. If the patient requires > 80 mg/day, consideration should be made to add another agent or to evaluate criteria for intrathecal baclofen delivery via a surgically implanted pump system.
4. **Valium** is a benzodiazepine effective for attenuating spasticity.
5. **Dantrolene** is the only peripherally acting antispasticity medication, which works by inhibiting calcium uptake at the sarcoplasmic reticulum. Liver function tests should be monitored regularly.

FDA, Food and Drug Administration; GABA, α-aminobutyric acid.

febrile episodes of UTI. Indwelling catheters increase the risk of UTIs and are also associated with an increased risk of calculi, epididymitis, fistula formation, and the development of bladder carcinoma. Prophylaxis with low dose of an antibiotic may be useful in reducing the incidence of UTI, but causes of recurrent UTIs should be sought before instituting antibiotic prophylaxis. Antibiotic prophylaxis is not recommended for hospitalized patients.

Chronic Pain

Another common complication is the development of chronic pain. This may be sensed at the level of the injury as well as below the level of the injury. The incidence of chronic pain has been estimated to be about 69%. Two major categories of pain are neuropathic and musculoskeletal. Neuropathic pain includes four types of pain: pain produced by the SCI and sometimes referred to as central pain or SCI pain, which occurs below the level of the injury; transitional zone pain, which occurs at the level of the injury and is sometimes called segmental pain; radicular pain, which may occur at any dermatomal level and is usually unilateral; and visceral pain, which is perceived in the abdomen.

Treatment of neuropathic pain in SCI is largely empirical. Drugs that have been used include narcotics, antidepressants, anticonvulsants, and others. Of the antidepressants, amitriptyline was not found effective in pain relief in a recent double-blind, placebo-controlled trial of patients with SCI and chronic pain. The newer SSRIs may produce an increase in spasticity and do not seem clinically effective for treatment of chronic SCI pain. Gabapentin has been found beneficial in SCI pain and has a better side effect profile than carbamazepine (Tegretol), a similar but older drug used for chronic neuropathic pain. The dose of gabapentin must be started low, 100 to 300 mg each night to avoid unpleasant side effects but then should be gradually increased to a maximum of 2,700 mg per day in divided doses or until complete pain relief. About a third of those patients treated with gabapentin who tolerate the medication find some pain relief.

Although narcotics are addicting, there are patients who must be maintained on chronic narcotics. It is important to establish a strict agreement with the patient regarding dosing because tolerance may develop and the patient may seek more medication. Generally combining types of drugs is helpful in reducing the need for higher doses of narcotics whenever pain is exacerbated. Any increased stress or illness may increase neuropathic pain and efforts should be made to reduce the stressors that occur in the life of the patient, as well as nociceptive stimuli such as calculi and UTIs. Nonpharmacologic modalities such as acupuncture, relaxation techniques, exercise, and self-hypnosis are useful to varying degrees.

Posttraumatic Syringomyelia (PTS)

The development of a syrinx, a fluid-filled cavity within the spinal cord, can be a devastating late complication of SCI. PTS is estimated to occur in 3% to 6% of SCI individuals, and the pathogenesis is unclear. The cavity develops within the initial injury site, followed by enlargement and extension above and below the level of injury. The cavity usually develops in the relatively hypovascular area of the cord in the gray matter between the dorsal horns and posterior columns, and may progressively expand with resulting loss of sensory and/or motor function. Extension may occur from pressure pulses within the epidural venous system, exacerbated by certain activities that cause Valsalva (e.g., coughing, sneezing, straining at stool, exercising). Ascending sensory level or change in neurologic examination consistent with ascending neurologic level should alert the clinician to the possibility of PTS.

Diagnosis is ascertained by a comprehensive physical examination followed by MRI. A cyst at the level of injury only is not considered PTS. There is no definitive correlation between the size of the syrinx and severity of deficit. Once PTS is diagnosed, each patient must be individually considered regarding follow-up and treatment. Any neurologic changes should be followed by serial clinical examination and repeat MRI scans. Electrodiagnostic testing is of significant value in following the progression of PTS. Conservative medical treatment consists of avoidance of straining and pain control. Surgical treatments include shunts and duraplasty; however, they are not always successful.

Cardiovascular Complications

Because of loss of function below the level of the lesion and resulting difficulty in exercising, SCI individuals have difficulty maintaining cardiovascular fitness. This relatively sedentary lifestyle promotes obesity, glucose intolerance, elevated cholesterol, and low levels of high-density lipoprotein (HDL). Cardiac causes are second only to pulmonary causes as causes of death in chronic SCI. Studies show a 16.9% incidence of ischemic heart disease in the SCI population, compared with 6.9% in age matched controls. Silent ischemia may occur with higher level of lesions. Hypertension is also more prevalent in the SCI population, and is related to increasing age as well as lesion level. Before initiating treatment of hypertension, secondary causes such as AD, renal artery stenosis, and renal insufficiency should be ruled out.

Hypotension is also a complex complication in acute and chronic SCI. Many factors are responsible for chronically lower baseline blood pressure, including decreased venous return, venous pooling in lower extremities, and loss of sympathetic peripheral vasoconstriction. Decreased stroke volume and left ventricular atrophy also contribute to a lower baseline blood pressure. In addition to low baseline blood pressure, acute SCI individuals are particularly prone to significant orthostatic hypotension. Multiple approaches may be used to compensate for loss of sympathetic reflex peripheral vasoconstriction on arising. Nonpharmacologic methods include compression stockings, abdominal binders, and the use of tilt-in-space or recliner wheelchairs. Pharmacologic interventions may include administering sympathomimetic agents before arising, administering salt tablets, or giving a mineralocorticoid. Midodrine is a selective alpha-1 agonist and is the preferred sympathomimetic agent over ephedrine, which has alpha as well as beta properties. Small doses of fludrocortisone acetate, a mineralocorticoid, may enhance blood pressure through volume expansion.

Endocrine Complications

Studies have shown that the SCI population has significantly increased risk for developing type II diabetes mellitus, likely resulting from insulin resistance. The cause of insulin resistance includes muscle wasting, adiposity, and relative inactivity. Prompt diagnosis and treatment is important to prevent both microvascular and macrovascular complications.

Male SCI patients may acutely or chronically develop low endogenous testosterone levels, because of suppression of gonadotropins and impairment in thermoregulation. Hypogonadal men may develop further muscle wasting, osteoporosis, decreased skin integrity (increasing the risk for developing pressure ulcers), and depression. Before initiation of androgen replacement therapy, prostate cancer should be ruled out.

Antidiuretic hormone (ADH) is secreted in response to hypovolemia and increased serum osmolality. In normal individuals it is secreted in diurnal surges with highest levels at night, thus preventing nocturnal diuresis. In some SCI individuals, the diurnal rhythm may be impaired, and exogenous ADH therapy may be beneficial at night. This is especially important if large nocturnal urine volumes are precluding a successful ICP for bladder management.

SCI individuals with concomitant brain injury may develop adrenal insufficiency, resulting in hyperkalemia, hyponatremia, and hypotension. Acute glucocorticoid treatment immediately after SCI may exacerbate this tendency, and it may be difficult to distinguish orthostatic hypotension from impaired sympathetic tone from that of adrenal insufficiency. Patients with dual diagnoses of SCI and brain injury may also develop the syndrome of inappropriate antidiuretic hormone (SIADH).

Osteoporosis below the level of the lesion develops immediately after SCI and may result in impaired calcium metabolism. Acutely injured individuals should receive increased fluids to deter the development of immobilization hypercalcemia. Nausea, abdominal pain, and elevated ionized calcium should alert the clinician to this diagnosis. Treatment should be initiated with intravenous fluids but may require biphosphanate medication.

Neurogenic factors affect hypothalamic temperature regulation, and individuals with higher lesion levels may be poikilothermic. The body takes on the temperature of the environment, and this places the SCI patient at risk for hyperthermia in warm weather and hypothermia in cool weather.

Depression

The loss of function with a SCI is associated with a profound change in lifestyle, body image, and relationships with others. It is not surprising that depression is common in acute and chronic SCI patients. Clinicians should be alert for signs and symptoms of depression. There are many choices of antidepressant medications, and the choice should be carefully considered based on side effect profiles.

PROGNOSIS, OUTCOME, AND FOLLOW-UP

The prognosis of improvement and functional outcome following SCI is complex and multifaceted, extending beyond the scope of this chapter. The most accurate way to predict recovery is the standardized physical examination as endorsed by the International Standards for Neurological and Functional Classification of Spinal Cord Injury Patients. This comprehensive examination determines the initial level and classification of the injury. Other diagnostic tests such as MRI may be helpful in further determination of prognosis. The presence of extensive cord edema and hemorrhage are poor prognostic indicators. The initial strength of a muscle is a significant predictor, at any level of injury, of achieving functional antigravity strength caudal to the neurologic level of injury. Other factors, such as preservation of pin-prick sacral sensation or volitional anal contraction, also portend an improved prognosis. Rate of improvement is another important factor, with most motor recovery occurring in the first 3 to 6 months. Incomplete injuries have a better prognosis overall for ambulation and functional outcome than complete injuries.

Charts have been published that correlate the neurologic level of injury with functional outcome, delineating expected independence with activities of daily living as well as mobility. These charts are useful; however, each injury is different, and factors such as patient motivation and family support must be considered. A thorough understanding of the pathophysiology of the injury and factors affecting neurologic recovery will assist in predicting ultimate functional capability. Patients should receive optimal pharmacologic and therapeutic interventions to enhance recovery. Patient education about recovery mechanisms, as well as methods used in determining prognosis, is an essential component of the rehabilitation process.

SUGGESTED READINGS

American Spinal Injury Association and the International Medical Society of Paraplegia. *International standards for neurological classification of spinal cord injury,* revised 2000. Chicago: American Spinal Injury Association and the International Medical Society of Paraplegia, 2000.

Cardenas DD, Mayo ME. Management of bladder dysfunction in physical medicine and rehabilitation. In: Braddom RL, ed. Philadelphia: WB Saunders, 2000.

Frost FS. Spinal cord injury medicine in physical medicine and rehabilitation. In: Braddom RL, ed. Philadelphia: WB Saunders, 2000.

Hammond MC, guest ed; Kraft GH, consulting ed. Topics in spinal cord injury medicine. *Phys Med Rehabil Clin North Am* 2000;38:182–191.

Kirshblum SC, O'Connor KC. Predicting neurologic recovery in traumatic cervical spinal cord injury. *Arch Phys Med Rehab* 1998;79: 1456–1466.

Nesathurai S, ed. *The rehabilitation of people with spinal cord injury,* 2nd ed. Blackwell Science, 2000.

Staas WE Jr, Ditunno JF Jr, guest eds; Kraft GH, consulting ed. Traumatic spinal cord injury. *Phys Med Rehabil Clin North Am* 1992.

Staas WE Jr, Freedman MK, Fried GF, et al. Spinal cord injury and spinal cord injury medicine. In: DeLisa JA, Gans BM, eds. *Rehabilitation medicine: principles and practice,* 3rd ed. Philadelphia: Lippincott Williams & Wilkins, 1998.

Sports Injury

John Cianca

This chapter introduces the basic principles of musculoskeletal medicine related to sports and human performance. It provides the essentials of the assessment and treatment of any injury that falls into this category. It is not a comprehensive review of treatment protocols or a discussion of all sports injuries.

FACTORS THAT LEAD TO INJURY

Injuries can be caused by either of two sets of factors. The first set are intrinsic factors; the second are extrinsic factors. Intrinsic factors are those elements that are readily ascribable to the athlete. These include tissue weakness, inflexibility, or overload; biomechanical errors; and lack of conditioning. They also include overall body size, performance ability, and playing style.

Extrinsic factors include faulty equipment, externally driven forces such as other athletes or playing surfaces, and coaching or the lack thereof. See Table 20.1.

Acute injuries are usually the result of sudden tissue overload and tensile failure. Chronic injuries occur most often from biomechanical and/or training errors. Chronic injuries may be insidious and slowly progressive or may follow a waxing and waning course with acute exacerbations.

PRINCIPLES OF BIOMECHANICS

The musculoskeletal system is designed to affect the movement of the body. The means by which it does this is referred to as biomechanics. Movement is a function that is intricate, yet appears smooth and simple when performed efficiently with respect to biomechanical principles. Unfortunately, for most people refinement of movement patterns is at best trial and error, if it is attempted at all.

Few people understand or consider how or why their body moves a certain way; the outcome is all that matters. Biomechanical errors of movement are often not considered if the intended outcome is achieved. Therefore, people develop bad habits in movement and in static posture. This often results in injuries, particularly those that are more severe than would be expected given the nature of the circumstances.

There is little or no isolated movement in the body. Because ultimately all structures in the musculoskeletal system are connected, the entire body is affected by dysfunction in a particular area. The connection between the axial and appendicular skeleton occurs at the shoulder and hip; these are the critical points of energy transfer. The scapulae and both sides of the pelvis form the four cornerstones of the musculoskeletal system; through these areas, force to accomplish movement is transferred from the axial to the appendicular skeleton and vice versa. These are critical regions and, thus, areas where many biomechanical errors occur. As a result, many injuries have their origin in these regions.

Table 20.1. Factors that Lead to Injury	
Intrinsic	**Extrinsic**
Tissue: weakness, inflexibility, overload	Faulty equipment
Biomechanical errors	Other athletes
Lack of conditioning	Playing surfaces
Body size	Coaching
Performance ability	Weather
Playing style	

People rely on distal limb function to accomplish tasks that are uniquely human. However, safe and efficient distal function is predicated on proximal control. Unless the cornerstones are correctly stabilized before distal function occurs, distal movements become inefficient, eventually leading to fatigue and injury.

A good example of this is the overhand throwing motion. Ground reactive forces are translated through the lower extremities and amplified as they pass through the hip into the spine. From here they are further amplified and transferred through the shoulder into the upper limb. The scapula and its musculature control this transfer, leading to useful force generation in the arm that is moved distally to the wrist, the fingers, and, finally, the ball.

Scapular stability controls the efficiency of glenohumeral kinematics. As stability breaks down proximally, distal structures in the kinematic chain are subjected to greater strain and are more vulnerable to injury. The same phenomenon occurs in the lower limb at the sacroiliac joint.

Biomechanical analysis uncovers the layers of dysfunction present in a given movement pattern. Tissue injury complex refers to the area of the body that is disrupted, dysfunctional, or both. Specifically, this would be the area of the body that is directly related to the presentation of symptoms. The clinical symptom complex is the constellation of symptoms that arises from an acute injury. This complex can involve pain, swelling, bruising, or any of the other descriptors that accompany the clinical injury. The functional biomechanical deficit refers to the combination of weakness and flexibility that leads to biomechanical errors in movement patterns. This is in essence a description of the factors that led to the tissue injury complex and the clinical symptom complex. The functional adaptation complex is a set of substitutions that are employed to compensate for the injured tissues' loss of function. These compensations are not optimal and tend to perpetuate and amplify already inefficient and unsafe movement patterns. This generally occurs in the more chronic situation. A clear example of this would be the limp that develops in a person with a chronic injury to a lower extremity. It allows the person to continue ambulating but in a faulty fashion that can lead to further injury. Tissue overload complex refers to structures that are vulnerable because of overwork; as a result, subsequent injuries may develop. It is not unusual for this complex to be the precipitating cause of the presenting illness. Such tissues need to be treated and rehabilitated to ensure complete resolution of the problem.

BASIC PHYSIATRIC TENETS OF SPORT MEDICINE

The eight basic tenets of sports medicine that form the physiatric frame of reference are listed in Table 20.2. They are the essential elements in treatment of any musculoskeletal injury. Each is described in the following.

1. Control of inflammation

The inflammatory process begins at the onset of injury. It is important in the initial stages of damage control and repair by the body; however, if left unchecked, it can impede and prolong injury repair and rehabilitation. Effective control of inflammation begins at the time of the injury with compression at the injury site and prompt application of ice. Icing should be done for 15 to 20 minutes at least two to three times daily for the first 48 to 72 hours. If the injury is severe and is accompanied by ecchymosis and profound edema, ice should be applied as frequently as every hour for 15 to 20 minutes during the first 24 to 48 hours. Be careful to protect the skin from thermal injury by application of a towel or cloth. If using ice massage, the layer of water that forms between the skin and the ice should be sufficient to protect the skin from injury. Compression of the injury, along with rest and elevation, decreases swelling. The use of antiinflammatory agents is an effective and sometimes powerful adjunct in the control and reduction of inflammation. Nonsteroidal antiinflammatory drugs (NSAIDs) are the first line of pharmacologic intervention. Local and systemic glucocorticoids are often very effective, but these should be used judiciously and reserved for refractory and/or severe inflammation.

2. Pain control

Pain also begins with the injury and progresses during the ensuing 24 to 48 hours. It is during the initiation of the pain process that intervention is critical. If pain is left uncontrolled, limitation of movement can become prolonged and severe. However, pain is an indicator of injury severity; absolute ablation of pain can be counterproductive, by providing a false sense of security to the patient. It is important that the patient be comfortable, yet still aware that there is an injury present.

Musculoskeletal injury pain control can be accomplished in several ways. Limiting inflammation reduces tissue distension, thus making the injured area less tender. Compression and rest

---

Table 20.2. Basic Tenets of Sports Medicine

1. Control of inflammation
2. Pain control
3. Restoration of joint ROM and soft tissue extensibility
4. Restoration of muscular strength
5. Restoration of muscular endurance
6. Retraining in biomechanics
7. Maintaining cardiovascular fitness
8. Development of programs to maintain strength, flexibility, conditioning, and skills

ROM, range of motion.

decrease inflammation and promote healing of the injured tissue. Icing limits pain by reducing reactive muscle hypertonus and providing superficial analgesia. Ice also causes vasoconstriction, which slows hemorrhage and decreases metabolic activity, thereby decreasing inflammation and pain.

NSAIDs are effective in pain control by reducing inflammation and decreasing pain. Refer to Chapter 2. Modalities such as transcutaneous electrical nerve stimulation (TENS) serve as a counterirritant and, therefore, block perception of pain. Limitation of weight bearing and the use of splints, braces, and taping serve to protect the injured area by limiting potentially unstable movement and controlling edema. This allows rest of the injured area and prevents the perpetuation of pain.

Pain and inflammation control is an interrelated process essential to the initiation of healing and rehabilitation. Once pain and inflammation are controlled, the next phase of rehabilitation can begin. This initial phase is the foundation of later phases and provides for repair of damaged tissue.

3. Restoration of joint range of motion (ROM) and soft tissue extensibility

Pain-free full-joint active range of motion (AROM), as well as soft tissue extensibility surrounding the joint, must be restored before initiating strengthening or endurance exercise. AROM prevents joint contracture and resulting functional limitation. Failure to reach full AROM before strengthening may lead to reinjury and/or biomechanical error.

Passive range of motion (PROM) techniques are used first, followed by active assisted range of motion (AAROM) and then AROM. PROM does not require muscle activation and, therefore, can be used very early in the rehabilitation process. It can help reduce edema and promote early return of joint function. The muscles and supporting structures are allowed to rest, resulting in less pain and edema.

4. Restoration of muscular strength

Once pain-free full AROM is restored, strengthening can begin. It is initiated with isometric exercises and progresses through manual resistance, elastic tubing (Theraband), isotonic, then isokinetic, and finally functional testing. Isometric exercises protect injured joints and antagonist muscles because they do not cause movement. They can actually be started before restoration of full ROM because of the lack of movement production. Elastic tubing exercises are an excellent way of introducing strengthening via AROM because they provide minimal, yet constant, resistance. There are several grades of tubing resistance, typically categorized according to color by the specific manufacturer. Isotonic exercise involves the use of machines or free weights that provide greater amounts of resistance and also require more skill in integrating other body parts to varying degrees in any given exercise. Isokinetic strengthening incorporates changing rates of speed in the movement arm, making the exercise more functionally based. Functional testing uses the actual activity to be performed; it is, therefore, the most challenging to the recovering athlete because strength is required in specific movement patterns. Coordination is much more important in these exercises.

Resistance exercise consists of sets of repetitions. Sets that consist of 15 to 30 repetitions are used to develop muscular endurance. Sets that consist of 10 repetitions or less are used to enhance power. Generally speaking, there should be a day of recovery between resistance workouts to allow muscles to rebuild. If muscle soreness lasts beyond 24 hours after exercise, the next resistance session should be delayed until the soreness has abated.

5. Restoration of muscular endurance including unloading

This tenet is reached with strengthening. Generally speaking, low-weight, high-repetition weight sets develop muscular endurance. Isometric sets can also increase a muscle's endurance. Variable resistance aerobic equipment is useful in developing muscular endurance in limb muscles, as well as in promoting cardiovascular fitness. Water exercise therapy, such as swimming or aqua running, is very useful in maintaining fitness and enhancing endurance, especially in injuries that necessitate weight-bearing restrictions. This type of treatment is called unloading. It can also be land based, through the use of pulleys and harnesses to counter the effect of body weight to varying degrees.

6. Retraining in biomechanics; activity-specific movement patterns

At this stage of treatment the patient has regained full ROM and functional strength in the affected area. Muscular endurance has also returned and injured tissue is responsive to the demands of sustained activity. Retraining the athlete in a sports-specific fashion has several advantages. The adage "practice makes perfect" is correct. The more a specific skill is performed, the more ingrained it becomes, in a process known as engram formation. The need for correct technique is obvious. The muscle is repetitively taken through motion and force requirements when a specific task is performed. Sport-specific retraining allows for proper biomechanical function, thereby preventing the development of substitution patterns that can lead to reinjury. By the end of the program the athlete has become more efficient in the activity, resulting in a safer, more effective performance.

7. Maintaining cardiovascular fitness

As an injury is treated, generalized conditioning can be advanced as soon as the athlete is able to tolerate sustained activity. This may be almost immediately if the affected area can be protected or rested during aerobic activity. Cross training is a valuable addition to rehabilitation programs for this reason. As the injured area recovers, it can be incorporated into the fitness program. Eventually, the athlete functions at full capacity in an aerobic program; cardiovascular fitness can be improved and subsequently maintained. (Refer to Chapter 7.)

8. Development of programs to maintain strength, flexibility, conditioning, and skills

These programs are integrated into the rehabilitation program as soon as active teaching is completed in a given area. At this point the athlete assumes responsibility for ongoing function beyond the rehabilitation program. It is an absolutely essential step in the return to safe, effective, independent function. Flexibility, strength, and aerobic fitness all must be incorporated into maintenance programs.

PHASES OF REHABILITATION
See Fig. 20-1.

Reduction (Acute) Phase
This phase includes inflammation and pain control; it centers on the control of the acute signs and symptoms of an injury. In an acute injury such symptoms include pain and inflammation as a result of local tissue injury. This injury can involve macro and/or micro trauma. The PRICE principle—protection, rest, ice, compression, and elevation—is an effective means of implementing intervention. Such measures should be used as soon as possible following injury.

In a chronic injury, signs and symptoms are not as apparent; however, protection, rest, and icing are still important measures. Much of the damage is at a micro level and is due to repetitive overload and secondary compensations that lead to inefficient and faulty biomechanics. This in turn can lead to further tissue injury, dysfunction, or both.

Restorative (Subacute) Phase
This phase includes the restoration of joint ROM and soft tissue extensibility and restoration of muscular strength and endurance, including unloading. The injury is now subacute in nature, having been treated when acute in the reduction phase. Therapy is designed to prepare tissues for return to integrated function in a specific task. Flexibility (ROM) is restored first, followed by strength, and then endurance. The tenets can overlap

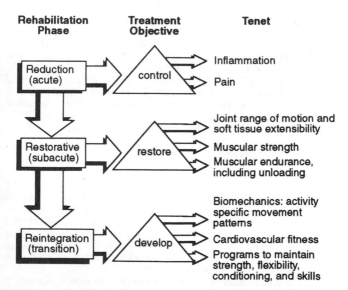

Fig. 20-1. Phases of rehabilitation as related to the tenets of sports injury.

somewhat, but generally it is best to advance rehabilitation through these tenets sequentially.

This phase may take the greatest amount of time and effort in therapy. Advancement to the next phase is predicated on successful restoration of flexibility, strength, and endurance. For this reason it is important to maintain cardiovascular fitness by means that still allow for restoration of injured tissue. For instance, if there is an ankle injury that precludes weight bearing during the restoration phase, fitness can be maintained by an arm ergonomer or by aqua running, which is nonweight bearing.

Encourage the patient to take a more active role in recovery. The transition toward self-care is an important step in prompt return to independent function and can best be accomplished by development of a home exercise program that mimics or supplements what has been taught in therapy. It then becomes the patient's responsibility to comply with the exercise program.

Finally, this phase serves as an initiation of the transition to coordinated tissue function. As flexibility is restored, strengthening begins. As strength returns, endurance training can be instituted. By the completion of this phase, the patient is ready to begin retraining in sport-specific tasks.

Reintegration (Transition) Phase

This phase consists of graded retraining in function. It begins with low-speed sport-related drills. Once a task is accurately performed, repetitions are increased and then the speed of performance of the repetitions is increased. The drills are then grouped into sessions. Once sessions are mastered in a similar fashion as the individual drills, the athlete is advanced to sport-specific maneuvers or activities.

When the athlete has mastered the skills necessary to perform the sport in safe and efficient form, practice of the activity on a regular basis begins. Concomitantly, cardiovascular fitness that has been developed is maintained. These two activities merge as the athlete begins performance of the sport for extended periods. At this point, rehabilitation moves into maintenance programs, and the athlete progresses to independent function in activities. Thus, rehabilitation is completed. The maintenance program is the most important aspect of the entire rehabilitative process, because it ensures ongoing independence and prevention of reinjury.

HISTORY AND PHYSICAL EXAMINATION

History

History includes a description of the current dysfunction and any similar previous occurrences. A thorough pain description should be obtained, including the location, frequency, and intensity of the pain. Pain descriptors pertaining to pain quality, radiation, and time of occurrence are appropriate. A rating of the pain such as from 1 to 10 can be helpful as a means of evaluating pain intensity from visit to visit. Attempts to elucidate what relieves, exacerbates, or worsens the pain are also important.

Obtain a description of the events leading up to and occurring during the actual injury. The mechanism of injury is the process of mechanical disruption or compromise that causes the injury. Ask questions that help recreate the scene. Have the patient describe what was happening when the injury occurred and describe in what position the injury began. See Table 20.3 for common sports-related injuries. If there was outside force, attempt to quantify its magnitude and from what direction it came. Record any other descriptors, such as an audible pop or snap, that might contribute to an understanding of the injury.

Once the mechanism of injury has been identified, the tissue or structures involved should be more obvious. This helps direct the physical examination and contributes to an understanding of the severity of the injury. However, often there is no discrete point of injury; therefore, a mechanism of injury is not as clear. In these cases, it is still helpful to have the athlete describe activities that seem to exacerbate the injury. This helps develop a functional picture of the injury.

Table 20.3. Common Injuries in Selected Physical Activities

Sport	Injury
Running	Plantar fasciitis
	Iliotibial band friction syndrome
	Patellofemoral dysfunction
	Hamstring tightness
	Low back pain
	Ankle sprains
	Achilles tendinitis
	Shin splints
	Stress fractures
Racquet sports	Lateral epicondylitis
	Rotator cuff impingement
	Muscle strains
Football	Mild head injury
	Ligamentous injury to the knee
	Dislocations and fractures
	Muscle strains
	Joint dislocations (shoulder, knee)
Basketball	Ankle sprains
	Muscle strains
	Jumper's knee (patellar tendinitis)
	Ligamentous injuries to the knee
Throwing sports	Rotator cuff impingement
	Lateral epicondylitis
	Shoulder instability
Skiing	Mild to severe head injury
	Shoulder dislocation
	Clavicular fracture
	Knee ligament injuries
	Lower limb fractures
	Skier's thumbs
	Patellofemoral dysfunction

It is also very useful to know about previous injuries, because they can shed light on preexisting dysfunctions or methods of biomechanical compensation. Frequently the current injury is directly related to previous injuries or indirectly a result of trauma from other activities.

Recent treatments can also provide clues to the process. These might include other physician visits, allied health interventions, or self-administered treatment. This information can also help to direct the treatment plan once the injury has been clearly defined.

Physical Examination

The area in question must be clearly visible. Have as much of the body exposed as necessary, but protect the patient's modesty; clothe the patient in a pair of shorts and a T-shirt or jog bra to begin the examination. As the examination progresses, these articles can be removed as indicated.

Begin the examination with visual inspection of posture, noting the condition of the axial skeleton. Inspect the area of complaint for deformities, erythema, or asymmetry. Compare this area to the other side of the body, if appropriate.

Palpate contiguous structures and proceed centrally to the area of injury. Initially, palpate lightly to obtain a general feel for the tissue and the surrounding structures, then deeper and more localized, noting areas of tension or asymmetry.

The passive portion of the examination consists of manual muscle testing, ROM testing, neurologic assessment, and provocative testing to elicit tissue dysfunction.

Dynamic assessment is necessary to obtain a functional diagnosis. It involves biomechanical evaluation during movement pertinent to the injury.

ASSIMILATION AND DIFFERENTIAL DIAGNOSIS

Formulate a differential diagnosis after considering the data and a biomechanically reasonable hypothesis. Identify all involved structures and their roles in the injury process so that the underlying cause, as well the presenting injury, can be corrected.

Use the components of soft tissue injury as outlined earlier in this chapter for a broader and more in-depth understanding of the biomechanical process of injury as it relates to particular athletes. This contributes to the formation of a differential diagnosis. The differential diagnosis then sums up all the clinical entities that contribute to or involve pathologic conditions in any of the five components of soft tissue injury. More traumatic acute processes or injuries may not have this depth of involvement and may be described and understood by simpler terminology. In the end, the differential diagnosis becomes an aid in the process of treating any given injury.

THERAPY PRESCRIPTION

Writing a prescription for physical therapy should be a precise means of communication from the physician to the therapist. Simply writing "evaluate and treat" nullifies the time and effort of the physician's evaluation and gives the therapist no helpful information in the attempt to treat the patient. It is ineffective and inadequate communication.

**Table 20.4. Example of a
General Sports Medicine Prescription**

Diagnosis: Right supraspinatus impingement with underlying
  scapular instability.
Treatment: (Note: A, B, and C are prescribed sequentially as
  the athlete advances through the three phases of rehabilitation over several weeks to months.)
A. *Acute:* Treat supraspinatus muscle with phonophoresis and
  range of motion; progress to strengthening program for all
  rotator cuff muscles.
B. *Restorative:* Begin scapular stabilizer muscle program with
  myofascial release techniques for the superior trapezius and
  levator scapulae. Strengthen the middle and inferior scapular
  muscles, including the rhomboids, middle and lower trapezius, and the serratus anterior to promote balanced muscular
  stabilization of the scapula. Concurrently stretch the anterior
  chest wall, including the pectoralis major and minor.
C. *Reintegration:* As pain subsides and range of motion returns,
  reeducate the shoulder girdle muscles in proper firing
  sequence for upper extremity activities such as throwing.
Frequency/duration: Please treat 2–3 times weekly for
  1 month.
Special instructions: Please treat one-on-one during the acute
  phase of treatment and thereafter as closely as possible. Keep
  me updated with problems as they arise and with patient
  progress. The patient will see me again in 4 weeks.

Next Physician Visit: 4 weeks.

A proper physical or occupational therapy prescription contains
the complete diagnosis, with elaboration of the involved structures.
It also specifies the types of methods called for and the area to be
treated. The prescription gives a time frame for implementation of
the therapies and indicates the frequency and duration of therapy.
Finally, it includes special instructions for restrictions and variations in treatment. Table 20.4 is an example of a prescription for
sports medicine.

Pursue conservative treatment at the onset and for as long as
progress continues. Reserve surgical intervention for those cases
that are obviously unstable (such as an anatomic defect as a result of trauma), have demonstrated no progress, or have reached
an endpoint in conservative therapy.

TYPES OF THERAPIES

Sports medicine therapies are shown in Table 20.5. In addition,
modalities such as heat or cold, typically used for other rehabilitative problems, may be indicated. Refer to Chapter 2.

SPECIAL POPULATIONS

The pediatric population undergoes much of the same injury
processes as adults; however, there are specific issues that must

Table 20.5.   Typical Sports Medicine Therapies

Therapy	Description
Myofascial release	Deep massage to an area to free layers of tissue from movement restrictions, alleviating pain and promoting unified tissue function
Unloading	A method of relieving a portion of the patient's body weight (by means of pulleys or by water) to lessen the impact to a certain area during exercise, allowing the patient to exercise within the parameters of weight-bearing restriction
Stretching	Performed in either dynamic or static fashion Passive: Uses only external force Active assisted: Uses a combination of external and internal forces Active: Uses force provided by the participant alone Proprioceptive neuromuscular facilitation (PNF). The muscle antagonist is activated, then passive stretch occurs.
Strengthening	A program of muscle contractions Concentric: A shortening contraction Eccentric: A lengthening contraction Isometric: Activating the muscle without movement Isotonic: Moving a uniform load by muscle contraction Isokinetic: Moving a varying load by muscle contraction at a uniform speed
Proprioceptive	Exercises promoting position sense without visual input to enhance joint function.
Manual therapies	Articulation: A technique of rhythmic oscillation applied to a joint which attempts to restore neutral mechanics to that joint Muscle energy: The patient develops force through activating muscles used by the therapist to influence the bony structure to which the muscles are attached High-velocity/low-amplitude: A quick but forceful thrust applied externally by the therapist; used cautiously, particularly in older or frail patients

Table 20.5. *Continued*

Therapy	Description
Alternative therapies	Pilates: Exercise that promotes rhythmic movement through proximally based strength, flexibility, and coordination
	Feldenkrais: Use of movement to increase kinesthetic awareness, enabling more graceful, safer movement
	Alexander technique: Focuses on kinesthetic awareness, particularly of the head and neck, to improve posture during movement
	Water exercise therapy: Unloading that relies on submergence in water, that can accomplish greater levels of unloading than land-based therapy
	Plyometrics: Activities using rapid eccentric muscle contraction to facilitate a more powerful concentric contraction
	Work hardening: Therapy designed to reacclimatize the worker to the work environment in a safe, efficient fashion
	Open kinetic chain activities: Distal aspect of the exercised limb is nonweightbearing
	Closed kinetic chain activities: Distal aspect of the exercised limb is weightbearing during exercise, more functionally based than open chain activities

be addressed. The pediatric patient tends to lack stability and strength in tissues that are undergoing rapid growth. Typically, injury results at the sites of maximal growth. The epiphyseal regions of bones are particularly vulnerable. The apophyseal areas, where muscles attach to bone, are also at risk for overload or overuse injury. Children are particularly susceptible to injury during or just after a growth spurt, because of a lag in development of soft tissue tensile strength. Overuse and overload injuries diminish as children gain strength and stability in soft tissue structures and as epiphyses close. Acute injuries to growth plates typically require orthopedic attention. Use the recovery period as an opportunity for education in biomechanics, because during these formative years proper technique can be taught and integrated into the child's movement patterns. Therefore, emphasize proper technique and movement reeducation during the restorative phase of rehabilitation.

Women comprise a group of patients who have unique sports medicine issues, specifically the role of exercise as related to pregnancy, the menstrual cycle, and the prevention of osteoporosis.

The geriatric athlete also has special concerns, because aging tissues lose their resiliency to injury, becoming weaker and less pliable. As a result there is less room for error in exercise. Injuries take longer to rehabilitate and must be rehabilitated in a less vigorous fashion. Counsel the geriatric athlete about these issues. The same general rehabilitation principles that apply to younger adults also apply to the geriatric population, but the time frame of recovery tends to be longer.

PATIENT EDUCATION

The doctor-patient-therapist relationship is a dynamic working alliance. It demands the respect of all three parties. The doctor-patient relationship is one in which mutual responsibility is the rule. The doctor acts as the educator, to empower the patient in coming to a new understanding of the workings of the body. The patient must assume the responsibility for regaining health and then maintaining it. The therapist enters the picture to help the physician in the education process, by using therapeutic techniques to educate the patient in the reattainment of health. In working with the therapist, the patient takes on the responsibility of becoming an active participant in health care, first by attending therapy, then by actively participating in the process of moving through acute therapy into a home-based program. The physician and therapist should work together in one conjoined care plan.

One-on-one therapist-patient interactions are best, especially in the acute phase of therapy. Having multiple therapists for one patient tends to lead to variation in treatment methods, which can be less effective, can be disconcerting to the patient, and can decrease patient compliance.

Patient education and empowerment are the goals of this triad of treatment. As one becomes educated, the ability to make decisions and eventually to take action in a productive fashion increases. The patient regains control of the condition as understanding of the situation and its implications grows. The doctor and the therapist are the facilitators of this process. The patient ultimately determines if the situation will change, assuming that the doctor and the therapist have fulfilled their roles.

FOLLOW-UP AND DISCHARGE

Once the therapeutic program has begun, regular follow-up with the physician is needed to monitor progress and to make adjustments in the program. During these follow-up visits, the therapist's notes should be available for review. The patient should also provide an impression of progress. In this way, the physician can monitor the patient's progress and evaluate the effectiveness of the patient-therapist interaction.

Follow-up visits become less frequent as the rehabilitation program continues. However, additional visits may be necessary if complications arise. In general, though, the patient eventually visits with the doctor only for evaluation of progress. At this point, discharge from physician care should be considered.

SUGGESTED READINGS

Cailliet R. *Shoulder pain,* 2nd ed. Philadelphia: FA Davis, 1981.

Herring SA. Rehabilitation of muscle injuries. *Med Sci Sports Exer* 1990;22:453–456.

Hoppenfeld S. *Physical examination of the spine and extremities.* Norwalk, CT: Appleton Century Cross, 1976.

Kibler WB. Clinical aspects of muscle injury. *Med Sci Sports Exer* 1990;22:4:450–452.

Reid DC. *Sports injury assessment and rehabilitation.* New York: Churchill Livingstone, 1992.

Saal JA. Dynamic muscular stabilization in the nonoperative treatment of lumbar pain syndrome. *Orthop Rev* 1990;19:691–700.

Saal JA. Rehabilitation of the injured athlete. In: DeLisa JA, Gans B, eds. *Rehabilitation medicine: principles and practice,* 2nd ed. Philadelphia: JB Lippincott, 1993:1131–1164.

Strauss RH. *Sports medicine.* Philadelphia: WB Saunders, 1984.

Team physician course, Part I. Dallas: American College of Sports Medicine, February 9–23, 1994.

Stroke

Susan J. Garrison and Elliot J. Roth

DEFINITION

Stroke is the clinical presentation of focal or global deficits in neurologic functioning caused by nontraumatic brain injury resulting from vascular disease inside the brain or in vessels leading to the brain, in which the onset is sudden or relatively rapid and the duration is more than 24 hours. The neurologic deficits caused by a completed stroke persist, whereas those of a transient ischemic attack (TIA) resolve completely within 24 hours.

ANATOMIC BASIS OF STROKE SYNDROMES

The clinical findings that result from the stroke depend specifically on the location of the vascular insult to the brain. Symptoms of stroke may arise from the anterior circulation, involving the carotid artery and its main branches (the anterior and middle cerebral arteries) or the posterior circulation (including the vertebral basilar and posterior cerebral arteries). Eighty percent of strokes occur in the carotid distribution, resulting in weakness of one side of the body and involving the face, arm, or leg in any combination, depending on which part of the brain is affected. Most (but not all) infarction strokes cause arm more than leg and face weakness. Strokes caused by posterior circulation lesions often cause brainstem or cerebellar dysfunction, with balance deficits, cranial nerve palsies, and other similar problems. Deeper strokes tend to cause pure motor or sensory problems without higher level cognitive or language disorders, whereas cortical strokes are associated with cognitive-perceptual dysfunction or aphasia.

STROKE-RELATED IMPAIRMENTS

Although loss of motor control is the most common impairment, it is by no means seen in all patients. An estimated 80% of stroke patients have some form of weakness or paralysis, usually hemiparesis, although monoparesis or quadriparesis are also seen. Aphasia, cognitive deficits, dysphagia, dysarthria, and other neurologic deficits are seen in roughly one third to one half of stroke patients.

NATURAL RECOVERY

Most patients with stroke demonstrate some degree of natural recovery of their deficits. The course, pattern, and outcome of recovery is highly variable. For most patients with classical middle cerebral artery stroke, spontaneous improvement in leg functioning tends to occur earliest, most frequently, and most completely. Return of arm control tends to be slower and more limited. Motor recovery tends to start with onset of spasticity, mostly distally first, then evolve into the presence of synergy or stereotypical movement patterns, and finally demonstrate isolated voluntary movement of limbs usually proximally first. However, this course can stop at any time. Improvement in cognition and language function tends to be the slowest to improve, but recovery of these functions tends to continue for longer periods, even long after motor recovery has ceased. Most (but not all) recovery occurs within the first 6 to 12 months following stroke, but it is possible to have improvements later. Although hemorrhagic strokes tend to be associated with more acute illness and a higher mortality rate, survivors often have more complete recovery, probably because of resorption of the blood. It is likely that a combination of factors explain the presence of spontaneous recovery, including resolution of edema, reversibility of injured but not infracted brain cells, and plasticity in which alternative neurons or pathways take over lost functions and new neural pathways form.

EPIDEMIOLOGY

Stroke ranks behind heart disease and cancer as the third most common cause of death in the Western world. Although past statistics placed the incidence at approximately 500,000 new strokes per year in the United States, more recent evidence suggests that the number is closer to 750,000; the upwardly revised figure is thought to be due to improved case finding rather than to increase in the actual new strokes per year. It is estimated that about one fifth of these are fatal (about 150,000 deaths per year in the United States) and that about 50% to 75% have some residual neurologic deficit, perhaps one half of whom require some type of rehabilitative services for their deficit. The prevalence of stroke, or the number of people alive today who sustained a stroke at some time in their past, is thought to be increasing to more than 4 million people in the United States. The likely reasons given for the increasing prevalence is the possibility that patients with stroke are surviving for longer periods following stroke.

Stroke is more common in older adults, but an estimated one third of all strokes occur in people younger than 65 years. Men have a higher incidence than women, and African-Americans have a higher incidence than whites. Other risk factors for stroke include hypertension, heart disease, diabetes, hypercholesterolemia, obesity, sedentary lifestyle, cigarette smoking, history of prior stroke or TIA, and family history.

ETIOLOGY AND PATHOPHYSIOLOGY

Strokes can be divided into hemorrhagic and ischemic types (Table 21.1). Ischemic strokes account for about 85% of all strokes and cause their brain injury through lack of blood supply. These are caused most often by atherosclerotic stenosis or occlusion

Table 21.1. Types of Stroke

Ischemic	85%
–Thrombotic	
–Embolic	
–Lacunar	
Hemorrhagic	15%
	100%

of the carotid, middle cerebral, or other cerebral artery. Embolic strokes, in contrast, occur abruptly as platelets, cholesterol, fibrin, or other blood components float in the circulation until they occlude small distal cortical vessels. Making up about 15% of all strokes, those strokes that occur in the setting of myocardial infarction, valvular heart disease, or cardiac arrhythmia such as atrial fibrillation usually are the result of cardiac emboli. Although thrombotic stroke tends to present with a slower, fluctuating, "stuttering" clinical course, embolic strokes tend to be more sudden and abrupt in onset. An estimated 15% of infarction strokes can be called "lacunar strokes," which result from small deep infarctions, usually less than 1 cm^3, occurring where small perforating arterioles branch directly off large vessels. Because of their deep brain location, these strokes usually cause motor deficits without cognitive or communicative problems. Hemorrhagic strokes, accounting for about 15% of all strokes, occur when blood is extruded from the vessel into the brain tissue and are divided roughly equally between subarachnoid hemorrhage (in which the blood enters the cerebrospinal fluid space) and intracerebral hemorrhage (in which the blood enters the brain parenchyma). Hemorrhagic stroke is the most catastrophic. Regions of the brain most commonly affected are similar to those affected in lacunar stroke, including the basal ganglia, internal capsule, and brainstem, although cortical hemispheric and cerebellar hemorrhages do occur. A small number of strokes are associated with other conditions, such as collagen vascular diseases, cerebral vasculopathies, coagulopathies, and substance abuse.

ASSESSMENT AND EVALUATION

Performance of a complete medical and neurologic evaluation, including history and physical examination at the time of presentation, is critical. Often this will need to be repeated frequently to assess whether the neurologic deficit progressed or improved. The history should document risk factors and associated medical conditions. Diagnostic evaluations may include computed tomography (CT) scan of the head; electroencephalogram (EEG); magnetic resonance imaging (MRI); carotid Doppler studies; cardiac evaluation, including two-dimensional echocardiograms and electrocardiogram (ECG); and routine laboratory evaluation of blood with clotting times. These studies are undertaken to determine cause of the stroke, the presence of associated medical conditions, and risk factors that may be addressed. See Table 21.2.

Table 21.2.   Risk Factors for Stroke
Age
Hypertension
Cardiac impairment
Previous CVA
TIAs
Diabetes

CVA, cerebrovascular accident; TIAs, transient ischemic attacks.

Typical patterns of deficits occur that may aid in localization of ischemic stroke. Lesions of the anterior cerebral artery usually result in paralysis and cortical hypesthesia of the contralateral lower limb, with mild involvement of the contralateral arm (Fig. 21-1). There may be impaired judgment and insight, incontinence of bowel and bladder, apraxia of gait, and sucking and grasping reflexes of the contralateral side. Middle cerebral infarction typically produces contralateral hemiplegia. Usually, the arm is more affected than the leg. Sensation is impaired in the same areas as motor loss (cortical sensory deficit or cortical hypesthesia). Blindness in one half of the visual field (hemianopsia), inability to recognize persons and things (agnosia), or difficulty in communicating (dysphasia) may occur. See Fig. 21-2. Posterior cerebral artery lesions result in mental change with memory impairment and inability to recognize or comprehend written words (alexia) or people and things (visual agnosia). The third cranial nerve may be paralyzed. Cortical blindness (unawareness by the patient that he or she cannot see) or hemianopsia may occur. See Fig. 21-3.

Brainstem strokes either leave minor deficits or are so severe that recovery is rare. Typical brainstem deficits include swallowing, visual, and balance problems.

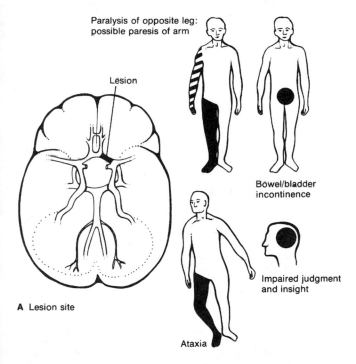

Fig. 21-1. Anterior cerebral artery. A: Lesion site. B: Typical deficits.

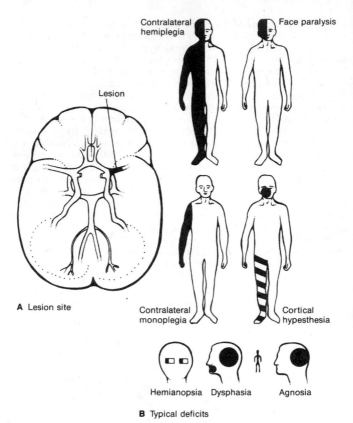

A Lesion site

Contralateral
hemiplegia

Face paralysis

Lesion

Contralateral
monoplegia

Cortical
hypesthesia

Hemianopsia   Dysphasia   Agnosia

B Typical deficits

Fig. 21-2.   **Middle cerebral artery. A: Lesion site. B: Typical deficits.**

REHABILITATION TREATMENT

The goals of rehabilitation are fivefold: (a) to prevent, recognize, and treat comorbid medical conditions including recurrent stroke and ongoing life functions, such as hydration and nutrition; (b) to maximize functional independence, through the use of functional training of daily skills and strengthening and flexibility exercises and by providing equipment and caregiver training as needed; (c) to facilitate psychologic and social adaptation and coping by the patient and family; (d) to enhance community reintegration and the resumption of prior life roles; and (e) to enhance quality of life for stroke survivors.

Traditional stroke rehabilitation employs the use of compensatory techniques for mobility, activities of daily living (ADLs), and communication while natural recovery, to the extent possible, occurs over time. A limited time trial of inpatient rehabilitation (2 weeks or less) allows a patient to demonstrate his or her appropriateness as a candidate for further inpatient rehabilita-

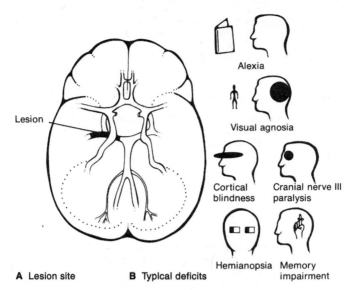

Fig. 21-3. Posterior cerebral artery. A: Lesion site. B: Typical deficits.

tion immediately following acute stroke. Poor prognostic indicators for stroke rehabilitation candidates are listed in Table 21.3.

Strokes are common events, yet stroke rehabilitation is complex. Although functional deficits appear to be similar, patients react individually. Therefore, each stroke rehabilitation program must be uniquely tailored. Even more important than physical deficits are the cognitive aspects affected by stroke. The left-brain injured, functionally right hemiplegic patient is much different with respect to communication and learning than the right-brain injured, functionally left hemiplegic patient. See Table 21.4. These differences must be recognized and addressed in treatment.

Table 21.3. Poor Prognostic Indicators for Stroke Rehabilitation Outcome

Severe memory problems
Inability to understand commands
Medical/surgical instability
Previous stroke
Advanced age
Urinary/bowel incontinence
Visual spatial deficits

Adapted from Jougblood L. Prediction of function after stroke: a critical review. *Stroke* 1986;17:765–776, with permission.

Table 21.4.   Characteristics of Right and Left Hemiplegic Patients

Right Hemiplegic (Left-Brain Injured)	Left Hemiplegic (Right-Brain Injured)
Communication impairment	Visual/motor perceptual problems
Learns by demonstration	Loss of visual memory
Will learn from mistakes	Left side neglect
May require supervision due to communication problems	Impulsive
	Lacks insight/judgment, requires supervision

From Garrison SJ. Learning after stroke: left versus right brain injury. *Topics in Geriatric Rehabilitation* 1991;6:3:45–52, with permission.

Rehabilitation of the stroke patient begins in the acute care setting. Timely intervention maximizes potential recovery and prevents problems resulting from immobility. See Chapter 10. Poststroke rehabilitation of the uncomplicated, medically stable patient is generally as follows. See Table 21.5. However, medical problems at any stage may slow the rehabilitation process (see the section on complications in this chapter).

Medical treatment of stroke consists of evaluation of the cause of the stroke and correction of underlying problems, if possible. One aspirin a day is the current accepted treatment for the patient who has sustained a thrombotic stroke. Dipyridamole (Persantine) has not been shown to be efficacious. Ticlopidine (Ticlid) 250 mg orally twice daily is indicated in thrombotic stroke if aspirin is not tolerated. Patients with embolic stroke should undergo thorough cardiovascular examinations and should be anticoagulated, long term, if indicated. Patients with lacunar and hemorrhagic stroke with elevated blood pressures may require antihypertensive medications.

COMPLICATIONS

Any patient who has sustained a stroke is at risk for further complications because of immobility, as well as from problems relating to his or her general medical condition.

Deep Venous Thrombosis (DVT)

DVT of the legs occurs in approximately 30% to 50% of stroke patients. It may not be detected clinically in the paralyzed leg. The risk of pulmonary embolism (PE) with DVT is approximately 10%. The lower extremities should be examined daily for discoloration, edema, or pain on movement. Noninvasive Doppler studies are diagnostic. Prevention includes antiembolic stockings, protection of the affected extremity, proper positioning, and ambulation as soon as appropriate. Use of minidose heparin is advocated. If DVT is suspected clinically, the patient should be adequately anticoagulated with heparin. A patient with a hemorrhagic stroke with

Table 21.5. Basic Guidelines for Poststroke Rehabilitation[a]

Day 1–3 (bedside)
Avoid positioning on affected limbs
Relieve common pressure areas, such as heels and sacral area
Document reflexes, tone, and muscular strength
Begin PROM & AAROM, daily by OT/PT or nurse
Dangle out of bed
Sit in chair
Document bowel/bladder function
Identify communication deficits
Implement dietary modifications
Assess social situation

Days 3–5 (to therapy department)
Send to PT/OT department by wheelchair
Use wheelchair cushion; avoid doughnut cushion
Evaluate ambulation potential in parallel bars
Baseline evaluations by PT/OT
Provide sling if shoulder subluxed
Remove indwelling catheter; begin timed voiding

Days 7–10 (acute inpatient rehabilitation)
Transfer activities (wheelchair to mat; wheelchair to bed)
Pregait activities
Admission to acute rehab unit
ADL practice: a.m. care and dressing
Psychologic evaluation
Strategies for communication
Swallowing addressed by speech/dietary therapy
Learning independence at wheelchair level

2–3 Weeks (acute inpatient rehabilitation)
Upgrade gait: assistive device/AFO
Team/family conference regarding prognosis and discharge
    planning
Therapeutic home evaluation
Upgrade from bedside commode to bathroom

3–6 Weeks (Acute Rehabilitation Discharge)
Family member/caretaker learns home program
Self-medications taught
Independent in dressing, grooming
Independent in wheelchair transfers and mobility
Bathroom and kitchen evaluations complete
Upgrade diet
Communication needs addressed

10–12 Weeks (outpatient physician office follow-up)
Review functional abilities
Discuss safety issues (falls)
Renew/adjust outpatient therapy orders
Renew medications
Obtain follow-up with other physicians, as indicated
Assess need for further patient/family counseling

AAROM, assisted active range of motion; ADL, activity of daily living; AFO, ankle foot orthosis; PROM, passive range of motion; PT, physical therapy.
[a]See Chapter 1 for specific orders and description of rehabilitation team.

onset longer than 3 weeks can generally be considered safe for anticoagulation.

Seizures

Seizures, more common following hemorrhagic and embolic strokes than thrombotic strokes, occur in 10% to 15% of stroke patients. One half of these occur in the acute period. Antiseizure medications should be tailored to the individual patient. Lethargy is a sign of overmedication.

Depression

Poststroke depression has both an organic basis, deriving directly from the brain injury, and a "reactive" basis, resulting from the new onset of disability and dependence. It appears to be more common in left hemisphere than right hemisphere injury. The depression may not become apparent until 6 months to 2 years following injury. Signs include poor cooperation, management problems, inconsistent recovery, or increasing neurologic deficit. Psychologic and psychiatric support should be given. Often, a trial of antidepressant medication is helpful.

Dysphagia

Evaluation and management of dysphagia may prevent aspiration pneumonia and helps ensure adequate nutrition. Swallowing problems, usually the result of the absence of or severe delay in the swallowing process, may be seen following brainstem stroke and unilateral cerebral lesions. Warning signs of swallowing impairment in the stroke patient include confused mental state, dysarthria, complaint of obstruction, weight loss, nasal regurgitation, and mouth odor. Dysphagia evaluation may be made at the bedside by the speech pathologist. A modified barium swallow may document abnormalities in the swallowing process. Treatment includes therapy to improve oral motor control and stimulate swallowing (thermal stimulation), as well as modification of the diet. Thickened liquids and altered consistency of food may be helpful. Nasogastric or gastrostomy feeding is recommended for patients at severe risk of aspiration. For those for whom little recovery is anticipated over 2 to 3 months, gastrostomy feeding with constant drip or bolus feeding is used. Bolus feeding should be avoided in any stroke patient who is at risk of aspiration, because stomach distension, regurgitation, and aspiration may occur.

Nutritional Status

Poor nutritional status is common in patients who are chronically ill or undergo prolonged hospitalizations. In addition to dysphagia, upper extremity paralysis, visual field neglect, communication impairment, and depression may decrease caloric intake. Calorie counts, weight records, total protein, serum albumin, and other laboratory indices of nutritional status should be monitored.

Incontinence

Urinary incontinence is common following stroke but is usually transient. A voiding trial (offering the patient the urinal or bedside commode on awakening, every 2 hours, and before sleep) will often solve the problem. Urinary tract infections should be treated. Fecal incontinence is generally related to immobility, change in diet, or fecal impaction. Continued incontinence of urine and feces may be indicative of bilateral or brainstem lesion and therefore is incurable.

Shoulder Hand Syndrome (SHS)

SHS, a type of reflex sympathetic dystrophy (RSD), is a well-recognized poststroke complication, although rare in carefully monitored patients. Characterized by painful active and passive range of motion at the affected shoulder, pain on extension of the wrist, edema over the metacarpals, and fusiform edema of the digits with pain on passive flexion of metacarpophalangeal (MCPs) and proximal interphalangeal (PIPs), SHS is commonly seen in the second to fourth month poststroke. The diagnosis is made clinically. Routine x-ray films show osteoporosis; delayed isotope scans may reveal increased uptake. Early recognition is necessary for appropriate treatment. The affected hand should be observed daily. Careful attention to positioning of the extremity is necessary to decrease edema and thereby decrease pain. Use of a compression glove may help decrease edema. The goal is to decrease pain so that passive stretching can be done to further decrease edema. This may be accomplished through application of a cold pack before stretching. Avoid contrast baths or application of warm water that may increase blood flow and thereby increase edema. In severe cases, a short course of oral steroids may be helpful. Use pillows, overhead sling, regular sling, arm trough, or lapboard with elbow pad. Low doses of antidepressant or antiepileptic medications may be helpful for the patient who cannot sleep because of shoulder pain at night. In severe prolonged cases, stellate ganglion blocks may be considered. Throughout SHS, the rehabilitation program should continue. If the problem recurs, the patient should undergo a second course of treatment.

Shoulder Subluxation

Shoulder subluxation, resulting from muscular weakness of the affected rotator cuff muscles and lack of tone, is a common finding poststroke. It is unclear whether subluxation leads to shoulder pain. The use of a standard sling is controversial. The ambulatory patient with a flaccid upper limb should use a sling when ambulating but should use an arm trough on the wheelchair. Nonambulatory patients should use a lapboard when seated.

Spasticity

Spasticity results from loss of cortical inhibitory influences. Usually, this can be treated with aggressive and consistent stretching exercises and proper positioning. Certain medications may be helpful, although side effects tend to limit their use. Injections of neurolytic medication such as botulinum toxin has been shown to have beneficial effect.

Other Complications

Other poststroke complications include overmedication, poor endurance secondary to cardiac complications, and falls. All medications should be reduced to the minimum and use of long-acting sedative-hypnotics should be avoided. Patients with known cardiac problems should be on appropriate medications. Nitroglycerin, if needed, should be available to the patient in therapy. Monitor blood pressures routinely. Observe for possible digitalis toxicity. Prevent falls by use of gait belts, restraints when necessary, close observation, and good transfer techniques.

The patient who has had a stroke is at increased risk for another. Note any new neurologic problem, especially refusal to eat, loss of speech, or focal motor deficit. Document the findings and investigate the cause.

PROGNOSIS, OUTCOME, AND FOLLOW-UP

Recovery from stroke is a natural process; rehabilitation techniques provide compensatory skills for functional deficits. In a typical pattern of recovery, muscular strength returns in a proximal to distal fashion, arm independent of leg. This accounts for the ability of most poststroke patients to ambulate eventually. When this typical pattern is not observed, the diagnosis of stroke must be questioned. In addition, other poststroke injuries such as fractured hip or brachial plexus injury must be ruled out.

From a functional standpoint, prognosis is related to prolonged flaccidity, late return of reflexes, late onset of motor movement, and lack of hand movement. Lack of sensory function is extremely debilitating in terms of activities of daily living and ambulation. A patient who has voluntary muscular movement but no sensation will not use the affected limb functionally.

Communication disorders and swallowing functions usually improve over months. Speech therapy will often be continued over a period of 1 to 2 years in severely aphasic patients who show improvement.

The "typical" patient with left hemiplegia requires a 3 to 4 week stay in acute care rehabilitation. The patient with right hemiplegia, with severe communication and swallowing problems, may require 4 to 6 weeks of inpatient rehabilitation.

All therapies should be continued at a less intense frequency (two to three times per week) after discharge from acute care rehabilitation for a period of 1 to 4 months or until the patient reaches established goals. Some patients initially require home care and advance to outpatient therapies as mobility improves. Outpatient physician follow-up visits should be scheduled every month or two to assess progress and renew therapy prescriptions. A patient who is nonambulatory because of hip weakness at the time of acute rehabilitation discharge may be considered for staged rehabilitation; when hip strength improves, he or she may be readmitted to learn ambulation. The patient who loses previous gains may also require readmission for assessment and remediation of problems.

On all office visits, equipment checks are made. Patients are instructed to keep the appropriate wheelchair prescribed while he or she was an inpatient so that it can be used for long-distance ambulation for up to several months.

SUGGESTED READINGS

Brandstater ME, Roth EJ, Siebens HC. Venous thromboembolism in stroke: literature review and implications for clinical practice. *Arch Phys Med Rehabil* 1992;73:S379–391.

Garrison SJ. Learning after stroke: left versus right brain injury. *Top Geriatr Rehabil* 1991;6:3:45–52.

Garrison SJ. Geriatric stroke rehabilitation. In: Felsenthal G, Garrison SJ, Steinberg FU, eds. *Rehabilitation of the aging and elderly patient.* Baltimore: Williams & Wilkins, 1994:175–186.

Garrison SJ, Rolak LA. Rehabilitation of the stroke patient. In: DeLisa JA, Currie D, Gans B et al, eds. *Principles and practice of rehabilitation medicine,* 2nd ed. Philadelphia: JB Lippincott, 1993.

Goodstein RK. Overview: cerebrovascular accident and the hospitalized elderly—a multidimensional clinical problem. *Am J Psychiatry* 1983;140:2:141–147.

The healing influence (videotape). Santa Fe, NM: Danamar Products, 1991.

Hurd MM, Farrell KH, Waylonis GW. Shoulder sling for hemiplegia: friend or foe? *Arch Phys Med Rehabil* 1974;55:519–522.

Jongblood L. Prediction of function after stroke: a critical review. *Stroke* 1986;17:765–776.

Moskowitz E. Complications in the rehabilitation of hemiplegic patients. *Med Clin North Am* 1969;53:541–558.

Orif R, Heiner S. Orthoses and ambulation in hemiplegia: ten year retrospective study. *Arch Phys Med Rehabil* 1980;61:216–220.

Robinson RG, Kubos KL, Starr LB, et al. Mood disorders in stroke patients: importance of location of lesion. *Brain* 1984;107:81–93.

Roth EJ. Medical complications encountered in stroke rehabilitation. *Phys Med Rehabil Clin North Am* 1991;2:563–578.

Roth EJ. Rehabilitation of the stroke patient. In: Rakel RE, ed. *Conn's current therapy, 1996.* Philadelphia: WB Saunders, 1996.

Roth EJ, Harvey RL. Rehabilitation of the stroke syndromes. In: Braddom RL, ed. *Physical medicine and rehabilitation,* 2nd ed. Philadelphia: WB Saunders, 2000.

Tepperman PS, Greyson ND, Hilbert L, et al. Reflex sympathetic dystrophy in hemiplegia. *Arch Phys Med Rehabil* 1984;65:442–447.

Traumatic Brain Injury

Cindy B. Ivanhoe and Gerard E. Francisco

DEFINITION

Traumatic brain injury (TBI) can be defined as injury to the brain caused by an external force. Severity can vary from mild to severe. The trauma causing the injury may be blunt, such as a blow to the head, or penetrating, as in missile injuries (Table 22.1). Movement of the brain within the skull can also cause injury. Damage may be manifested by loss of consciousness, posttraumatic amnesia (PTA), skull fractures, objective neurologic or neuropsychologic abnormality, or evidence of intracranial injury on neuroimaging. Varying degrees of physical and cognitive deficits may result, depending on the severity of damage, secondary complications, and associated injuries. Residual deficits range from negligible to severely disabling.

EPIDEMIOLOGY

In this country, TBI is the leading cause of death and disability for the 40 years and younger age group. The peak incidence of TBI occurs between the ages of 15 to 24 years, with males injured two to three times more often than females. There are two other smaller peaks in the incidence of TBI: one in children below 5 years and the other in the older than 75 age group. It is estimated that the annual rate of TBI in the United States is 100 per 100,000 persons. Each year, about 70,000 to 80,000 individuals with TBI demonstrate long-term functional loss. Most persons with TBI are unemployed and from lower socioeconomic groups. There is often a history of alcohol abuse, drug abuse, and/or psychiatric care. About one third of TBI survivors have had a previous head injury. Motor vehicle accidents are the leading cause of TBI in adolescent and adult populations. There is a high correlation with positive blood alcohol levels at the time of injury. Falls and sports-related injuries are common causes of TBI in the pediatric and adolescent population. In the United States, violence is responsible for about 20% of TBIs.

ANATOMY AND PATHOPHYSIOLOGY

Primary brain damage as a result of TBI occurs at the moment of impact. Refer to Fig. 22-1. Secondary damage occurs as a result of the subsequent pathologic complications arising from the intracranial and extracranial damage.

Primary Brain Damage

Linear acceleration and deceleration result in the relative movement between the rigid skull and the soft, incompressible brain. Contusions occur over the frontal lobes and the anterior tips of the temporal lobes; the occipital lobe is damaged less frequently. Hemorrhagic contusions can vary in extent from a superficial layer of blood (a subpial hemorrhage) to one that involves the whole depth of the cortex, causing necrosis and edema. The contusions may be bilateral and asymmetrical. Localized contusions under

Table 22.1. Terminology of Traumatic Brain Injury

Nonpenetrating brain injury	Traumatic brain injury in which the dura remains intact
Penetrating brain injury	Traumatic brain injury in which dural integrity is violated
Head injury/trauma	Inexact term, because head injury may occur in the absence of brain injury (e.g., scalp laceration)
Concussion	Inexact term and not recommended. Commonly used interchangeably with mild brain injury with transient impairment of consciousness. Actually describes causative mechanism of injury, i.e., a blow or punch to the head

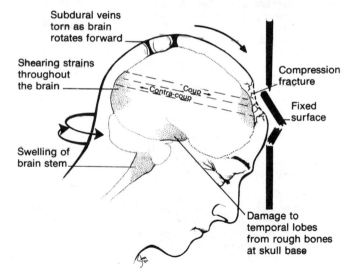

Fig. 22-1. Acceleration/deceleration injury.

the area of impact are seen with depressed skull fractures and gunshot wounds.

Rotational acceleration causes movement between the different components of the brain, resulting in diffuse axonal injury (DAI), thought to be due to shearing of nerve fibers in the white matter. The corpus callosum and upper brainstem are commonly affected. At autopsy, the brain appears grossly normal. There may be moderate ventricular enlargement resulting from axonal loss and atrophy. Microscopic examination reveals scattered axonal retraction balls, microglial stars, and, later, demyelination of the nerve processes distal to the point of injury. Apoptosis ("programmed cell death") and cell necrosis ("uncontrolled and abrupt cell death") are responsible for some histologic findings in the injured brain.

Secondary Brain Damage

Late coma in a previously conscious patient or deepening of coma is due to secondary brain damage. Factors leading to secondary complications can be divided into two categories—intracranial and extracranial. Intracranial hematomas (epidural, subdural, and intracerebral) and edema contribute to increased intracranial pressure (ICP), which causes tissue necrosis and obstruction of intracranial veins. Pressure is increased, thereby compromising cerebral blood flow. Watershed areas (boundary zones between adjacent major vascular territories) and the basal ganglia, hippocampus, and Purkinje cells of the cerebellum are most vulnerable to ischemia. Increased ICP can also cause various herniation syndromes (transtentorial uncal herniation and cingulate gyrus herniation) leading to compromised brainstem function, cranial nerve palsies, and contusion. Subarachnoid hemorrhage can lead to vasospasm and ischemia. The arachnoid villi may become blocked by cellular debris, leading to decreased absorption of cerebrospinal fluid (CSF) and a further rise in ICP.

The most common extracranial factor that contributes to secondary brain injury is hypoxemia. This may be caused by the head injury or by associated injuries. Hypotension, anemia, hyponatremia, and other metabolic abnormalities must also be monitored and appropriately managed.

ASSESSMENT

The Glasgow Coma Scale (GCS) is most commonly used to categorize patients' level of consciousness at the initial neurologic examination in the field and emergency room. It assesses the patient's ability to open the eyes, speak, and make motor responses to standard stimuli. The scale provides broad quantification of responsiveness but does not evaluate subtle changes that occur in patients' progression from coma. (See Tables 22.2 and 22.3.) Brainstem dysfunction in a comatose patient is evidence of great force at impact; the prognosis is worse. Pupillary responses, eye movements, and oculovestibular reflexes, as well as signs of autonomic dysfunction, posturing, and movement disorders, are helpful in determining prognosis. Document detailed neurologic evaluations and repeat sequentially. The Coma/Near Coma Scale rates reaction to pain, verbal commands, and sensory modalities and is one scale for quantifying minute changes in neurologic status.

Table 22.2.   Glasgow Coma Scale

Indicator	Category of Response	Grade
Eye Opening	Spontaneous	4
	When spoken to	3
	To noxious stimulus	2
	None	1
Verbal Response	Oriented to place and date	5
	Confused, disoriented	4
	Inappropriate words	3
	Incomprehensible words	2
	None	1
Motor Response	Obeys command	6
	Localizes noxious stimulus	5
	Withdraws from noxious stimulus	4
	Flexor posturing in response to noxious stimulus	3
	Extensor posturing in response to noxious stimulus	2
	No response	1

States of Severe Impairment of Consciousness (Tables 22.4 and 22.5)

The vegetative state describes the finding of wakefulness without awareness. A patient in coma will die, awaken, or become vegetative. The vegetative state is defined by the return of sleep-wake cycles and, therefore, eye opening. The patient may blink in response to threat and his or her eyes may move from side to side, seemingly following family members or staff. Observers frequently misinterpret the phenomenon of "tracking" as awareness of the environment. Patients may also exhibit primitive postural reflexes, including limb movements. These findings, which represent brainstem functioning, often make it difficult for observers to accept that the patient has no awareness of the environment. In the work of Jennett and Teasdale, no patient classified as vegetative 3 months after injury ever gained independence. Ten percent regained consciousness but remained dependent.

Table 22.3.   Classifying Severity of TBI based on Glasgow Coma Scale (GCS) and Radiographic Findings

Mild—GCS score of 13–15 at lowest point after resuscitation
   Uncomplicated—normal brain CT scan
   Complicated—CT scan evidence of brain injury
Moderate—GCS score of 9–12 at lowest point after resuscitation
Severe—GCS score of 3–8 at lowest point after resuscitation

CT, computed tomography; TBI, traumatic brain injury.

Table 22.4.   Terminology of States of Severe Alteration of Consciousness

	Coma	Vegetative	Minimally Conscious
Clinical Feature			
Spontaneous eye opening	None	Yes	Yes
Sleep-wake cycle	None	Resumes	Abnormal to normal
Arousal	None	Sluggish; poorly sustained	Obtunded to normal
Evidence of perception, communication ability, or purposeful motor activity	None	None	Reproducible but inconsistent
Visual tracking	None	None, but may have roving eye movements	Often intact
Yes/no responses, verbalizations and gestures	None	None	None to unreliable and inconsistent

Table 22.5.   Assessment Scales for Persons with TBI and Severely Impaired Consciousness

Coma-near coma scale
Rates reaction to pain; response to auditory, tactile, visual, and olfactory stimuli; and ability to follow command

Coma recovery scale
Evaluates arousal, visual, auditory, motor, oromotor/verbal, and communication abilities

Western neuro-sensory stimulation profile
Measures responses to sensory stimulation, visual tracking, object manipulation, arousal, and attention

Sensory stimulation assessment measure
An expansion of GCS, rating patient responses to standardized visual, auditory, tactile, gustatory, and olfactory stimulations

Individualized assessment using single-case experimental methodology
No limitation to items in a standardized battery because the assessment is tailored for each patient

GCS, Glasgow Coma Scale

Cognitive function is evaluated by a variety of tests, usually administered by neuropsychologists and speech pathologists, as in Table 22.6; the Disability Rating Scale and the Rancho Los Amigos Levels of Cognitive Functioning (Table 22.7) scale are widely used scales to describe the TBI survivor's level of functioning.

TREATMENT

General

Criteria for admission to a brain injury program vary with the program. Patients may be accepted for coma management, or they may need to be able to follow commands. Some programs accept patients while they are still ventilator-dependent.

Coma Management Programs

Coma management programs are available in a variety of settings. The goals are to facilitate arousal from coma, prevent complications of immobility, and educate and train families in the care of their loved one. Sensory stimulation programs have yet to be proven effective but are useful for monitoring responsiveness and involving family members. Medications can be adjusted to minimize clouding of the patient's already impaired sensorium. A few medications are proposed to increase arousal and recovery of consciousness (Table 22.8).

The Rehabilitation Team

The rehabilitation team assesses the patient's strengths and deficits and sets appropriate short- and long-term goals. In addition to a comprehensive history, and physical and neurologic examination (see Table 22.9), a functional evaluation is performed for formulation of appropriate treatment plan and goal setting. Types of evaluations performed vary based on individual patient abilities. There is often overlap in the evaluations, but, in general, team member responsibilities are listed in Table 22.10.

Posttraumatic Amnesia (PTA)

When admitted for rehabilitation many survivors are following commands but are confused and in a state of PTA. PTA is defined as the length of time until the return of continuous memory. At this stage, patients are often confused and agitated, as they try to make sense of an environment that they no longer understand. If behavioral interventions and reassurance are not adequate, pharmacologic interventions may become necessary. Use of an antidepressant, psychostimulant, or mood stabilizer in an agitated patient is preferable to a tranquilizer or neuroleptic medication (see later).

COMPLICATIONS

Agitation

Agitation is best described as an excess of a certain behavior. It is a common occurrence during recovery from TBI. As the patient's confusion resolves, there is a parallel decrease in agitation. Thus, tranquilizers and neuroleptics, often given in acute care settings, may increase confusion and worsen agitation. The use of these

Table 22.6. Some Cognitive and Neuropsychologic Tests

Domain	Test
Depth of coma Neuropsychologic examination	Glasgow Coma Scale (GCS)
Orientation/PTA	GOAT COAT Oxford/Westmead Scale
Language	Token Test Controlled Oral Word Association (COWA) Boston Naming Test
Attention	Digit Span Paced Auditory Serial Addition Test (PASAT) Digit Cancellation Symbol Digit Modalities Test
Learning and memory	Rey Complex Figure Logical memory (Subtest of Wechsler Memory Scale) Selective Reminding Test Continuous Recognition Memory Test
Motor skills	Finger Tapping Grooved Pegboard Grip Strength
Mental flexibility and concept format	Trail Making Wisconsin Card Sorting Test
Personality/ psychopathology MMPI	Category Test
Emotional, social, and behavioral impairment	Neurobehavioral Rating Scale General Health Questionnaire (GHQ) Katz Adjustment Scale/Relative Form Portland Adaptability Index
Disability/impairment	FIM FAM (FIM + cognition, psychosocial adjustment, communication) Sickness Impact Profile
Handicap	CHART Community Integration Questionnaire (CIQ)
Global	Glasgow Outcome Scale (GOS) Disability Rating Scale (DRS) Glasgow Outcome Scale-Extended (GOSE) Rancho Los Amigos Level of Cognitive Functioning Scale

Table 22.6. *Continued*	
Domain	Test
Multidimensional	Portland Adaptability Index (PAI)
	Functional Independence Measure (FIM)
	Functional Assessment Measure (FAM)
	Program Evaluation Conference System (PECS)
	Sickness Impact Profile (SIP)

drugs may delay motor and cognitive recovery. Behavioral and environmental measures (Table 22.11) should be employed. Medical conditions that may cause agitation, such as pain and electrolyte abnormalities, also need to be ruled out. If nonpharmacologic measures do not adequately control agitation, pharmacologic medications can be considered. Mood stabilizing, activating, and psychostimulant drugs (Table 22.12) are preferred over tranquilizers or neuroleptics. Restraints should be avoided if possible, because these patients may hurt themselves more in their attempts to break free.

Swallowing

Swallowing disorders or dysphagia after brain injury are usually the result of damage to the brainstem or anterior cortical areas. Evaluation includes an assessment of reflexes (cough, bite, gag, rooting, suck); head, tongue, and jaw control; taste; and pulmonary function. The patient may pocket oral contents or demonstrate drooling and choking. Use of video fluoroscopy, also known as the "cookie swallow" or modified barium swallow, documents the presence or absence of aspiration and allows a more accurate determination of food consistencies that the patient can safely swallow (Fig. 22-2). The patient may require insertion of a gastrostomy tube to ensure proper nutrition with minimal risk of aspiration.

Seizures

Approximately 5% of all TBI patients develop posttraumatic seizures. The risk is greatest in patients who have depressed skull fractures, acute intracranial hematomas, or early seizures (occurring within the first week after injury). Patients are often started on phenytoin (Dilantin) or phenobarbital in the acute neurosurgical setting because these drugs are easily administered parenterally and have been in use for a long time. The literature suggests that prophylaxis is probably not necessary after the first week. There is a trend to treat only patients who have had seizures. Carbamazepine (Tegretol) and valproic acid (Depakene, Depakote) appear to have the fewest cognitive and behavioral side effects. The most significant side effect of carbamazepine (Tegretol) is bone marrow suppression. If the leukocyte count falls below 3,000 cells with less than 50% neutrophils, this medication should be discontinued.

Table 22.7.   Rancho Los Amigos Scale

I	No response Unresponsive to any stimulus
II	Generalized response Limited, inconsistent, nonpurposeful responses, often to pain only
III	Localized response Purposeful responses; may follow simple commands; may focus on presented objects
IV	Confused, agitated Heightened state of activity; confusion, disorientation, aggressive behavior, unable to do self-care, unaware of present events, agitation appears related to internal confusion
V	Confused, inappropriate Nonagitated; appears alert; responds to commands; distractible; does not concentrate on task; agitated responses to external stimuli; verbally inappropriate; does not learn new information
VI	Confused, appropriate Good directed behavior, needs cueing; can relearn old skills as activities of daily living; serious memory problems; some awareness of self and others
VII	Automatic, appropriate Appears appropriate; oriented; frequently robot-like in daily routine; minimal or absent confusion; shallow recall; increased awareness of self, interaction in environment; lacks insight into condition; decreased judgment and problem solving; lacks realistic planning for future
VIII	Purposeful, appropriate Alert, oriented; recalls and integrates past events; learns new activities and can continue without supervision; independent in home and living skills; capable of driving; defects in stress tolerance, judgment, abstract reasoning persist; many function at reduced levels in society

Table 22.8.   Neurostimulant Medications

Methylphenidate (Ritalin)
Dextroamphetamine (Dexedrine)
Bromocriptine (Parlodel)
Amantadine (Symmetrel)
Levo/Carbidopa (Sinemet)
Some tricyclic antidepressants
Selective serotonin reuptake inhibitors

Table 22.9. Rehabilitation Admission Information

At rehabilitation admission record the following information:
History
Loss of consciousness
Initial and postresuscitation Glasgow Coma Scale (GCS) score
Length of coma
Secondary complications, such as intracranial hypertension or
   hypoxia
Associated injuries
Diagnostic studies
Surgeries
Social history
Premorbid personality
Family support
Financial issues
Educational level
History of substance abuse
Examination
Physical examination
Emphasize neurologic examination

Posttraumatic Hydrocephalus

Symptoms range from deep coma to the triad of dementia, ataxia, and incontinence. Presentation may be atypical, with emotional disturbances, seizures, spasticity, or subtle cognitive changes. Diagnosis is based on radiographic evidence on computed tomography (CT) scan in conjunction with clinical assessment. When there is a question as to the significance of CT findings, serial CT scans may be helpful. Hydrocephalus should be suspected when recovery is slower than expected, progress slows or halts, or function regresses. Hydrocephalus can develop anytime after a TBI.

Spasticity

Spasticity is usually defined as a velocity-dependent increase in muscle tone, resulting from upper motor neuron disease. It can limit function, cause pain, result in deformities, and prevent progress in therapies. Unless it causes pain, interferes with hygiene, limits function, or causes contractures, spasticity may not need to be treated. In some instances, spasticity is beneficial, in that it maintains muscle bulk, assists patients with marginal motor strength in transfers and standing, and helps prevent osteoporosis and deep venous thrombosis.

Management using physical modalities includes the application of cold or heat, stretching, splinting, casting, positioning, functional electrical stimulation (FES), relaxation, and motor reeducation. Serial application of casts allows for sustained muscle stretch and provides a warm environment that affects soft tissue pliability. Positioning techniques reduce hypertonicity. For example, abduction of the thumb can result in easier extension of fingers that are otherwise tightly flexed. Nerve blocks and botulinum toxin injections, both local treatments, are preferable to systemic

Table 22.10.   Functional Evaluation of Person with TBI by Rehabilitation Team Member

Team Member	Task
Neuropsychologist	Employs battery of psychologic tests, which vary according to patient's level of functioning. To assess intellectual functioning, judgment, attention, concentration, language, and memory for incorporation into aspects of the patient's program
Physical therapist	Identifies gross movement patterns (synergy) and develops program to normalize movement and decrease tone
Occupational therapist	Assesses through functional tasks: evaluates postural reflexes, tone, coordination, and range of motion (ROM). Records reactions to pain, tactile, auditory, gustatory, and olfactory stimuli. Head control is influenced by muscle weakness, abnormal reflexes, and tone
Speech pathologist	Evaluates language, communication, speech, cognition, hearing, swallowing; uses battery of tests, including: Woodcock-Johnson Psychoeducational Battery Ross Information Assessment Processing Detroit Test of Learning Aptitude There is no standard battery of speech tests for the TBI population
Recreational therapist	Designs a program of leisure activities to help carry over skills from other therapies; aids in reintegration into community
Rehabilitation nurses	Carry over therapy programs, train caregivers/family members, provide nursing care, develop bladder and bowel programs, monitor oral intake
Music therapist	Develops plan to increase attention, encourage verbal expression, increase upper extremity activity and carry over goals of other therapies in an engaging setting

TBI, traumatic brain injury.

Table 22.11. Nonpharmacologic Management of Agitation

Manage level of stimulation in the environment
Rule-out medical conditions that may increase confusion or present as agitation, such as pain, nonconvulsive seizure, infection, or electrolyte abnormalities
Reduce the patient's confusion
Protect the patient from harming himself, herself, or others
Tolerate restlessness as much as possible

---

medications that have central nervous system (CNS) depressant effects. Injection techniques usually yield the best results when combined with the previously mentioned techniques and motor reeducation. Although frequently used in many settings, oral spasmolytics cause significant problems with sedation in TBI survivors. Intrathecal baclofen therapy provides great relief of spasticity that involves multiple muscle groups, without causing sedation. It requires implant of a pump into the lower abdominal area and routine follow-up for pump refills. Its greatest effects are on the lower limbs with less predictable effects on the upper limbs. All modalities for spasticity management are best used in conjunction with each other.

Heterotopic Ossification (HO)

HO is ectopic bone formation around joints. Risk factors include coma longer than 2 weeks, spasticity, long bone fractures,

---

Table 22.12. Pharmacologic Agents for Agitation

Beta-blockers
Anxiolytics
  Buspirone
  Benzodiazepines[a]
Antipsychotics
  Haloperidol[a]
  Risperidone[a]
  Quietapine[a]
  Olanzapine[a]
Antiepileptics
  Valproic acid
  Carbamazepine
Dopamine agonists
  Bromocriptine
  Amantadine
Tricyclic antidepressants
  Amitriptyline
  Nortriptyline

---

[a]Use judiciously, if at all.

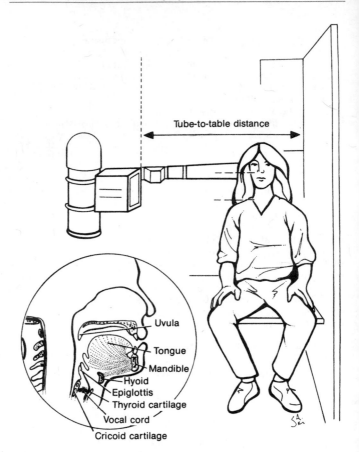

Fig. 22-2.   Modified barium swallow ("cookie swallow") procedure, performed under fluoroscopy.

or decrease in range of motion. Incidence ranges from 11% to 76%. The most commonly involved locations are the shoulder, elbow, and hip. Diagnosis is usually made when there are clinical findings of limited range of motion, pain, and swelling. An elevated alkaline phosphatase level is suggestive of HO but is nonspecific in patients who have sustained trauma. Triple-phase bone scans are most sensitive for early diagnosis of HO. Nonsteroidal anti-inflammatory drugs (NSAIDs) are sometimes used acutely to decrease pain and swelling. Continue aggressive range of motion. Etidronate (Didronel) 20 mg/kg in a single daily dose for 3 months, followed by 10 mg/kg daily for 3 months, may inhibit bone formation. The most common side effects are gastrointestinal but usually do not mandate cessation of the medication. Long-term treatment with etidronate can lead to osteomalacia.

Endocrine Abnormalities

The syndrome of inappropriate antidiuretic hormone secretion (SIADH) is most frequently seen. This results in dilutional hyponatremia and is, therefore, managed with fluid restriction. SIADH generally resolves during the acute neurosurgical phase of treatment. Another condition, also characterized by hyponatremia, is cerebral salt wasting. This condition must be distinguished from SIADH, because treatment differs. Diabetes insipidus (DI) is less commonly seen. It results in a failure of antidiuretic hormone (ADH) secretion with resultant diuresis of dilute urine and hypernatremia. SIADH and DI are managed the same way as in other patient populations. Menstrual irregularities are frequent. Menstruation usually resumes around 6 to 12 months postinjury. Studies suggest that up to 20% of persons with severe brain injuries have one or more disturbances of anterior pituitary hormones; the clinical significance is unclear.

Injuries and Fractures

Up to 89% of patients have one or more extracranial injuries, which must be identified early to minimize long-term disability. Always evaluate patients for cervical spine injuries. Peripheral nerve injuries may result from initial trauma, compression resulting from poor positioning or restraints in the acute setting, or HO.

Autonomic Disturbances

Systemic hypertension, which may result from high ICP and catecholamine release, is frequently seen. Increased cardiac output and tachycardia are also common in the acute care setting. Focal injuries near the hypothalamus can result in hypertension. β-blockers, indicated in the hyperdynamic state, may later impair the patient's cognitive functioning. Hypotension is usually orthostatic. Central fevers, although uncommon, are seen in patients with lesions of the anterior hypothalamus or generalized decerebration. Hypothermia, secondary to lesions of the posterior hypothalamus or resulting from endocrine dysfunction, may occur.

Respiratory Complications

Pneumonia is common, as is bacterial colonization of tracheostomy sites. Decannulation is indicated when the need for mechanical ventilation has resolved, the proximal airway is intact, there is no further need for pulmonary toilet, and the patient can swallow safely. Abnormalities seen before decannulation include vocal cord paralysis, tracheal stenosis, subglottic stenosis, glottic stenosis, and tracheomalacia. These may be due to intubation, head injury, or a combination of the two.

Gastrointestinal Complications

The patient with TBI is hypermetabolic, with high caloric needs. Gastrostomy tube feedings are preferable to hyperalimentation if the need is long term; observe for changes in weight and serum albumin level. The risk of gastrointestinal bleeding secondary to stress ulcers is increased and histamine H_2-receptor antagonists are frequently prescribed. Omeprazole (Prilosec) or famotidine (Pepcid) are preferable to cimetidine (Tagamet), which may cause behavioral disturbances (Table 22.13). Metoclopramide (Reglan),

**Table 22.13.   Suggested Alternatives
to Sedating Medications**

Drug Class	Sedating Medications	Alternative
Antidepressants	Tricyclics	SSRIs
Antispasticity	Baclofen (oral), tizanidine	Botulinum toxins, motor point blocks, intrathecal baclofen (ITB)
Antiepileptics	Phenytoin	Carbamazepine, valproic acid, gabapentin
Pro-gastric motility	Metoclopramide	Erythromycin
H₂-blockers	Cimetidine	Omeprazole, famotidine

SSRIs, selective serotonin reuptake inhibitors.

frequently used to improve gastric motility, is related to the phenothiazines; it can cause sedation, extrapyramidal symptoms, restlessness, and movement disorders acutely and as a delayed effect. Decrease gastric reflux by using a feeding jejunostomy tube, specific positioning, and small bolus or continuous tube feeding rather than simply medicating with metoclopramide (Reglan).

Genitourinary Complications

Neurogenic bladder is rare following head injury. If present, there is usually uninhibited detrusor hyperreflexia. Use an external collecting device for males and diapers for females. A hyporeflexic bladder with resultant overdistension may also occur. Bladder training should begin once the patient is aware of his or her surroundings. There is a high incidence of urinary tract infection in patients arriving on the rehabilitation unit, usually secondary to prior instrumentation. Obtain a screening urinalysis, culture, and sensitivity at the time of rehabilitation admission. Cognitive dysfunction plays an important role in incontinence.

PROGNOSIS AND OUTCOME

Most patients who remain unconscious 1 month following brain injury will either recover or die within the first year. Consciousness is usually regained within 3 months. Twenty percent to 30% of patients who do not regain consciousness will die within the first year. Age is a powerful predictor of outcome; the pediatric population demonstrates a better outcome than the adult. Common negative prognosticators include a low GCS, impaired eye movements and pupillary responses, surgical mass lesions, and unconsciousness longer than 3 months. Apolipoprotein E₄, previously linked to Alzheimer's disease, is believed to be a susceptibility marker for unfavorable outcome after TBI.

Psychosocial aspects of patients' lives also influence outcomes. Emotional disturbances and changes in behavior frequently accompany TBI. A lack of self-awareness and the disinhibition that often

Table 22.14.   Glasgow Outcome Scale

1 Dead
2 Vegetative
3 Severe disability
4 Moderate disability
5 Good recovery

accompany brain injury can lead to increasing isolation from friends and family. It is generally easier for family members to accept their loved one's physical disability than change in personality.

A number of scales and tests exist that provide valuable information about the degree of a patient's injury. Numerous physical findings are interpreted as good or bad prognosticators. However, patients have varying combinations of factors contributing to disability; accurate predictions are difficult. The Glasgow Outcome Scale (Table 22.14) is widely used for categorizing late outcome after traumatic and nontraumatic coma. It reflects the patient's social dependency by placing him or her in one of the following categories: vegetative state, severe disability, moderate disability, and good recovery.

FOLLOW-UP

Following discharge from acute rehabilitation, patients with TBI may be treated in comprehensive outpatient services, day treatment, residential programs, transitional or skilled living facilities, or home. Goals are for them to eventually participate in a rewarding lifestyle, within their functional limitations. This may include supported or sheltered employment. For many TBI survivors, some degree of dependence on others remains. Ideally, there should be access for continued support. The difficulties are dynamic and continue to present physical, social, cognitive, and behavioral challenges to patients and families. Although many patients require minimal follow-up, others will always require frequent medical rehabilitative support.

SUGGESTED READINGS

Giacino JT, et al. Aspen Neurobehavioral Conference. Development of practice guidelines for assessment and management of the vegetative and minimally conscious states. *J Head Trauma Rehabil* 1997.

Boake C, Francisco GE, Ivanhoe CB, et al. Brain injury rehabilitation. In: Braddom R, et al., eds. Philadelphia: WB Saunders, 2000: 1073–1116.

Guidelines for the Management of Severe Head Injury, American Academy of Neurological Surgery, 1996 American Academy of Physical Medicine and Rehabilitation Practice Parameter (Brain Injury Special Interest Group). *Arch Phys Med Rehabil* 1998.

Horn LJ, ed. Pharmacology and brain rehabilitation. *Phys Med Rehabil Clin North Am* 1997.

Horn LJ, Zasler ND, eds. *Medical rehabilitation of traumatic brain injury.* Philadelphia: Hanley & Belfus, and Mosby, 1996.

Multi-society Task Force Report on the Persistent Vegetative State, American Academy of Neurology. *N Engl J Med* 1994.

Narayan RK, Wilberger JE, Povlishok JT, eds. *Neurotrauma.* McGraw-Hill, 1996.

Rappaport M, Herrero-Backe C, Rappaport ML et al. Head injury outcome up to ten years later. *Arch Phys Med Rehab* 1989;70:885–892.

Rehabilitation of persons with traumatic brain injury. NIH consensus statement, Vol 16, Number 1, 1998.

Rosenthal M, Griffith ER, Bond MR et al., eds. *Rehabilitation of the adult and child with traumatic brain injury,* 2nd ed. Philadelphia: FA Davis, 1999.

Whyte J, Hart T, Laborde A, et al. Rehabilitation of the patient with traumatic brain injury. In: DeLisa J, et al., eds. Philadelphia: Lippincott–Raven, 1998:1191–1240.

Yablon SA. Post-traumatic seizures. *Arch Phys Med Rehabil* 1993; 74:983–1001.

Wheelchairs

Charles E. Levy, Theresa Frasca Berner,
and Michael L. Boninger

DEFINITION

Wheeled mobility in its broadest sense includes any device with wheels that helps a person get around. Conceivably this could include items such as riding lawnmowers, golf carts, roller skates, and wheeled carts. In a rehabilitation context, wheeled mobility refers to wheeled walkers, manual and power wheelchairs, and scooters.

EPIDEMIOLOGY

As of 1996, there were 1,363,000 manual wheelers, 93,000 power wheelchair users, and 64,000 scooter users in the United States. In 1998, wheelchairs accounted for 38% of the home medical equipment market, the single largest category (home care beds 27%, bathroom safety supplies 15%, ambulatory aids 10%, and miscellaneous patient aids 10%).

ASSESSMENT AND EVALUATION

The history and physical examination are directed at achieving three critical goals: determining or confirming the diagnosis, assessing the patient's functional abilities and limitations, and identifying the resources available to procure an appropriate device.

History

First the physician must establish the diagnosis and understand the prognosis. Most patients present with a known diagnosis, and it is usually not necessary to recapitulate the workup. However, the clinician must scrutinize the medical history sufficiently to screen for alternative diagnoses that might change the patients' treatment plan. For example, a patient with Guillain-Barré syndrome may present with similar limitations in strength and endurance as another patient with amyotrophic lateral sclerosis. Because the former would usually be expected to regain abilities whereas the latter would be expected to decline, their wheelchair prescriptions would be markedly different. If the diagnosis is uncertain but the workup is complete, a reasonable prescription can be generated by extrapolation based on the past course of the disease.

The next questions to be answered are "Will the patient be enabled by a wheeled mobility device, and, if so, what kind of device would be appropriate?" These questions demand consideration not only of the patient's immediate motor and cognitive abilities but also of issues of transport and environment. A power chair that is too heavy to be transported or too wide to fit in the office or home will not be used, despite the fact that patient may have been able to sit with an improved posture and maneuver the device in the clinic.

Next to be considered is how the device will be procured. The typical list price in the United States in 1997 for a new lightweight foldable wheelchair was $1,100 to $2,500. Power wheelchairs commonly list between $4,000 to $18,000. This does not include additional costs of adaptive seating or assistive technology systems such as environmental control units, augmentative communication systems, or computer jacks. Most patients are not prepared to pay list price out-of-pocket for a new wheelchair, and there are usually restrictions to the aid provided by public and private insurance. Alternatives include buying used or floor models, trade-ins, or using community resources such as the Multiple Sclerosis Society. State bureaus dedicated to vocational rehabilitation often help purchase equipment deemed necessary as part of efforts to return a client to work. When any single source fails, a combination of resources may succeed. The American Medical Association publishes a book that describes essential components of a letter of medical necessity and sources of funding on a state-by-state basis.

Because most insurers, both private and public, provide only one chair every 5 years, it is paramount that the physician provides an accurate prescription the first time. The ideal device would maintain or improve the patient's best posture, be easy to operate and maneuver in the intended environments, be mechanically sound and backed by reliable and accessible sales and manufacturer's representatives, and be aesthetically pleasing. Unfortunately, for many patients, the ideal device does not exist. In these cases the knowledgeable physician is indispensable in helping to guide the patient to an acceptable compromise.

Physical Examination

The physical examination in the context of a wheelchair seating and positioning clinic must aid in the determination of the patient's capabilities and limitations in regards to propelling or guiding a wheelchair. The exam focuses on the patient's cognition, judgment, safety awareness, vision, strength and coordination of the limbs, stability and balance of the trunk, posture, and the patient's body proportions.

A thorough assessment of the patient's posture is integral to crafting a successful wheeled mobility prescription. Proper seating and positioning preserves or expands the patient's ability to participate by minimizing pain; correcting or accommodating postural deformities; protecting skin integrity; promoting full chest expansion during respiration; increasing reach; easing transfers, self-care and toileting; and presenting the user in the most attractive manner possible. The specific goals of seating are to maintain good pelvic position, optimize spinal alignment, provide pressure relief, and provide a stable base of support from which to work.

After the medical, functional, psychosocial, and cognitive/communicative needs are determined the physical evaluation can begin. If the client enters the clinic in a wheelchair, the patient's sitting posture should be noted. Poor habits such as sitting with crossed legs (decreasing the available weight-bearing surface) may be observed. Slouching may indicate that the patient has knee flexion contractures or hypertonicity. If a knee flexion contracture or hypertonicity is found during the physical examination, the hanger angle of the wheelchair may need to be increased (Fig. 23-1).

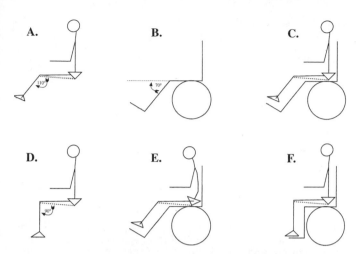

Fig. 23-1. A: Person with normal posture, able to extend knees to 110 degrees. Hamstrings represented by dashed line. Pelvis represented by triangle. B: Standard wheelchair configuration with 70-degree hanger angle. C: Normal posture is maintained when person A sits in standard wheelchair. D: Person with knee flexion contractures at 90 degrees because of shortened hamstrings. Hamstrings represented by dashed line. Pelvis represented by triangle. E: When person with knee flexion contractures is placed in wheelchair with 70-degree hanger, the pelvis is pulled into a posterior tilt resulting in kyphosis of the spine. F: Patient is able to sit with erect upright posture in a wheelchair with a 90-degree hanger angle. (Illustration courtesy Charles E. Levy, MD.)

Important information can also be gleaned by watching the manner in which a patient transfers. Clumsy or careless transfers can contribute to the development of pressure sores and may be improved with training or proper equipment.

The examination of patients with normal posture, flexibility, and balance may only require a series of measurements taken in a seated position. Typically all that is entailed to define the dimensions of the wheelchair are popliteal fossa-to-floor height, popliteal fossa-to-posterior buttocks length, hip width, and shoulder width. The physical examination for a person suspected of having significant postural abnormalities is much more complex, often demanding that at least two examiners work together. One holds the patient in a particular position while the other measures physical dimensions and range of motion. Although these types of assessments may actually be conducted by physical and/or occupational therapists, the physician should understand how the examination is performed and be able to independently judge the outcome. The physician is ultimately responsible for the prescription and should be an active participant in determining seating solutions.

The examination begins with the patient in a supine position and then progresses to an examination of seated posture. The supine posture is examined first to help the examiner appreciate postural deformities separate from how they manifest in an upright position. After the patient transfers onto a mat table and is lying supine, lumbar and pelvic ranges of motion are established. Because the position of the pelvis is a prime determinant of the curvature of the spine, pelvic mobility is noted as the pelvis is rocked in an anterior and posterior direction and rotated in the transverse plane. Asymmetries and obliquities may be noted. Next, hip range of motion is measured. The pelvis must be stabilized while the hip is flexed and extended. While measuring the hip range of motion, the knee is maintained in a flexed position to eliminate the influence of the hamstrings.

Once the supine evaluation is completed, a seated evaluation commences. The patient is positioned at the edge of the table with his or her feet resting on the floor or a platform. At this point, sitting posture and balance, orientation in space, and the need for posterior and lateral supports are noted. Lumbar and pelvic ranges of motion are determined through observation and palpation. With one examiner supporting the client in the back and the other kneeling in front, notations are made of the degree of pelvic obliquity, pelvic rotation, and the extent of leg-length discrepancy if any of theses conditions are present. The position of the pelvis in the anterior-posterior plane is also recorded. The therapist sitting behind the client notes the presence of scoliosis, kyphosis, lordosis, and/or any posterior rib deformities. The extent of lateral flexibility and the shape of the trunk are examined, as are the positions of the shoulders and head. Hamstring length should always be measured with the hips flexed at or as close as tolerated to 90 degrees. As long as an individual can reach 110 degrees or greater of knee extension, with hips at 90 degrees, standard legrests with a 70-degree hanger will fit. However, if an individual with a knee flexion contractures of less than 110 degrees is placed in a wheelchair with a standard 70-degree hanger angle, then he or she will continually be scooting out of the chair and sitting with their pelvis in posterior pelvic tilt (Fig. 23-1). This will place the client at risk for pressure sores. A patient who cannot tolerate sitting at 90 degrees of hip flexion may require a wheelchair with an increased seat-to-back angle. Finally, the range of motion of the ankles and feet are evaluated; inspection to detect ulcers and/or calluses also takes place. If an individual is contracted in plantar flexion, adjustable footplates may be indicated to allow the foot to make full contact with the footplate, minimizing the risk for pressure sores.

At this point an interventional examination begins. By selectively supporting the pelvis, a stable pelvic base is created. Besides hands-on support, materials such as foam wedges may be used. Once this base is established, the modifications for trunk, back, and head support may be modeled (i.e., hands beneath the axilla may replicate the effects of lateral supports attached to the wheelchair back uprights). The appropriate hanger angle, legrests, and footplates are determined depending on the flexibility and range of motion of the lower limbs once the optimal seated position has been established. Depending on the availability of equipment, the patient can be placed in a wheelchair in which different wheelchair cushions and backs can be tried and modified.

If the patient's posture is sufficiently flexible, then the wheelchair prescription should be designed to correct any positioning problems. If the posture includes fixed deformities, the prescription should take this into account to accommodate these needs to provide the patient the most comfortable and practical seating. This may involve modifying the chair by increasing the seat-to-back angle, providing customized cushions and backs, or modifying legrests or footplates. For patients who are prone to worsening posture and deformities (i.e., Duchenne's muscular dystrophy) all efforts should be made to prevent or slow further physical deformity. The ultimate goal is to find the least obtrusive combination of equipment that will provide as much freedom and independence as possible for any specific patient. If the final prescription includes specialized communication devices or environmental control units, these too must be mounted in accessible locations that cause the least unwanted restriction of movement and comfort.

Physical therapists and **occupational therapists** often direct the wheelchair seating and positioning clinic. These therapists contribute valuable expertise in the evaluation of the patient's range of motion, strength, and posture. Physical and occupational therapists can also provide valuable information about the client's functional level, which may affect the appropriateness of certain components. Functional areas include capability to use power or manual mobility, ability to perform pressure relief, ability to transfer to and from the wheelchair, and ability to ambulate. Often the therapist has already developed a trusting working relationship with the patient. In these cases the therapist is in an ideal position to function as an advocate for the patient and ensure that all questions and concerns have been addressed. If therapists are unavailable to perform such services, the responsibility defaults to the physician. In some settings the physician will rely on vendors or manufacturer's representatives for help. Rehabilitation technology engineers, speech language pathologists, nurses, social workers, case managers, vocational rehabilitation counselors, peer counselors, and educational professionals may also play important roles on the wheeled mobility team.

TREATMENT

Rational decision making for the wheeled mobility prescription can be accomplished by asking a series of questions in an orderly fashion (Fig. 23-2, Table 23.1). In the following discussion, the general terms *wheelchair* or *powered wheelchair* include scooters unless otherwise noted. Likewise, the term *chair* is used as shorthand for wheelchair.

It is obvious that those with bilateral lower limb paralysis require wheelchairs, whereas those with sufficient endurance and functional gait do not. On occasion, however, patients present with limited ability to ambulate. For these patients the key is to determine what limits their walking. A psychologic or medical approach may be in order if fear, pain, or vertigo limit ambulation. Gait instability may be best treated with a directed course of physical therapy or bracing. Patients who can maintain an upright posture will more easily access counters and navigate tight corners (i.e., bathrooms). They will retain the psychologic benefit of engaging others face to face at a standing level. Upright posture offers advantages such as better maintenance of bone density. Reasonable

(text continues on page 349)

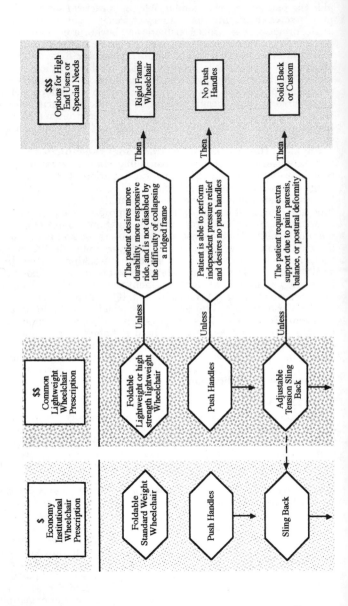

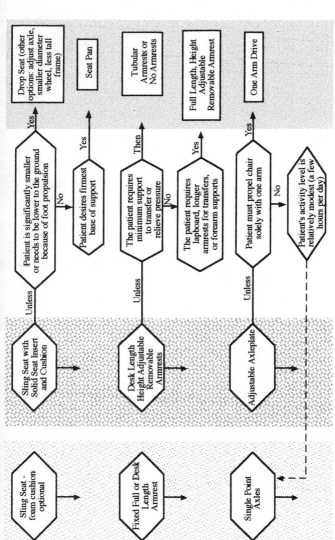

Fig. 23-2. *Continued.*

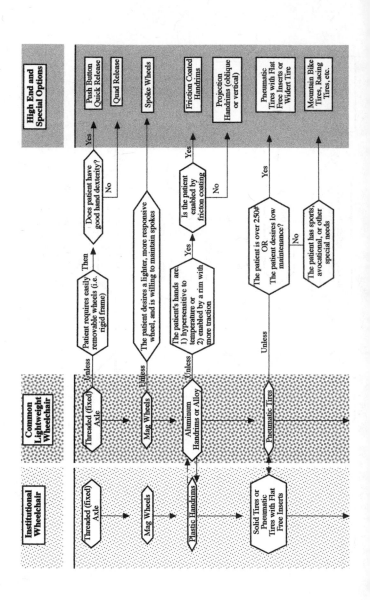

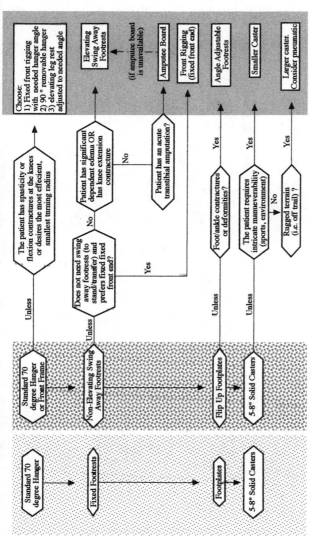

Fig. 23-2. Algorithm for manual wheelchair options. (Adapted from Levy CE, Boninger M, McDermott M et al. Wheeled mobility. In: Grabois M, ed. *Physical medicine and rehabilitation: the complete approach.* Blackwell Science, 2000:685–711, with permission.)

Table 23.1. Manual Wheelchair Prescription Form

Physician _____   Date of Rx _____   Measurements: Hips _____ Shoulders _____
Pt. Name _____   Seat to Mid Scapula _____   Knee to Heel _____
Diagnosis _____   Back to Knee _____

1. **Construction**
   ☐ Standard ☐ Lightweight ☐ Lightweight high strength ☐ Ultra lightweight
   ☐ Heavy duty ☐ Extra heavy duty ☐ Hemiheight ☐ Other _____

2. **Frame**
   ☐ Folding ☐ Rigid ☐ Hybrid

3. **Push Handles**
   ☐ Yes ☐ No

4. **Back**
   ☐ Sling ☐ Adjustable tension ☐ Solid Brand _____ Size _____ ☐ Custom molded
   ☐ Sling with solid seat insert ☐ Solid pan seat ☐ Adjustable tension sling Size _____

5. **Seat**
   ☐ Sling ☐ Solid Brand _____ Size _____ ☐ Custom molded

6. **Cushion**
   ☐ Foam ☐ Contoured foam ☐ Fluid filled ☐ Air filled ☐ Honeycomb ☐ Other Brand _____ Size _____

7. **Armrest**
   ☐ Tubular OR a) ☐ Full length vs. ☐ Desk length ☐ Flip back
   b) ☐ Fixed vs. ☐ Detachable
   c) ☐ Fixed height vs. ☐ Adjustable height

8. **Chair Axle**
   ☐ Single point ☐ Adjustable ☐ Other

9. **Wheel Axle**
   ☐ Threaded ☐ Quick release ☐ Quad release

10. **Wheels**
    ☐ Mag ☐ Spoke

11. **Hand rims**
    ☐ Plastic ☐ Aluminum/Alloy ☐ Friction coated ☐ Projections (oblique or vertical) ☐ None
    ☐ One-arm hand drive ☐ Right / ☐ Left

12. **Tires**
    ☐ Solid ☐ Pneumatic tires ☐ Pneumatic tires with flat-free inserts
    ☐ Mountain tire ☐ Racing tire ☐ Other _____

13. **Hanger Angle**
    ☐ 60° ☐ 70° ☐ 80° ☐ 90° ☐ Other _____

14. **Calf Pad**
    ☐ Yes ☐ No

15. **Legrest**
    ☐ Fixed ☐ Swing away detachable ☐ Folding front rigging ☐ Elevating ☐ Amputee board
    ☐ Fixed front rigging (rigid chair)

16. **Footplates**
    ☐ Flip up ☐ Angle adjustable ☐ Rigid platform ☐ Detachable platform

17. **Casters**
    ☐ Solid ☐ Pneumatic ☐ 3" ☐ 5" ☐ 7" ☐ 8" ☐ 9" ☐ Other _____

18. **Safety Features**
    ☐ Positioning belt ☐ Antitips ☐ Wheel locks: ☐ Push-to-lock, ☐ Pull-to-lock, ☐ Scissor
    ☐ Grade Aids ☐ Wheel locks Location: _____

19. **Accessories**
    ☐ Full lap tray ☐ Half lap tray (Right or Left) ☐ Lumbar support Brand: _____
    ☐ Lateral support(s) Location: _____
    ☐ Manual recline ☐ Manual tilt-in-space

20. **Misc.**

options should be explored to preserve walking in those who are capable. Gait aids that should be considered include canes, axillary and forearm crutches, orthoses, and static and wheeled walkers. Four-wheeled walkers that feature hand brakes, seats, and baskets can be very helpful. These are equipped with large wheels that allow travel over deep carpets and mildly uneven terrains. However, the physician should not be reluctant to recommend a wheelchair or scooter for the marginally ambulatory. The proper device can enhance mobility and preserve energy, expanding participation in desired activities.

After it has been determined that a seated mobility device is necessary, then one must choose between manually propelled and power wheelchairs. Because manual chairs are lighter, less mechanically complex, easier to transport, provide continued cardiovascular challenge, and are less expensive, they are preferred over power chairs for those capable of manual propulsion. For those who lack the endurance or strength necessary for self-propulsion and possess the requisite cognitive and perceptual skills, powered mobility is appropriate.

Manual Wheelchair Prescription

Medicare has classified manual wheelchairs as follows from the heaviest to the lightest: standard (more than 36 lb), lightweight (36 lb), high-strength lightweight (less than 34 lb with a lifetime warranty on the side frames and cross braces and a sectional or adjustable back), and ultra lightweight chair (less than 30 lb with an adjustable axle and a lifetime warranty on the side frames and cross braces). Almost all rigid frame chairs are ultra lightweight chairs. All of these types of wheelchairs are warranted for patients up to 250 pounds. The previous order also reflects the relative cost of each class of chair, from least to most expensive.

Standard wheelchairs are more difficult to propel and transport; they offer little in terms of adjustability and are often manufactured with fixed armrests and footplates and less-expensive materials. Their sole advantage is that they are less expensive. They may be adequate for some patients who need a chair only temporarily, for example, following a hip replacement. To take advantage of the full spectrum of adjustability and options, one must look to high-strength lightweight and ultra lightweight chairs.

Medicare, to contain costs, demands that patients meet an escalating set of criteria to be vended a lighter, stronger chair. The patient's functional status must be verified on a form signed by a physician. As an example, a Medicare enrollee is eligible to receive a standard wheelchair if the individual would be bed or chair confined without a wheelchair. To receive a lightweight chair, the user must be bed or chair confined without a wheelchair and unable to propel a standard chair but be able to propel a lightweight chair. For a high-strength lightweight chair, the patient must self-propel "while engaging in frequent activities that cannot be performed in a standard or a lightweight wheelchair" or "require a seat width, depth, or height that cannot be accommodated in a standard, lightweight or hemi-wheelchair and spends at least 2 hours per day in the wheelchair." A high-strength lightweight wheelchair is seldom approved if the duration of need is less than 3 months. Although ultra lightweight chairs may be the most desirable because of their ease of wheeling, durability, and styling, they are generally also the most expensive. Medicare approves ultra lightweight wheelchairs only on a case-by-case basis. Vendors can improve their chances of getting approval by documenting the need of the patient with a physical or occupational therapist's evaluation. A letter from the actual user may also be helpful. Medicare policy does allow a patient to upgrade equipment by paying the difference between the prescribed and desired item. For example, a person who qualifies for a high-strength lightweight chair may receive an ultra lightweight chair if he or she is willing to pay the difference in cost between the two chairs. There is no set formula that other insurers follow. Some policies allocate a set allowance, others allow negotiation, and others provide no payment for durable medical equipment.

The vendor is required to follow a physician's prescription and cannot legally substitute. However, if the physician prescribes an item that is beyond the profit margin that the vendor will accept, the vendor can refuse to fill the prescription. Knowledgeable physicians, particularly those who may refer many patients, may influence the vendor to liberalize policy.

Active patients exceeding 225 pounds may put such wear and tear on a lightweight frame, that a heavy-duty frame is indicated. Heavy-duty frames are warranted up to 300 pounds; beyond 300 pounds, an extra-heavy duty wheelchair is recommended. Physicians and vendors place themselves at risk for legal liability if they prescribe or provide frame that does not meet the patient's weight requirements. Extra cross bracing and gusseting (reinforcement) may be available from some manufacturers to upgrade the weight tolerance of a specific frame.

After the weight tolerance of the frame has been chosen (standard, lightweight, high-strength lightweight, ultra lightweight, heavy duty, or extra heavy duty), the next decision is "foldability" of the frame.

Frames come in two types of configuration—foldable and rigid. Most foldable frames chairs have an "X" brace underneath the seat and fold like an accordion (Fig. 23-3). In rigid frame wheelchairs, the back folds forwards and the wheels pop off (Fig. 23-4). Most users describe the ride and the "feel" of a rigid chair as more responsive. This has been attributed to the fact that there is inherently some "flex" in folding frame chairs to allow them to collapse. Rigid chairs are generally more durable and slightly lighter than the comparable foldable chair. It takes skill to learn to breakdown a rigid chair. The back must be folded to the seat, and then the wheels are usually removed. Many less active users or those who have an able-bodied assistant prefer the simplicity of folding frame chairs. Conversely, those who value performance at a premium will choose rigid frames. There are a few hybrid chairs that fold by unconventional means to offer some of the convenience of X-brace chairs with some of the desired wheeling characteristics of rigid frame chairs.

The prescription can now be organized sequentially from the push handles (the posterior-superior corner) to the front casters (the anterior-inferior corner). Decisions are guided by the goal of maximally enhancing a client's mobility and function, with the least amount and least expense of equipment (Fig. 23-2, Table 23.1).

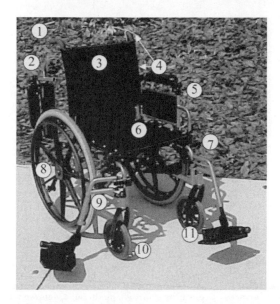

Fig. 23-3. Common components found on a foldable wheelchair. 1, Push handle; 2, flip-back armrest; 3, sling back; 4, cane; 5, desk length height-adjustable armrest; 6, sling seat; 7, push-to-lock wheel lock; 8, mag wheel with single-point axle; 9, 70-degree swing away detachable legrest; 10, caster; 11, flip-up footplate and heel loop. (Illustration courtesy Charles E. Levy, MD.)

Push handles, as their name suggests, can be used by a helper to push the chair.

Other uses for push handles or canes are as follows:

- To allow a helper to negotiate stairs
- As a fulcrum for those with poor trunk balance: one arm wraps around the handle to stabilize the body while the other hand reaches
- As a place to suspend backpacks

The sling back is the most common wheelchair back. A fabric is simply suspended between the canes. Lower end chairs may feature a back constructed of a nonbreathable synthetic material that is bolted to the chair. A better alternative is an easily removable washable nylon. Sling backs are prone to fatigue over time, which can promote kyphosis and place the shoulders at a biomechanical disadvantage. An adjustable-tension sling back (which incorporate horizontal straps at preset intervals) is often preferred. Besides combating material fatigue, these can be loosened and tightened to provide lumbar support and to increase trunk stability. When more support is needed, a solid back may be the solution. Prefabricated solid backs come in a variety of heights, depths, and contours. Most can be easily mounted and removed. Custom backs

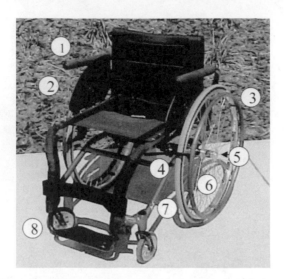

Fig. 23-4. Common components found on a rigid wheelchair.
1, Tubular armrest; 2, clothing guard; 3, pushrim; 4, scissor wheel
lock; 5, quick-release button; 6, spoke wheels; 7, rigid box frame;
8, fixed front end (fixed front rigging). (Illustration courtesy
Charles E. Levy, MD.)

are individually fabricated for the hard to fit (i.e., fixed spinal deformities). Lateral supports can be attached to the canes to add
further trunk stability.

Most folding chairs come with sling seats; some rigid chairs
come equipped with a solid seat pan. Like sling backs, sling seats
fatigue over time. This can cause internal rotation and adduction
of the femurs. To prevent this, a solid seat insert (often a wooden
board) can be added beneath the cushion. Alternatively, a cushion
with a stiff, bowed under-surface can be selected that is manufactured to accommodate the sagging of the sling seat. Adjustable
tension seats, which can aid in positioning the ischial tuberosities,
pelvis, and femurs, are also available from some manufacturers.

Armrests come in three basic configurations, from which a few
variations can be generated. Tubular armrests are found almost
exclusively on rigid chairs. Because tubular armrests tend to
bend under the pressure, they are most appropriate for those with
adequate trunk balance and abdominal strength to transfer without totally relying on a push-off from the armrest.

Height-adjustable detachable desk length armrests are standard equipment on most lightweight folding wheelchairs. They
allow a wheeler to approach a table almost as closely as an able-
bodied person sitting on a static chair. They provide a stable surface for push-offs and can be detached for side-to-side transfers.
The height adjustable feature provides for elevation or depression of the arm pad depending on a given user's stature. A few

patients require a full-length armrest for better leverage, fore-arm support, or as a surface from which equipment such as arm troughs or lap trays can be attached. A flip-back armrest is a kind of detachable armrest that pivots at the posterior post. This is usually more convenient than complete removal of the standard removable armrest.

A half lap tray is helpful in positioning the shoulder in hemiplegia to decrease pain and the extent of subluxation. A full lap tray allows placement of environmental control units and can function as a gentle restraint.

Most ultra lightweight chairs are equipped with an adjustable axle in the vertical and horizontal positions. A properly aligned axle improves the efficiency of propulsion, eases wheelies (for hopping curbs and other obstacles), and provides stability while also minimizing the turning radius.

For users who have control of one upper limb only (the other limb and both lower limbs are nonfunctional) one-arm drive is available. Unfortunately, with only one upper limb active, the user must both propel and steer with one hand. This is often too difficult to be practical, in which case a power wheelchair may be more appropriate.

Starting from the center of the wheel and working outward, the important considerations are type of axle (threaded or removable), type of strut (mag or spoke), type of pushrim, and type of tire.

The wheel axle is the shaft on which the wheels rotate. Axles can be threaded (standard on foldable chairs) or quick release (standard on rigid chairs to a permit easier transport in cars). As their name implies, quick-release axles allow the wheel to be detached with a push of a button. For those with reduced finger dexterity, a lever release consisting of a looped nut that is attached to the axle (a "quad release") may be enabling.

Wheels may be attached to the rim with either a metal spoke as seen on most bicycles or by several struts made of plastic or composite (mag wheel). Spoke wheel rims are generally lighter than comparable mag wheels and may provide a smoother ride. However, spokes tend to loosen and break more easily than the struts of a mag wheel and thus require more maintenance. The central hub of a mag wheel is typically narrower than a spoked hub. This is a consideration for when trying to minimize the width of the chair to fit through doorways.

Pushrims are usually made of aluminum or a similar alloy, plastic, or a plastic composite. Smooth metal pushrims can be coated with rubber or vinyl. This option offers the advantage of making the chair easier to push by increasing traction between the hand and the pushrim. Unfortunately this increases friction, which can lead to burns when the wheeler uses his or her hands to slow down the chair (i.e., when the chair is going down hill). Coated pushrims also tend to chip and tear with everyday use. One manufacturer offers a pushrim with a friction coating that only covers a portion of the rim surface to allow the user the option of gripping either a smooth or rubberized surface. Gloves keep hands clean and protected and can increase traction between the hand and the rim.

Projections ("quad knobs"), which can be vertically or obliquely oriented, are typically used to improve rim traction for those with poor handgrip (i.e., individuals with a C6 tetraplegia). However, even with quad knobs, manual wheelchair use is not practical for most individuals with a C6 tetraplegia, because of limitations in strength, balance, and endurance.

Tires can be air-filled (pneumatic), filled with a foam insert (flat-free), or solid. Pneumatic tires are lighter, more responsive, and provide the best cushioning from impact. Unfortunately, they demand periodic attention to maintain proper inflation and are also prone to punctures. Pneumatic tires can come in wide variety of sizes, diameters, and treads similar to those available for bicycles. Tires that feature flat-free inserts, although heavier and less shock absorbent, require very little upkeep. The solid polyurethane tire requires the least maintenance but also lacks tread. It is suitable for predominantly indoor, noncarpeted, (i.e., institutional) surfaces.

The hanger attaches the leg rest to the chair. At a hanger angle of 0 degrees, the knee is extended; a hanger angle of 90 degrees causes the knee to be bent at a right angle to the thigh, as seen in normal sitting. 70 degrees is the hanger angle common to most foldable chairs. The knee is placed in a relatively neutral position while the feet are positioned such that they avoid colliding with the casters when the chair is turned. A 60-degree hanger may be necessary to accommodate knee extension contractures but increases the turning radius. A hanger of 90 degrees or greater can accommodate hamstring contractures and allow a tighter turning radius and require less effort in turning. Bending the knees beyond 90 degrees places the feet underneath the user.

The legs and feet can be supported either on a swing-away removable footrest (the only option for most foldable chairs) or a front rigging (the usual option for most rigid chairs). The swing-away removable footrest can be rotated away from or entirely removed from the frame of the chair. This allows the feet to touch the ground, which eases stand pivot transfers or foot propulsion. A common option is flip-up footplates to allow the user to reach the floor without having to move the leg rest. Heel loops limit the posterior excursion of the foot; foot straps can help to position the foot on the plate but must be released for transfers. Footplates may also be made angle adjustable to accommodate plantar-flexion contractures.

Elevating leg rests usually come with a calf pad and can be helpful to control edema, to accommodate knee extension contractures, or to avoid knee-flexion contractures (i.e., in a patient with a new transtibial amputation).

Front rigging requires the user to lift his or her legs beyond the footplates when transferring. Front rigging can be adapted with a one-piece swing away footplate, but this requires the user to bend forward to detach the footplate.

Most manual wheelchairs are equipped with solid casters. Solid casters are preferred to air-filled because the air-filled caster is large and bulky and deflates frequently. However, large air-filled casters may be helpful to negotiate uneven terrains. One great advantage of the air-filled caster is that they reduce the amount of impact absorbed by the frame and thus may extend the frame's life. Standard caster sizes of 6 to 8 inches in diameter allow easy rolling over a variety of terrains, while still fitting with a standard 70-degree hanger. Smaller casters (available as small as 2 in. "Roller Blade" wheels) allow steeper hanger angles and also turn more sharply. Although they function well in the gym, they are more easily caught in grates, deep carpets, and uneven or muddy surfaces.

Standard safety features include a positioning belt, wheel locks and antitip devices. The physician may be legally liable if these are not included in the prescription and the patient subsequently comes to harm that might have been prevented were these items present. The positioning belt for most users is a simple lap belt with a push button or airline buckle, although Velcro closures may be needed for those with insufficient finger dexterity. Patients with significant spasticity may require elaborate chest straps to control posture. Wheel locks hold the chair in position and prevent rolling. Locking requires more effort than releasing; for those with marginal strength, the locks can be set as either push-to-lock or pull-to-lock, depending on the user's preference. Brake extensions can increase leverage to ease locking and unlocking and to facilitate reaching to the opposite side in hemiplegia. Scissor locks are located on the frame tubing that runs anterior posterior and have the advantage of being completely hidden when disengaged. These locks, which are more difficult to reach and require more effort to engage, are useful during vigorous wheeling in which the thumb might be caught in standard wheel locks. Grade aids are small spring-loaded mechanisms that attach to the wheel near the wheel lock and, when engaged, prevent the wheel from slipping backwards. This option can ease propulsion up longer inclines. Antitip devices prevent the chair from toppling backwards. Unfortunately, they also block wheelies, which may be required to jump curbs or to climb inclines.

Adjusting a Manual Chair for Specific Patient Needs

Wheelchairs should be adjusted to fit individual users. Ultra lightweight chairs offer the maximum in flexibility of adjustment. A number of studies have shown that adjusting the setup of a wheelchair affects the efficiency of propulsion, as well as the forces born by the upper limbs, and probably reduces the risk of upper limb injury. Features that can be modified include the seat angle, seat-to-back angle, axle position, camber, and footrest height. In general, a posture of 90 degrees between spine and femur and 90 degrees between femur and tibia is encouraged. Fixed deformities or poor abdominal tone (i.e., lower to middle thoracic spinal cord injuries and above) can demand that the seat-to-back angle be opened. Certain solid backs come with hooks that allow an extra 25 degrees in recline. Some chairs offer adjustable positioning for the canes. In other instances, bent canes can be obtained. The angle of the seat can be adjusted so that the sacrum sits lower than the knees ("dump"). This can combat the tendency to slide out of a chair and can prevent the pelvis from falling into a posterior tilt. As the pelvis tilts posteriorly, the lumbosacral spine falls into kyphosis. Chest expansion is limited leading to restricted inspiration and the shoulders are put into a position of mechanical disadvantage confining reach.

Positioning the axle properly in relationship to the patient's seated center of gravity (COG) is critical for safety and best propulsion. As the axle is moved anteriorly, a shorter wheelbase is provided offering advantages such as decreased rolling resistance, decreased downhill turning tendency, improved maneuverability, improved efficiency of propulsion, and usually improved portability. However, this comes at a price. The chair will lose stability and tend to tip backwards. Conversely, placement of the axle posteriorly away from the COG increases stability but also makes popping wheelies more difficult (which are often necessary to negotiate curbs) and increase the turning radius and rolling resistance. Patients with lower limb amputations experience a posterior shift of their seated COG when they lose any part of the lower limb. Some require that the axle be repositioned posteriorly to compensate. Vertical repositioning of the axle is valuable for individuals of shorter or taller stature and those who require the wheelchair to be close to the ground for effective foot propulsion. In general, the height of the axle should be adjusted so that with the hands on the top of the pushrims the elbow is at a 90-degree angle.

Wheels also may be angled away from the wheelchair on a vertical axis. This is referred to as camber. Increasing the camber (changing the wheel's vertical orientation so that the top of the wheel is tilted toward the user while the bottom is tilted away) increases the ease of propulsion, as well as the mediolateral stability of the wheelchair. Because of improved responsiveness of wheelchairs with camber, larger camber angles are often used in sports. Although there are several advantages to increased camber, it does increase the overall width of the wheelchair and the turning radius.

Ultimately, there is more to optimal performance than finding, fitting, and adjusting manual wheelchairs for specific users. An often-overlooked area is manual wheelchair propulsion technique. Based on the latest research and sound ergonomic principles, wheelchair users should be instructed to use long propulsive strokes that maximize the amount of time the hand is in contact with the pushrim. Wheelers should be instructed to avoid excessive initial impact at the start of a propulsive stroke. Finally, during recovery it is better to let the hand drift below the pushrim at the end of the stroke. There are also a host of everyday skills that wheelers must obtain such as how to perform wheelies to help hop curbs, how to fold and load a wheelchair in a car by oneself, and so forth. A course of physical or occupational therapy may be indicated to assess deficiencies and teach skills.

Adjustments to minimize chair width:

1. Wrap around armrests that offer structural placement of the posterior upright of the armrest behind the canes of the chair
2. Mag wheels tend to be narrower than spoke wheels
3. Placement of the wheels closer to the center of a threaded axle
4. Relocation of the axle plate from the exterior to the interior of the frame
5. Replacement of the pushrim brackets with shortened ones or removing the pushrim entirely
6. For foldable chairs, a device exists that attaches to the armrest and to the seating tube underneath the fabric of a sling seat. When the wheeler twists a handle, the distance between the seating tube and the armrest is shortened, which has the effect of partially folding the chair with the user in it, thus making the chair less wide

Power Wheelchairs and Scooters

Problem solving for powered mobility is very similar to that for manual chairs, except that there are generally less factors from which to choose. The largest consideration is whether to prescribe a scooter, a power chair with easily detachable batteries and motor, or power-base power wheelchair. As always, patient participation and choice are essential to generating a successful prescription.

Four criteria should be met before power mobility is authorized. First, the physician must be convinced that the patient's needs cannot be met with lesser equipment. Manual wheelchairs and walkers are lighter, easier to transport, and, by virtue of their relative simplicity, may be less vulnerable to malfunction. Next, the patient (or caregiver) must demonstrate sufficient vision and judgment to guide the chair safely. Third, the patient must be enabled by powered mobility in the intended environment. A scooter that works well in the clinic may be too long to fit in the office. Lack of proper ramps may make it impossible for the power chair to enter or leave the home. In some instances, vendors can lend an appropriate device for a few days to see if the expected benefit is achieved. Finally, a plan should be in place to transport the device to the intended environment. If public transportation is impractical or unavailable, the patient or caregiver may have to invest in an adapted van.

Scooters

Of the three power mobility options, scooters are the least expensive but also least adaptable if specialized seating is required (Fig. 23-5). They are said to carry less of "the stigmata of disability." They come in three- and four-wheel designs; three-wheel designs are most common. Four-wheel designs offer increased

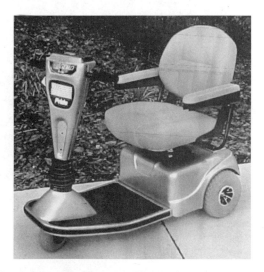

Fig. 23-5.   A three-wheel scooter. (Illustration courtesy Charles E. Levy, MD.)

stability and power but at the cost of increased price, weight, and turning radius. The typical scooter seat is a swiveling bucket seat or captain's chair. One common scooter option is a powered elevating seat (usually 2 to 7 inches), which can aid transfers and reach. This option is also available on some power wheelchairs. Many scooters can be disassembled for transport in a car. The heaviest part, the transaxle, typically weighs 35 to 40 pounds, which will present a challenge to some users. Appropriate larger cars may be equipped with a trunk lift, a power-assistive device. Because of their length, scooters may not fit on some public transportation (buses, vans) that accept power chairs. The longer wheelbases found on scooters translate to a longer turning radius. The tiller steering mechanism is mechanically similar to handlebars on a bicycle, demanding coordinated bimanual strength. Despite these negatives, for patients who are able to ambulate short distances, the scooter offers a well accepted, less expensive alternative to the power chair. A typical scooter user would be a patient with peripheral vascular disease, multiple sclerosis, arthritis, pulmonary, or cardiac disease whose ambulation is limited by endurance or ataxia.

Scooters are not practical for the nonambulatory. These individuals are most enabled by power wheelchairs. One option is the choice of power wheelchair with an integrated seat and base (folding frame power chairs with detachable batteries or rigid frame power chairs with detachable modular motors) eliminates many options available in power-base power wheelchairs (Fig. 23-6). The

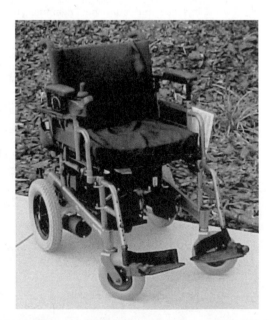

Fig. 23-6.   A folding frame rear wheel drive power wheelchair. (Illustration courtesy Charles E. Levy, MD.)

options jettisoned include powered recline, tilt-in-space, and a ventilation tray for those that must rely on mechanical ventilation. Because the electronics on folding frame power wheelchairs are usually less sophisticated, drive options beyond a standard joystick are limited as are options for environmental control units. As in manual chairs, folding frames tend to be less durable. The main advantage of the folding frame is that the power chair can be transported in many ordinary automobiles with simple disassembly provided there is someone to lift the weight of the batteries and the chair. The rigid frame chairs with the modular motors are likely to be more durable but more difficult to transport in a car. Whether the frame is foldable or rigid, these chairs offer virtually all of the static seating options found in manual chairs. The profile of a folding frame power chair user overlaps that of the scooter user, except that he or she might require a smaller turning radius (i.e., in home use), greater posture control, or improved accessibility for public transportation. Many of these users are nonambulatory.

Virtually all folding power chairs are directed by joysticks. Typically this is attached to the left or right armrest, to be guided by the least impaired or the dominant hand. A few patients are best served by a drive placed in a central position on a lap tray. Although a standard joystick topped with a ball can be easily manipulated by a normal hand, a T-bar or a custom-made hand piece may be necessary for those with reduced grip. Tires and casters may be true pneumatics or filled with a flat-free insert. If a user has a particular need for increased traction, a wider tire may be ordered with the caveat that wheelchair width will increase. Beyond this, the folding wheelchair prescription should include the back angle if different than standard, type of back and cushion, specification of armrest, specification of footrest, and standard safety features such as positioning belt and antitip devices (see manual wheelchair prescription discussed previously for a description of some of these options). Wheel locks are usually unnecessary because a power chair is always "in gear" unless the motor is manually disengaged.

Power-base power wheelchairs are made up of a power base consisting of the motor, frame, rear wheels, and front casters to which a seating system is then chosen and attached, which includes the seat, back, arm rests, controller, and footrests. Most power-base chairs cannot be easily broken down to component parts by users and most of the time are transported as a whole requiring a power lift or a ramp to be added to the vehicle. It is generally believed that power-base chairs are more rugged and durable than folding frame chairs. The motorized wheels may be located in the rear, center, or front of the wheelchair. The popularity of midwheel-drive wheelchairs for a variety of patients is testimony to their suitability to a variety of patient needs (Fig. 23-7). By locating the wheels in the center, a smaller turning radius is achieved and better traction results from having the patient's body weight directly over the drive wheels. Front-wheel drive offers easier operation when turning corners and in tight maneuvers when one is trying to get close to a surface and may be able to scale taller obstacles. Rear-wheel drive chairs offer the greatest stability; the fastest chairs tend to have rear-wheel drive (Fig. 23-8).

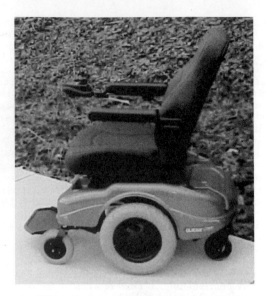

Fig. 23-7.   A midwheel or center-wheel drive power chair.
(Illustration courtesy Charles E. Levy, MD.)

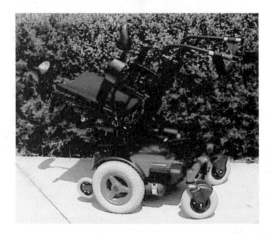

Fig. 23-8.   A rear-wheel drive power-base power wheelchair with a
60-degree power tilt. (Illustration courtesy Charles E. Levy, MD.)

Power-base wheelchairs offer an array of adjustability. They can accommodate those who are ventilator dependent with a vent tray; those who need power recline, tilt-in-space (Fig. 23-8), or both; and those who need complex electronics to best operate environmental control units or to guide the chair without a hand-operated joystick. Patients with sufficiently progressive diseases (i.e., amyotrophic lateral sclerosis) are often better served with a power-base chair even if they do not need the previously mentioned options at the time of evaluation.

Patients who cannot perform their own pressure relief are at risk for developing pressure ulcers. For these, low-shear power recline offers periodic repositioning to avoid skin breakdown. Power recline is also a means of postural realignment for those who are in their chairs for many hours or sleep in their chairs. Automatic power elevating foot rests or manual elevating foot-rests usually accompany power recline. Although it may seem counterintuitive, manual elevating legrests operated by a helper may be preferred to automatic power legrests, which elevate every time the back is lowered. This automatic elevation can greatly increase the length of the chair, and users may prefer to be able to exert choice as to when this occurs. Tilt-in-space can also accomplish pressure relief and is particularly useful for those with contractures or hypertonicity who cannot tolerate power re-cline. The greatest disadvantage of tilt-in-space is the potential back flow of urine into the bladder if the tubing or the leg bag of an indwelling bladder catheter is raised above the height of the bladder. A few patients have spasticity that is best treated with a combination of power tilt and recline. Patients using either tilt-in-space or recline systems almost certainly need a headrest added to the chair.

With modern technology, virtually any body movement that is under voluntary control can serve to operate a power chair. Navigation can be guided with modified joysticks, fiberoptic switches, or laser switches that are activated when a laser beam is interrupted by a specific body movement (i.e., finger or head movement). These can be throughout the wheelchair frame to exploit available movement. Still, most of those unable to oper-ate a hand-controlled joystick are fit with controls at chin first, then the head, and then mouth if the preceding option is not fea-sible. Chin controls can either be proportional or microswitch operated, with proportional being easier to learn but requiring more endurance than latched controls. A variety of devices can be fit at the end of the chin control joystick; ups are easy to op-erate, but experienced users may prefer a simple thin rod that extends horizontally to the chin, which is less cosmetically ob-trusive. Head controls can receive their input by a rear-mounted joystick, by sensors sensitive to motion as detected by perturba-tion of magnetic field, or by laser light switches. An advantage of head control is a relatively unobstructed view of the face. For those with no usable head movement, mouth controls can be used. The sip and puff system is the established standard but is latch controlled. Pneumatic switches activated by small changes in mouth pressure control speed and direction. The switches can be operated those with little breath support, even by those on ventilators.

Aesthetics

It may be impossible for the able-bodied to truly understand the meaning of a chair to the rider. Wheelchairs, so critical in everyday mobility, quickly become an extension of the user. Users are attracted to the image that they perceive the chair projects. Some opt for an attention grabbing style with bright colors and bold styling, whereas others look for a chair that blends into the background. As is true in so much of rehabilitation, patient happiness and compliance is often proportional to the patient's sense of involvement and control over his or her recovery.

Pediatric Wheelchairs

For children mobility represents more than the method in which one travels; mobility also is a component of development. When not otherwise contraindicated, children should be placed in mobility devices that allow them to explore their environment as soon as possible. Parents and caregivers should be prepared that such exploration may disrupt established routines. Seating for the child is a much more dynamic process than with adults. Even in nonprogressive conditions such as cerebral palsy, as the child grows the wheelchair and seating system must be adapted or replaced. Because of this constantly changing picture, pediatric power chairs more commonly use power bases, enabling seating components to be changed. Manual wheelchairs are also designed to accommodate growth. A multidisciplinary approach, often with the involvement of educational professionals, is essential.

Expense limits most wheelers to use only one chair to meet all of their mobility needs. However, to fully participate to the extent that physical limitations allow, many wheelers require more than one chair. A manual wheeler using an unobtrusive folding frame chair in a business setting might need the following:

- A power chair to access uneven terrain for outdoor recreational activities
- Sports chairs specific for tennis, quad rugby, racing, and basketball
- A colorful rigid frame manual chair for socializing

Standing Wheelchairs, Power-Assist Wheelchairs, and Beyond

Manual and power wheelchairs are available that allow a user to stand. In the power chairs, the stand function is activated by a switch and powered by the battery. Manual standing chairs rely on a mechanical mechanism powered by the user, although add on power is available in some models. The extra weight of the manual standing chairs makes them a less than optimal choice for everyday active wheeling. However, for someone that must reach above the waist, they can be invaluable. Power standing chairs are more expensive than conventional chairs power chairs. The potential benefits of standing include improved bone mineral density, decreased incidence of contractures, reduction of spasticity, improved bladder emptying, improved bowel function, and pressure relief. There are also psychologic and social benefits to meeting others face-to-face in a standing position.

Power-assist is an emerging technology in power chairs. Power-assist chairs are manual chairs that have been fitted with, or mod-

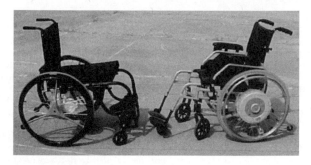

Fig. 23-9.   Two power-assist wheelchairs. On the left, a prototype of a variable ratio power-assist wheelchair. On the right, the batteries and motor are in the hub of the wheel. (Illustration courtesy Charles E. Levy, MD.)

ified to accept, small batteries and motors (adding approximately 30 to 50 lb to the chair) (Fig. 23-9). The motor is activated briefly when the pushrim is stroked. In this way, wheeling is made much easier. The addition of power assist can be helpful for those who must push long distances, who have low endurance, or for those who have or wish to avoid upper limb musculoskeletal pain or dysfunction. Unlike joystick-controlled power chairs or scooters, power-assist chairs demand some amount of large muscle effort from the user. This can be beneficial by allowing the user to get a limited amount of exercise while wheeling. Because power-assist units are relatively small and lightweight, they may allow the chair to be transported without the addition of a specialized lift.

A myriad of other wheelchair and wheelchair-related devices are available. These include geared wheels for manual wheelchairs that decrease the resistance the wheeler encounters when pushing and power devices that can be attached to a manual wheelchair to help a caregiver transport a wheeler up and down stairs. A power wheelchair with four-wheel drive that has the capacity to stand on two wheels and climb stairs has been developed but is not available to the general public at the time of this publication.

Wheelchair Cushions

Wheelchair cushions perform three vital functions. They provide protection against the occurrence of skin ulceration, they provide seating stability, and they provide comfort. Cushions can be classified into several categories based on materials, cost, complexity, or ability to diffuse pressure. Simple foam cushions are inexpensive and provide only a modest amount of pressure relief. These are generally appropriate for users who are at low risk for ulceration such as those still capable of limited ambulation or those who will use a wheelchair for a brief period before resuming ambulation. Cushions capable of greater pressure relief incorporate various fluids, gels, foams, air bladders, or plastic polymer honeycomb materials into their designs. Air-flotation systems generally provide the greatest amount of pressure relief but at the price of decreased seating stability. These cushions also require periodic maintenance to ensure proper inflation. The typical user would be someone in whom the risk of ulceration was high such as an individual with C6 complete tetraplegia. For users at a moderate risk for ulceration, such as a person with paraplegia that can perform independent pressure relief, cushions that incorporate fluids, higher density "memory" foams, or a honeycomb may be appropriate. Each of these cushions provides a relatively stable base of support, with reasonable durability and low maintenance. Gels tend to make cushions heavier. Certain cushions can be easily modified with wedges, hip guides, or other forms of alteration to accommodate postural deformities. For patients who are hard to fit or especially vulnerable, pressure mapping can be helpful to determine the optimal seating system. A variety of manual and computer-aided systems are available to precisely measure the patient's contours. From this a custom carved or poured wheelchair cushion and back can be fabricated.

GLOSSARY

Adjustable axle plate—Axle plate that allows for anterior/posterior adjustability or upward/downward adjustability or a combination of both. Adjusting the position of the wheel allows the chair to be fit to the user for the best position for propulsion and stability.

Adjustable tension back—A sling back that uses a series of adjustable horizontal straps to provide better, more customized support and to resist material fatigue.

Amputee axle plate—A particular kind of adjustable axle that allows the wheel to be repositioned posteriorly to accommodate for posterior shift in the center of gravity that accompanies lower limb amputations.

Amputee board—A board that can be inserted on the seat to keep the knee extended, typically used for patients with transtibial amputations.

Antitip devices (antitippers)—A safety feature that consists of small wheels placed on posts extending from the rear of the wheelchair that limit the distance the wheelchair can tip backwards.

Armrest—A platform or surface designed to support the forearm during rest. This surface is often used to push against in pressure relief maneuvers and in transfers.

Brake extensions—Tubes that extend from the wheel locks, which improve the leverage and increase the accessibility of the wheel locks typically prescribed for upper limb weakness or hemiplegia.

Camber—The angle the wheel is set in relationship to a vertical axis. Most manual wheelchairs are set at 0 degrees of camber. However, a greater camber angle can improve side-to-side stability and provide an ergonomic advantage for propulsion.

Casters—Small swiveling wheels that help to provide stability. These are almost always located at the anterior of a manual wheelchair.

Chin control—A joystick mechanism that allows the user to operate the wheelchair using his or her chin.

Desk length armrests—Armrests that are cut away to allow easy access to tables and desks.

Detachable armrests—Armrests that can be easily removed from the chair. This eases transfers.

Elevating leg rests—Adjustable height leg rests that can position the knee from 90 degrees of flexion to full extension. Common indications include positioning of a contracted or postsurgical knee to decrease edema.

Fixed armrests—Armrests integral with the wheelchair frame that cannot be removed.

Flat-free inserts—An inner liner that replaces the air-filled tube in pneumatic tires to increase durability of the tire.

Flip-up foot plates—A hinged footplate that can be rotated to allow the feet to touch the ground, which eases transfers and standing.

Foldable frame wheelchair—Wheelchair frame that collapses to ease transportation. By far the most common design employs an X-brace, although other designs exist.

Foot plates—A platform on which the foot rests.

Front rigging—The fixed front end, including a footplate, found on most manual rigid frame chairs.

Full length armrests—Armrests that extend from the back of the wheelchair to the front edge of the seat.

Grade aid—A spring-loaded mechanism with teeth that allows the wheel to move forward but not in reverse. This prevents the wheelchair from rolling backwards when on ramps or inclines.

Hanger—Attaches the legrest to the chair. Front hangers can be fixed, swing-away, or rigid. Removable hangers make transfers easier. Front hangers can be angled at 90 degrees or greater to 60 degrees, with 70 degrees being considered standard.

Joystick—A power wheelchair guidance device that is usually operated by hand, although it may be adapted to other body parts.

Lap tray—A surface (usually wood or a clear Plexiglas) attached to the armrests across the lap used to support one or both limbs and to provide a working surface. Typical users require extra support due to weakness, edema, or impairments of motor control. Plexiglas surfaces allow the user a greater view of their lower body. Full trays extend the entire distance across the armrests. Half trays are less cumbersome and often sufficient for those with hemiplegia.

Lateral supports—Guides that can be attached to either cane to position the trunk more securely.

Low shear power recline—A power recline system allows a user to change the back-to-seat angle when a switch is activated. In a low-shear system, either the seat or the back is constructed of two surfaces, which slide on one another while the angle is being changed to reduce shear.

Mag wheels—Wheels designed with a strut of a plastic type of material that connects the rim to hub.

Positioning belt—A lap harness that resembles an automobile safety belt. When properly aligned and tightened, a positioning belt can exert a positive influence on posture by securing the pelvis in an advantageous position. These belts prevent the user from accidentally exiting the chair.

Pneumatic tires—Tires with an air-filled inner tube such as those found on bicycles.

Power-base power wheelchair—A modular power wheelchair design in which the seating system is a completely separate system from the base. The base includes the frame, wheels, motor, battery, and drive.

Projections—See quad knobs.

Proportional drive—A type of switch mechanism on a power wheelchair, which responds proportionally to the amount of displacement of the joystick from a neutral position. Speed increases proportionally with the degree of displacement.

Pull-to-lock wheel locks—Wheel locks that are engaged with a pulling movement (elbow flexion). This configuration places the lock handle in a vertical position when the lock is engaged. The disadvantage of this is increased risk of scraping the buttock during a swing through transfer. See push-to-lock wheel locks.

Push handles—Handles projecting off the posterior rear of the wheelchair back posts. These allow a caregiver to push the wheelchair.

Pushrims—Rims attached lateral to the wheel. They are stroked by the wheeler for manual propulsion.

Push-to-lock wheel locks—Wheel locks that are engaged with a pushing movement (elbow extension). This configuration is easy to lock. However, in the locked position the lock handle protrudes from the wheel, and may be more likely to catch the thumb. See pull-to-lock wheel locks.

Quad knobs—Projections placed onto the pushrim of a wheelchair. They can be vertical or angled. They facilitate propulsion for those with poor grip such as those with tetraplegia.

Quad release axles—A type of removable axle that is attached to a looped nut that allows for quick removal of the wheels by an individual with poor manual dexterity.

Quick-release axle—Axles that allow the wheel to be removed from the frame using a push-button mechanism.

Rigid frame—A wheelchair frame that cannot be folded.

Scissor locks—A type of wheel lock usually found on sports chairs that are mounted under the seat. When disengaged, they are retracted under the seat and thus pose no hazard to the thumb during pushing. Because they are positioned under the seat, they require longer reach and greater sitting balance to operate compared with conventional locks.

Scooter—Three- or four-wheeled power mobility device guided by a tiller. The tiller serves the same function as a handlebar on a bicycle.

Sip and puff—A power wheelchair steering mechanism using a straw placed in the user's mouth. Through various combinations of "sips" and "puffs," the user guides the chair.

Sling back—Back of wheelchair consisting of a fabric suspended between the back rails (posts) of the chair.

Sling seat—A fabric suspended between the seat rails of the wheelchair.

Solid back—Back of wheelchair consisting of rigid material covered with foam that is placed between the back rails of the wheelchair.

Solid seat pan—As opposed to a sling seat, a wheelchair seat consisting of a rigid material, usually metal or wood, that spans the seat rails of the chair.

Solid seat insert—A board made out of a rigid material, often wood, that is placed between a sling seat and the wheelchair cushion to provide stiffer support.

Spoke wheels—Wheels designed with metal wire struts that connect the rim to hub.

Swing away foot rests—A footrest that swivels on the hanger to ease transfers and standing.

T-bar—A "T" shaped joystick used to improve grip.

Threaded axle—A nonremovable axle.

Tilt-in-space—A seating system in which the entire seat and back can be tilted as a single unit maintaining the back-to-seat angle.

Trunk lift—A mechanism to aid in the loading and unloading of wheelchairs. They are usually set up for car trunks and have a pneumatic mechanism for lifting the wheelchair.

Tubular armrest—One-piece nonadjustable armrests made from a bent tube. Tubular armrests lack an anterior attachment to the frame.

Wheel axle—Shaft on which the wheels rotate.

Wheel lock—Important safety feature of a wheelchair that allows the wheels to be fixed so the chair does not move.

Wheel lock extension—A tube placed on standard wheel locks to increase leverage and shorten the distance needed to reach the wheel lock.

Wrap-around armrest—An armrest in which its posterior post is seated behind the upright of the back. This decreases the overall width of the chair compared with standard armrests where the inferior post is located lateral to the upright of the back.

SUGGESTED READINGS

Axelson P, Minkel J, Chesney D. *A guide to wheelchair selection: how to use the ANSI/RESNA wheelchair standards to buy a wheelchair.* Washington, DC: Paralyzed Veterans of America, 1994.

Boninger ML, Baldwin MA, Cooper RA et al. Manual wheelchair pushrim biomechanics and axle position. *Arch Phys Med Rehabil* 2000;81:608–613.

Boninger ML, Cooper RA, Baldwin MA et al: Wheelchair pushrim kinetics: body weight and median nerve function. *Arch Phys Med Rehabil* 1999;80:910–915.

Boninger ML, Towers JD, Cooper RA et al. Shoulder imaging abnormalities in individuals with paraplegia. *J Rehabil Res Dev* 2001; 38:401–408.

Cooper RA. *Wheelchair selection and configuration.* New York: Demos Medical Publishing, 1998.

Davidoff G, Werner R, Waring W. Compressive mononeuropathies of the upper extremity in chronic paraplegia. *Paraplegia* 1991;29: 17–24.

Fitzgerald SG, Cooper RA, Boninger ML et al. Comparison of fatigue life for 3 types of manual wheelchairs. *Arch Phys Med Rehabil* 2001;82:1484–1488.

Kirby RL. Principles of wheelchair design and prescription. In: Lazar RB, ed. *Principles of neurologic rehabilitation.* New York: McGraw-Hill, 1997:465–481.

Levy CE, Berner TF, Sandhu PS et al. Mobility challenges and solutions for fibrodysplasia ossificans progressiva. *Arch Phys Med Rehabil* 1999;80:1349–1353.

Levy CE, Boninger M, McDermott M et al. Wheeled mobility. In: Grabois M, ed. *Physical medicine and rehabilitation: the complete approach.* Blackwell Science, 2000:685–711.

Subject Index

Page numbers followed by "f" denote figures; those followed by "t" denote tables.